FOURTH EDITION

Medical Law and Ethics

BONNIE F. FREMGEN, Ph.D.

Pearson

Boston   Columbus   Indianapolis   New York   San Francisco
Upper Saddle River   Amsterdam   Cape Town   Dubai   London   Madrid
Milan   Munich   Paris   Montreal   Toronto   Delhi   Mexico City   Sao
Paulo   Sydney   Hong Kong   Seoul   Singapore   Taipei   Tokyo

Library of Congress Cataloging-in-Publication Data

Fremgen, Bonnie F.
  Medical law and ethics / Bonnie F. Fremgen. — 4th ed.
     p. ; cm.
  Includes bibliographical references and index.
  ISBN-13: 978-0-13-255922-5
  ISBN-10: 0-13-255922-6
    1. Medical laws and legislation—United States.
2. Medical care—Law and legislation—United States.   3. Medical ethics.   I. Title.
    [DNLM: 1. Legislation, Medical—United States.
2. Ethics, Medical—United States. W 32.5 AA1]
   KF3821.F74 2012
   344.7304'1—dc22

                          2010044156

Notice: The material in this textbook contains the most current information about the topic at the time of publication. This text is not meant to be used in lieu of qualified legal advice for situations that arise in either one's professional practice or personal life. An attorney should always be consulted for legal advice. Since laws for healthcare professionals vary from state to state, it is always wise to consult specific laws within one's state of practice.

Note Re Case Studies: The names used in the case studies throughout the text are fictitious.

Publisher: Julie Levin Alexander
Publisher's Assistant: Regina Bruno
Editor-in-Chief: Mark Cohen
Executive Editor: Joan Gill
Assistant Editor: Nicole Ragonese
Editorial Assistant: Mary Ellen Ruitenberg
Director of Marketing: David Gesell
Senior Marketing Manager: Katrin Beacom
Marketing Specialist: Michael Sirinides
Marketing Assistant: Crystal Gonzalez
Managing Production Editor: Patrick Walsh
Production Liaison: Julie Boddorf

Production Editor: Bruce Hobart, Laserwords
Senior Media Editor: Amy Peltier
Media Project Manager: Lorena Cerisano
Manufacturing Manager: Ilene Sanford
Manufacturing Buyer: Alan Fischer
Senior Art Director: Maria Guglielmo
Cover Designer: Wanda España at wee design
Cover Image: iStockphoto
Composition: Laserwords
Printing and Binding: R.R. Donnelley/Willard
Cover Printer: Phoenix Color Corporation

Credits and acknowledgments borrowed from other sources and reproduced, with permission, in this textbook appear on the appropriate pages within text.

10 9 8 7 6 5 4 3 2 1

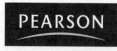

www.pearsonhighered.com

ISBN-13: 978-0-13-255922-5
ISBN-10:   0-13-255922-6

To my children, who have always been my inspiration for ethical behavior. And a special thanks to my husband for his continual support and help.

Brief Contents

1   Introduction to Medical Law, Ethics, and Bioethics   1

PART I   THE LEGAL ENVIRONMENT   29

2   The Legal System   29

3   Importance of the Legal System for the Physician and the Healthcare Professional   55

4   Today's Healthcare Environment   75

PART II   THE HEALTHCARE ENVIRONMENT   99

5   The Physician–Patient Relationship   99

6   Professional Liability and Medical Malpractice   131

7   Public Duties of the Physician and the Healthcare Professional   163

8   Workplace Law and Ethics   185

9   The Medical Record   217

10   Patient Confidentiality and HIPAA   239

PART III   MEDICAL ETHICS   263

11   Ethical and Bioethical Issues in Medicine   263

12   Ethical Issues Relating to Life   291

13   Death and Dying   321

Contents

Preface   xi

Letter to the Student   xv

How to Interpret Case Citations   xvii

About the Author   xix

Reviewers   xxi

1   Introduction to Medical Law, Ethics, and Bioethics   1

Why Study Law, Ethics, and Bioethics?   3

Medical Law   7

Ethics   8

Models for Examining Ethical Dilemmas   18

What Ethics Is Not   20

Bioethics   21

The Role of Ethics Committees   22

Quality Assurance Programs   23

Medical Etiquette   23

PART I   THE LEGAL ENVIRONMENT   29

2   The Legal System   29

The Legal System   31

Sources of Law   33

Classification of Laws   36

The Court Systems   44

The Trial Process   46

3   Importance of the Legal System for the Physician and the Healthcare Professional   55

Medical Practice Acts   57

Licensure of the Physician   58

Standard of Care   61
Confidentiality   62
Statute of Limitations   63
Good Samaritan Laws   64
Respondeat Superior   64
Risk Management   67

4   Today's Healthcare Environment   75
Today's Healthcare Environment   77
Types of Medical Practice   82
The Ethics of Fee Splitting   86
Medical Specialty Boards   86
Allied Health Professionals   89

PART II THE HEALTHCARE ENVIRONMENT   99

5   The Physician–Patient Relationship   99
Physician's Rights   101
Physician's Responsibilities   102
Professional Practice Responsibilities   103
Patients' Rights   112
Rights of Minors   119
Patients' Responsibilities   119
Role of the Healthcare Consumer   124

6   Professional Liability and Medical Malpractice   131
Professional Negligence and Medical Malpractice   134
The Tort of Negligence   135
Fraud   139
Office of Inspector General   141
Defense to Malpractice Suits   143
Professional Liability   145
Alternative Dispute Resolution   150
Liability of Other Health Professionals   151

Tort Reform   154

Malpractice Prevention   154

7   Public Duties of the Physician and the Healthcare Professional   163

Public Health Records and Vital Statistics   165

Controlled Substances Act and Regulations   174

Protection for the Employee and the Environment   177

8   Workplace Law and Ethics   185

Professionalism in the Workplace   187

Discrimination in the Workplace   188

Privacy and the Workplace   188

Cultural Considerations   189

Religious Considerations   190

Effective Hiring Practices   191

Legal and Illegal Interview Questions   193

Federal Regulations Affecting the Medical Professional   194

Equal Employment Opportunity and Employment Discrimination   194

Employee Health and Safety   200

Compensation and Benefits Regulations   203

Consumer Protection and Collection Practices   206

9   The Medical Record   217

Purpose of the Medical Record   219

Contents of the Medical Record   220

Ownership of the Medical Record   226

Confidentiality and the Medical Record   226

Retention and Storage of Medical Records   229

Reporting and Disclosure Requirements   232

Use of the Medical Record in Court   233

10   Patient Confidentiality and HIPAA   239

Confidentiality   241

Health Insurance Portability and Accountability Act (HIPAA) of 1996   244

Ethical Concerns with Information Technology (Informatics)   256

PART III MEDICAL ETHICS   263

11   Ethical and Bioethical Issues in Medicine   263

Early History   265

Ethical Standards and Behavior   266

Codes of Ethics   267

Codes of Ethics for Other Medical Professionals   269

Bioethical Issues   269

Ethical Issues and Personal Choice   274

The Ethics of Biomedical Research   275

Human Genome Project   278

Genetic Engineering   279

Healthcare Reform   282

12   Ethical Issues Relating to Life   291

Fetal Development   293

Assisted or Artificial Conception   294

Contraception   299

Sterilization   299

Abortion   302

Genetic Counseling and Testing   309

Wrongful-Life Suits   312

13   Death and Dying   321

The Dying Process   323

Legal Definition of Death   323

Stages of Dying   333

Quality-of-Life Issues   334

Use of Medications   334

Hospice Care   335

Palliative Care   336

Viatical Settlements   337

Advance Directives   337

Choices in Life and Death   338

Appendix A. Codes of Ethics   345

Appendix B. Case Citations   349

Glossary   353

Index   365

Preface

The allied health professional has always been an important member of the medical team. This team awareness is even more critical in today's healthcare environment, because the physician no longer practices medicine alone. Therefore, the text discusses medical law and ethics as it relates to allied healthcare professionals, as well as the physician's duties and responsibilities.

Medical Law and Ethics is written in straightforward language that is aimed at the nonlawyer health professional who must be able to cope with multiple legal and ethical issues. This text is appropriate for those studying in a college or university who are working toward careers in the allied health field in a variety of settings, such as medical offices, hospitals, clinics, laboratories, and skilled-nursing facilities. Because most allied healthcare professionals work either with or for a physician, it is important to understand the physician's responsibilities and duties to the patient. Therefore, they are covered in this book. Included are examples of common legal and ethical issues that affect those working in the healthcare field. A wide range of pertinent topics are discussed, such as the legal system, professional liability and medical malpractice, public duties of the physician, the medical record, and ethical and bioethical issues. There is an in-depth discussion of the regulations affecting the healthcare professional, including up-to-date information about the Health Insurance Portability and Accountability Act of 1996 (HIPAA). The intent is to help healthcare professionals to better understand our ethical obligation to ourselves, our patients, and our employers. A new addition to stimulate discussion is the Critical Thinking Exercise at the end of each chapter.

Many legal cases are sprinkled throughout the text to demonstrate the history of the law as it pertains to subjects such as patient confidentiality, managed care, federal regulations affecting the employee, death and dying, and abortion. In some examples, the cases may seem old, but because we as a country have a legal system based on case law, these laws are still pertinent today. A legal icon (scales of justice) appears in the margin to indicate legal case citations.

A special feature called Med Tips provides quick information about law and ethics. These brief scenarios and hints help to maintain interest in this vital subject. Each chapter includes glossary terms highlighted in bold on first reference, extensive end-of-chapter exercises, and one actual practice case. The appendices include a sample of codes of ethics that form a basis for current practice and legal case citations.

This text provides an overview of medical law and ethics. Practicing health care professionals should know the legal requirements in their own jurisdictions.

Finally, many educators have offered thoughtful comments as reviewers of this text. I am extremely grateful that they have shared their time and experience to help develop this textbook.

CHAPTER STRUCTURE

▶ **Learning Objectives.**   These include an overview of the basic knowledge discussed within the chapter and can be used as a chapter review.

▶ **Key Terms.**   Important vocabulary terms are listed alphabetically at the beginning of each chapter and printed in bold the first time they are defined in the text.

▶ **Introduction.**   Each chapter begins with an introductory statement that reflects the topic of the chapter.

▶ **Review Challenge.**   A selection of short answer, matching, and multiple-choice questions are included to test the student's knowledge of the chapter material.

▶ **Case Study.**   The case studies are based on real-life occurrences and offer practical application of information discussed within the chapter. These are included to stimulate and draw upon the student's critical-thinking skills and problem-solving ability.

▶ **Critical Thinking Exercise.**   These exercises at the end of each chapter challenge the student to answer the question "What would you do if . . ." relating to many current healthcare and legal dilemmas in today's environment.

▶ **Bibliography.**   These useful resources provide further information on the topics included within the chapter.

SPECIAL FEATURES

▶ **Med Tip.**   Med Tips are placed at strategic points within the narrative to provide helpful hints and useful information to stimulate the student's interest in the topic.

▶ **Legal Case Citations.**   Discipline-specific cases are used throughout the text to illustrate the topic under discussion. The cases reflect the many medical disciplines, including that of the physician, that come together in the care of the patient. While this book is not meant to be a law book, the cases cited in the book are meant to emphasize the importance of the law for the students.

▶ **Points to Ponder.**   Thought-provoking questions give students an opportunity to evaluate how they might answer some of the tough, medically related ethical dilemmas in today's society. These questions can also be used for critical debate among students during a class activity.

▶ **Discussion Questions.**   These end-of-chapter questions encourage a review of the chapter contents.

▶ **Put It into Practice.**   These thought-provoking activities appear at the end of each chapter. They provide a clinical correlation with the topics discussed in the chapter and stimulate the student's own contemplation of legal and ethical issues that are apparent in everyday life.

▶ **Web Hunt.** This end-of-chapter internet activity encourages the student to access the multitude of medical resources available through this medium.

▶ **Appendices.** Codes of Ethics are included in Appendix A; useful healthcare websites are listed online; the case citations used throughout the book are listed in Appendix B.
▶ **Additional Examination Review Questions.** These are included in the Instructor's Resource Manual.

ACKNOWLEDGMENTS

This book would not have been possible without the assistance and guidance of many people. I am grateful to the editorial and production staffs at Pearson Education for their skill and patience with this project. I thank Joan Gill, executive editor and Mark Cohen, editor-in-chief, for their leadership and guidance with this project; Nicole Ragonese and Melissa Kerian whose courtesy and thoroughness are greatly appreciated; Pat Walsh, managing production editor, whose calm presence is always available; Julie Boddorf, production liaison; and Bruce Hobart, Laserwords, whose skill and patience is remarkable, for their great attention to detail and all their hard work.

Letter to the Student

It's a natural tendency to read some of the case examples in this book and think that they must be fictional as no well-trained healthcare professional would ever be so negligent. However, the short ethics cases at the beginning of each chapter, with the exception of the historical cases, are indeed real. All of these cases are drawn from the author's experience.

Throughout the book there are numerous examples of actual legal cases that usually resulted in suffering for patients, as well as for physicians and other healthcare professionals. The cases discussed are not meant to focus on particular healthcare disciplines, nor to exclude any disciplines. And these cases are not meant to frighten but, rather, to alert all of us to the potential risks to patients when healthcare professionals are not diligent about the care they provide. Do not memorize the case citations, but rather try to understand the circumstances and why the case was included in this book.

I have a great respect for *all* the disciplines mentioned in this book. My intent is to prepare students to promote good patient care, as well as to protect themselves and their employers from lawsuits.

For a successful start to your study of medical law and ethics, consider following the ABCs of classroom success: **A**ctively participate, **B**enefit from the experience, and **C**ommit to learning. It is necessary for you to attend class to truly benefit from your ethics education. So much happens in the classroom—especially the interaction between you and your classmates. The discussion portion of an ethics class is one of the most important components. You must be present to contribute. The text serves as an information source and as the first step in your education—the dynamics of classroom interaction between you, your instructor, and the other students is critical for success in learning.

Actively participate when you attend class. It is necessary to absorb what takes place during the class session. Listen carefully to what your instructor and fellow students say. If you don't share your ideas, experiences, and questions, then the rest of the class is losing what you have to offer. The dialogue about ethics that you have with your instructor and fellow classmates can be one of the most meaningful learning experiences.

Benefit from the experience and ideas of your peers (classmates). Listen to the opinions of others during class discussions. Pay particular attention to the opinions that differ from your own. As a member of the healthcare team, you will frequently hear opinions that differ from your own—both from your coworkers and your patients. You do not have to change your opinions or beliefs, but try to keep an open mind to the opinions of others.

Commit to learning by carefully reading and analyzing the textbook material. Look for new information and also for discussion points that both agree and disagree with your own perspective. Take this course seriously so that it is not a waste of your time. In fact, your ethics class can be one of the most important classes that you take! Communicate what you have learned. Your perspective is important for others to hear. Use your time wisely in class, share your ideas, and listen to the thoughts of others.

The law is dynamic and often is revised as changes take place in society. For example, one of the newest laws affecting healthcare, the Healthcare Insurance Portability and Accountability Act of 1996 (HIPAA), has recently had an added impact regarding the necessity for healthcare organizations, including physicians' offices, to provide notice to all patients concerning their privacy practices. This textbook is not meant to be a study of the law, but rather to introduce students to the impact that law and ethics have on their professional lives.

Finally, our goal as teachers is to help our students learn how to judge themselves and their actions. Because you won't have us with you in the workplace, we want you to be able to evaluate your own actions in light of their ethical and legal impact on others.

How to Interpret Case Citations

Selected legal cases are used in this textbook to illustrate various legal principles. At the end of each case summary is a citation such as, *Moon Lake Convalescent Center v. Margolis,* 433 N.E.2d 956 (Ill. App. Ct. 1989). This citation, similar to a street address, tells you where you can find this case among the many sets of reported cases (called *reporters*) in the library. Most case citations end with information in parentheses, such as (Ill. App. Ct. 1989), which tells you what court (the Illinois Appellate Court) decided the case and the year (1989) of the decision, but you do not need that information when you are simply trying to locate a particular case in the library. The small *v.* between the litigants' names stands for "versus." A case citation consists of

▶ The italicized case name—usually the name of the plaintiff and the defendant. In our example, *Moon Lake Convalescent Center* (defendant) and *Margolis* (plaintiff).
▶ The name of the reporter(s) where the case is published (Northeast Reporter, 2d series).
▶ The volume number(s) of the reporter(s) where the case is published (433).
▶ The page number of the volume where the case begins (956).
▶ The year the case was decided (1989).
▶ For federal Court of Appeals cases, a designation of the circuit; for federal District Court cases, the state and judicial district where the court is located; for state cases, an indication of the state if it is not apparent from the name of the reporter (Illinois Appellate Court).

Therefore, our example case between Moon Lake Convalescent Center and Margolis is found in volume 433 of the Northeast Reporter, 2d series, on page 956.

Abbreviations for other reporters (books) are:

A (Atlantic Reporter)
P (Pacific Reporter)
U.S. (United States Reporter)
F.Supp. (Federal Supplement)
F (Federal Reporter)
NE (Northeast Reporter)
NW (Northwest Reporter)
NYS (New York Supplement)
So (Southern Reporter)
SW (Southwestern Reporter)

Most reporters have been published in two or more series, such as 2d, meaning second series. The student should not be concerned with memorizing the names of the reporters. The abbreviations for them are found at the beginning of most of the legal research publications that we use. As you do research within your own state, you will become familiar with the abbreviations that are most commonly used. Legal research can be done through a law library or via the Internet from Lexis-Nexis, which is a subscription service used by law firms and libraries.

About the Author

Bonnie F. Fremgen, Ph.D., is a former associate dean of the Allied Health Program at Robert Morris College and was vice-president of a hospital in suburban Chicago. She has taught medical law and ethics courses as well as clinical and administrative topics. She has broad interests and experiences in the healthcare field, including hospitals, nursing homes, and physicians' offices. She currently has a patent pending on a unique atrophy-reducing wheelchair.

Dr. Fremgen holds a nursing degree as well as a master's in healthcare administration. She received her Ph.D. from the College of Education at the University of Illinois. She has performed postdoctoral studies in medical law at Loyola University Law School in Chicago.

Dr. Fremgen has taught ethics at the University of Notre Dame, South Bend, Indiana; University of Detroit, Detroit, Michigan; and Saint Xavier University, Chicago, Illinois.

Reviewers

FOURTH EDITION REVIEWERS

Rosana Darang, MD
Bay State College
Boston, Massachusetts

Amy DeVore, CPC, CMA (AAMA)
Butler County Community College
Butler, PA

Candace Lynn Doyle, M.S.Ed.
Midlands Technical College
West Columbia, South Carolina

Gail High, CMOA
YTI Career Institute - Altoona Campus
Altoona, Pennsylvania

Cecelia Jacob, MA
Southwest Tennessee Community College
Memphis, Tennessee

Ana M. Linville, M.Ed. BAAS,
   MT(AMT), MLT(ASCP)
University of Texas at Brownsville/Texas
   Southmost College
Brownsville, Texas

Michelle Lovings, MBA
Missouri College
Brentwood, Missouri

Lorraine Papazian-Boyce, MS, CPC
Colorado Technical University Online
Hoffman Estates Illinois

Donna M. Rowan, MAT
Harford Community College
Bel Air, Maryland

George W. Strothmann, CPhT
Sanford Brown Institute
Fort Lauderdale, FL

Lori Warren Woodard, MA, RN, CPC,
   CPC-I, CCP, CLNC
Spencerian College
Louisville, Kentucky

Mindy Wray, BS, CMA, RMA
ECPI - Greensboro Campus
Greensboro, North Carolina

PREVIOUS EDITION REVIEWERS

Frank Ambriz, PA-C, MPAS
University of Texas–Pan Am
Edinburg, Texas

Theresa Allyn, BS
Edmonds Community College
Lynnwood, Washington

Anne M. Arto
Pasco-Hernando Community College
Brooksville, Florida

Deborah Bedford, AAS, CMA
North Seattle Community College
Seattle, Washington

Norma Bird, MEd, BS, CMA
Idaho State University College of
   Technology
Pocatello, Idaho

Susan J. Burnham, RNC, CLNC, IBCLC
Renton Technical College
Renton, Washington

Rafael Castilla, MD
Hohokus School of Business and
  Medical Sciences
Ridgefield, New Jersey

Kat Chappell, CMA, BS
Highline Community College
Des Moines, Washington

Michael W. Cook, MA, RRT
Mountain Empire Community College
Big Stone Gap, Virginia

Tonya Hallock
Concorde Career Institute
Garden Grove, California

Mack Henderson, PhD, MEd,
  CPC, CCS-P
Durham Technical Community College
Durham, North Carolina

Janice C. Hess, MA
Metropolitan Community College
Elkhorn, Nebraska

Robert K. Johnson, JD
Ivy Tech Community College
Greenwood, Indiana

Jennifer Lame, BS, RHIT
Idaho State University
Pocatello, Idaho

Vivian C. Lilly, PhD, MBA, MS, BS, RN
North Harris College
Houston, Texas

Sharon Tompkins Luczu, RN, BA,
  MA, MBA
Gateway Community College
Phoenix, Arizona

Christine Malone, BS
Everett Community College
Everett, Washington

Betsey Morthland, MS
Black Hawk College
Moline, Illinois

Lisa Nagle, CMA, BSEd
Augusta Technical College
Augusta, Georgia

Michael O'Sullivan, DPH
University of Massachusetts–Lowell
Lowell, Massachusetts

Helen W. Spain, BSEd, MSEd
Wake Technical Community College
Raleigh, North Carolina

Susan Stockmaster, MHS
Trident Technical College
Charleston, South Carolina

Lenette Thompson
Piedmont Technical College
Greenwood, South Carolina

Valeria Truitt, BS, MAEd
Office Administration
Craven Community College
New Bern, North Carolina

Lori Warren, MA, RN, CPC, CCP, CLNC
Spencerian College
Louisville, Kentucky

Amy L. Wilson, BS, RT(R), RDMS, RVT
University of Southern Indiana
Evansville, Indiana

Introduction to Medical Law, Ethics, and Bioethics

Learning Objectives

1. Define the glossary terms.
2. Describe the similarities and differences between laws and ethics.
3. Discuss the reasons for studying law, ethics, and bioethics.
4. Describe how to apply the three decision-making models discussed in this chapter.
5. Explain why ethics is not *just* about the sincerity of one's beliefs, emotions, or religious viewpoints.

Key Terms

Amoral
Applied ethics
Bioethicists
Bioethics
Comparable worth
Compassion
Cost/benefit analysis
Due process
Duty-based ethics
Empathy
Ethics
Fidelity

Indigent
Integrity
Justice-based ethics
Laws
Litigious
Medical ethics
Medical etiquette
Medical practice acts
Morality
Precedent
Principle of autonomy

Principle of beneficence
Principle of justice
Principle of nonmalfeasance
Quality assurance
Rights-based ethics
Sanctity of life
Sexual harassment
Sympathy
Tolerance
Utilitarianism
Virtue-based ethics

THE CASE OF JEANETTE M. AND THE PHONE CALL

Jeanette, an 80-year-old widow, called her physician early one morning complaining of shortness of breath. She spoke to the office receptionist who asked if she was having any other difficulty. Jeanette said no. The receptionist said she would give the message to the doctor.

The doctor's office was extremely busy that October day giving out flu shots. The receptionist immediately became busy answering telephone calls and admitting a long line of patients waiting for their annual flu shot. The telephone message from Jeanette was left unnoticed on the front office desk for several hours and was then placed on the physician's desk with other messages.

Jeanette became so exhausted from her shortness of breath that she fell asleep. When she awoke in the afternoon she could not catch her breath. She called her neighbor and just said, "Help." Paramedics arrived at Jeanette's home shortly after the neighbor called 911 and found Jeanette to be unresponsive. She was taken to the local emergency room where she was diagnosed and treated for pneumonia and congestive heart failure. The emergency room staff tried to determine who her personal physician was, but Jeanette had no personal belongings or medical information with her. She never regained consciousness and died that evening.

When her neighbor went over to Jeanette's home that evening to feed the cat, she noticed the light on the phone's answering machine. The doctor had returned Jeanette's call at 5:00 P.M. She apologized for not calling sooner.

1. Do you believe that this case presents a legal or an ethical problem or both?

2. In your opinion, is anyone at fault for Jeanette's death?

3. Is anyone on the physician's staff at fault? Is the physician at fault?

4. What could have been done to prevent this problem?

I long to accomplish a great and noble task, but it is my chief duty to accomplish humble tasks as though they were great and noble. The world is moved along, not only by the mighty shoves of its heroes, but also by the aggregate of the tiny pushes of each honest worker.

Helen Keller

Introduction

Medical professionals encounter healthcare dilemmas that are not experienced by the general population. They are faced with individual choices that must, of necessity, always take into consideration the common good of all patients. Medical–ethical decisions have become increasingly complicated with the advancement of medical science and technology. The topics of medical law, ethics, and bioethics, while having very specific definitions, are interrelated. One cannot practice medicine in any setting without an understanding of the legal implications for both the practitioner and the patient. Medical ethics is an **applied ethics,** meaning that it is a practical application of moral standards that are meant to benefit the patient. Therefore, the medical practitioner must adhere to certain ethical standards and codes of conduct. **Bioethics,** a branch of applied ethics, is a field resulting from modern medical advances and research. Many medical practitioners, patients, and religious organizations believe that advances in bioethics, such as cloning, require close examination, control, and even legal constraints.

One teacher of medical law and ethics clearly stated that our primary goal is to teach students to think independently and become sensitive to the risks and issues that pervade the field. The ultimate goal in teaching this topic is that students will be able to understand complex healthcare public policy from all sides of an issue, regardless of personal beliefs. We want our students to be able to conduct themselves in a manner that is ethical, legal, and exemplary.

WHY STUDY LAW, ETHICS, AND BIOETHICS?

Without a moral structure for their actions, people would be free to pursue their own self-interests. In many cases, people would behave in a moral fashion within the constraints and framework of their culture and religious beliefs. However, upon closer examination of living without the constraints and limitations imposed by moral standards and laws, a state of hostility may arise in which only the interests of the strong would prevail. The words *justice* and *injustice* would have little meaning. We all believe we know the difference between right and wrong. We may firmly believe that while some decisions are difficult to make, we would intuitively make the right decision. However, there is ample proof in medical malpractice cases that, in times of stress and crisis, people do not always make the correct ethical decisions. Because what is illegal is almost always unethical, it is important to have a basic understanding of the law as it applies to the medical world.

MED TIP

We must always remember that our primary duty is to promote good patient care and to protect our patients from harm.

We should also understand that we live in a **litigious** society in which people have become excessively inclined to sue healthcare practitioners. In addition, healthcare agencies, hospitals, nursing homes, and manufacturers of medical products and equipment are all at risk of being sued by patients and their families. In fact, in our society anyone can sue anyone else. Lawsuits take a great toll in terms of stress, time, and money for all parties involved. While being sued does not indicate guilt, nevertheless it can affect the reputation of a person or an institution even if judged to be innocent in a court of law.

MED TIP

A basic understanding of law and ethics can help protect you and your employer from being sued.

Another reason for studying ethics and the law is that people often convince themselves that what they are doing is not wrong. For example, plagiarism, which is using someone else's words or ideas, may be both unethical and illegal, depending on the circumstances. It's understandable that an author who has worked hard to write a book would not want another author to use his or her written material without permission and proper credit. In fact, lawsuits have been won when plagiarism is proven to have occurred. In this case, it is both illegal and unethical. But what happens when a student has someone else do his or her work? Or if students lift passages from another book and then claim the words as their own? Is this also illegal and unethical? It may be both. A student entering the medical field is held to a high standard. Strong ethical values can begin with something as simple as turning in honest papers. There have been numerous examples of people lying on their job resume by embellishing duties and achievements on past jobs, stretching employment dates to cover gaps between jobs, inflating salaries, and even omitting criminal convictions. Many healthcare employers are sensitive to this problem and use consulting firms to perform background checks on potential employees. These examples illustrate current ethical, and even some illegal acts.

Medicine is based on the professional skills of many persons, including physicians, nurses, physician assistants, medical assistants, radiology technicians, pharmacists, surgical technologists, phlebotomists, reimbursement specialists and coders, pharmacy technicians, and a multitude of other allied health professionals. The healthcare team, composed of these professionals, with the addition of healthcare administrators, often must decide on critical issues relating to patient needs. In some cases, the decisions of these professionals are at odds with one another. For example, when an obstetrician withholds resuscitation attempts on a severely handicapped newborn, such as one born without a brain (anencephalic), he or she may be acting in opposition to the law in many states and the ethics of many people. Does a nurse have an ethical responsibility to override this order if he or she believes it to be wrong? Is there a better way to handle such an ethical dilemma without the patient's suffering in the process? It is generally understood that nurses and other allied healthcare professionals carry out the orders of their employer/physician. However, as illustrated in the above case, in some situations, confusion arises about what is the right thing to do. In the Jeanette M. case at the beginning of the chapter, does the physician's receptionist have any responsibility for the physician's delay in returning the patient's call?

It is generally accepted that some behavior, such as killing, is always wrong. But even this issue has been in the news when, as Hurricane Katrina roared through New Orleans in 2005, several critically ill hospital patients who could not be moved, and would certainly die, were allegedly given a lethal injection of morphine by a doctor and two nurses. In 2007 a grand jury determined not to indict the physician and cleared her of all accusations. There have been 194 Katrina-related claims filed by a Louisiana state agency that manages malpractice lawsuits. There is a concern, resulting from this case, that prosecutions against hospitals and medical staff could prevent doctors from helping in times of a disaster. As a result, two state laws were passed in 2008 protecting medical staff during states of emergency.

MED TIP

A study of law, ethics, and bioethics can assist the medical professional in making a sound decision based on reason and logic rather than on emotion or a "gut feeling."

Ethics asks difficult questions, such as "How should we act?" and "How should we live?" The answers to such questions are often subjective and can change according to circumstances, so it is realistic to ask, "Why study ethics?" The short answer is that in spite of the many gray areas of ethics, we are expected to take the right action when confronted with an ethical dilemma. We must consider the consequences of wrongdoing. We must learn how to think about the ethics of an action and then how to translate those thoughts into action. So, even if the "right thing" isn't always clear, we can prepare our minds to think about an action and to see how the experiences of others can influence our own actions. The important thing is to be able to think and then take action!

Of course, not all illegal or unethical cases end up with a lawsuit or in a court of law. However, brief descriptions of actual court cases are sprinkled throughout the book to illustrate the topics that are discussed in the chapter. These cases alert us to the variety of situations that have negatively affected the careers of physicians and healthcare professionals, as well as the patients who were harmed.

While studying ethics, ask yourself the following questions. Do you know what you would do in each of the following situations? Do you know whether you are exposing yourself to a lawsuit?

- A fellow student says, "Sure, I stole this book from the bookstore, but the tuition is so high that I figured the school owed me at least one book." What do you do? (Chapter 1, Introduction to Medical Law, Ethics, and Bioethics)

- An orderly working in a skilled-nursing facility is left alone in the dining room in charge of a group of elderly residents who are finishing their dinner. One of the residents does not want to eat but wishes to go back to his own room, which he cannot find by himself. The orderly has been instructed never to leave patients alone. Because he cannot leave the dining room full of patients, nor can he allow the one elderly resident to find his own room, the orderly locks the dining room door. The elderly resident claims he has been falsely imprisoned. Is he correct? (Chapter 2, The Legal System)

- You are drawing a specimen of blood from Emma Helm, who says that she doesn't like having blood drawn. In fact, she tells you that the sight of blood makes her "queasy." While you are taking her blood specimen, she faints and hits her head against the side of a cabinet. Are you liable for Emma's injury? If you are not liable, do you know who is? (Chapter 3, Importance of the Legal System for the Physician and the Healthcare Professional)

- You are a recently hired registered nurse working in the office of an internist. You have agreed to answer the phone calls in a physician's office while the receptionist is having lunch. A patient calls and says he must have a prescription refill order for blood pressure medication called in right away to his pharmacy, because he is leaving town in 30 minutes. He says that he has been on the medication for four years and that he is a personal friend of the physician. No one except you is in the office at this time. What do you do? (Chapter 4, Today's Healthcare Environment)

▶ Terry O'Rourke, a 25-year-old female patient of Dr. Williams, refuses to take her medication to control diabetes and is not following her dietary plan to control her disease. After repeated attempts to help this patient, Dr. Williams has decided that she can no longer provide care for Terry. The office staff has been advised not to schedule Terry for any more appointments. Is there an ethical or legal concern (or both) regarding this situation? Is there anything else that either Dr. Williams or her staff should do to sever the patient relationship with Terry? (Chapter 5, The Physician–Patient Relationship)

▶ You drop a sterile packet of gauze on the floor. The inside of the packet is still considered sterile; however, the policy in your office is to re-sterilize anything that drops on the floor. This is the last sterile packet on the shelf. The chances are very slight that any infection would result from using the gauze within the packet. What do you do? (Chapter 6, Professional Liability and Medical Malpractice)

▶ The pharmaceutical salesperson has just brought in a supply of nonprescription vitamin samples for the physicians in your practice to dispense to their patients. All the other staff members take samples home for their families' personal use. They tell you to do the same, since the samples will become outdated before the physicians can use all of them. It would save you money. What do you do? Is it legal? Is it ethical? (Chapter 7, Public Duties of the Physician and the Healthcare Professional)

▶ You feel a slight prick on your sterile glove as you assist Dr. Brown on a minor surgical procedure. Dr. Brown has a quick temper, and he will become angry if you delay the surgical procedure while you change gloves. As there was just a slight prick and the patient's wound is not infected, will it hurt to wear the gloves during the procedure? Who is at fault if the patient develops a wound infection? Is this a legal and/or ethical issue? (Chapter 8, Workplace Law and Ethics)

▶ Demi Daniels calls to ask you to change her diagnosis in her medical record from R/O (rule out) bladder infection to "bladder infection" because her insurance will not pay for an R/O diagnosis. In fact, she tested negative for an infection, but the physician placed her on antibiotics anyway. What do you do? Is this legal? Is it ethical? (Chapter 9, The Medical Record)

▶ A physician from another office steps into your office and asks to see the chart of a neighbor whom he believes may have an infectious disease. He states that the neighbor is a good friend and that she will not mind if he reviews her medical chart. Is it legal for you to give the chart to this physician? (Chapter 10, Patient Confidentiality and HIPAA)

▶ A well-known baseball Hall of Fame fielder received a liver transplant in 1995. It took only two days for his hospital's transplant team to locate an organ donor for this national hero when his own liver was failing due to cirrhosis and hepatitis. The patient was a recovering alcoholic who also had a small cancerous growth that was not believed to be life-threatening. Because there are relatively few liver donor organs available, there were mixed feelings about speeding up the process for a famous person. He subsequently died a few years later from cancer. What are the ethics of giving a scarce liver to a recovering alcoholic? What are your thoughts about the statement "People should not be punished just because they are celebrities?" (Chapter 11, Ethical and Bioethical Issues in Medicine)

▶ Your neighbor's 18-year-old unmarried daughter has just given birth to a baby boy. The neighbor is concerned that neither she, nor her daughter, can take care of this baby. She asks you what you can suggest. Is it a violation of ethics to tell her about the Safe Harbor Law? (Chapter 12, Ethical Issues Relating to Life)

▶ An elderly widow is rushed to the hospital in the middle of the night with a massive heart attack. She is in need of an emergency treatment which requires the services of a special surgical team. It takes almost two hours to gather the entire team back together as they have all left for the day. This patient has a good chance of recovering if the procedure is done within six hours after the heart attack occurs. But, as soon as the surgical team is together and the operating room is ready, another patient, a 45-year-old woman, is brought into the emergency room in need of the same procedure to save her life. It is agreed that the 45-year-old woman will receive the treatment first, but the procedure takes longer than expected. This procedure could not be performed on the widow because the six hour "window of opportunity" to do the procedure had passed. The younger woman lives, and the elderly widow dies the next day. Is the decision on who will receive the procedure an ethical or legal one, or both? (Chapter 13, Death and Dying)

These situations, and others like them, are addressed throughout this book.

MEDICAL LAW

Laws are rules or actions prescribed by an authority such as the federal government and the court system that have a binding legal force. Medical law addresses legal rights and obligations that affect patients and protect individual rights, including those of healthcare employees. For example, practicing medicine without a license, Medicaid fraud, and patient rape are violations of medical laws that are always illegal and immoral or unethical.

It is easy to become confused when studying law and ethics, because, while the two are different, they often overlap. Some illegal actions may be quite ethical—for example, exceeding the speed limit when rushing an injured child to the hospital. Of course, many unethical actions may not be illegal, such as cheating on a test. Law and ethics exist in everyday life and, thus, are difficult to separate. An insurance company denying payment for a life-saving heart transplant on a 70-year-old male is not illegal in most cases, but it may well be unethical.

MED TIP

In general, an illegal act, or one that is against the law, is always unethical. However, an unethical act may not be illegal. For instance, a physician traveling on a plane does not have a legal obligation to come forward when an announcement is made requesting a doctor to assist with an emergency. But it may be an unethical action if the passenger dies without the help of an available doctor.

There is a greater reliance on laws and the court system, as our society and medical system have become more complex. In fact, some physicians have been practicing a form of medicine called "defensive medicine." This means that they may order unnecessary tests and procedures in order to protect themselves from a lawsuit; because then they can say "I did everything that I could to treat the patient." This type of preventive medicine is not only costly but also may put the patient through needless and uncomfortable tests and procedures. In some cases, physicians may even avoid ordering tests or procedures that may carry a risk for the patient because they do not want to take a chance that a lawsuit may result if the patient outcome is poor.

The law provides a yardstick by which to measure our actions, and it punishes us when our actions break the laws. Many of the actions punishable by law are considered morally wrong, such as rape, murder, and theft. The problem with measuring our actions using only the law, and not considering the ethical aspects of an issue, is that the law allows many actions that are morally offensive, such as lying and manipulating people. Laws against actions such as adultery, which most people agree is immoral, exist, but they are rarely enforced. Some situations involving interpersonal relationships between coworkers, such as taking credit for someone else's work, are difficult to address with laws. Other work issues such as lying on job applications, padding expense accounts, and making unreasonable demands on coworkers are usually handled on the job and are typically not regulated by laws.

A further caution about relying on the law for moral decision-making: the requirements of the law often tend to be negative. The standards of morality, on the other hand, are often seen to be positive. The law forbids us to harm, rob, or defame others; but in most states it does not require us to help people. Morality would tell us to give aid to the drowning victim even if the law does not mandate that we do so.

Many people believe that something is wrong, or unethical, only if the law forbids it. Conversely, they reason that if the law says it's all right, then it is also ethical. Unfortunately, these people believe that until the law tells them otherwise, they have no ethical responsibility beyond the law. Finally, laws are often reactive and may lag behind the moral standards of society; slavery is the most obvious example. Sexual harassment and racial discrimination existed as moral problems long before laws were enacted to suppress this behavior.

There are a multitude of laws, including criminal and civil statutes (laws enacted by state and federal legislatures) as well as state medical practice acts that affect healthcare professionals. **Medical practice acts,** established in all 50 states by statute, apply specifically to the way medicine is practiced in a particular state. These acts define the meaning of the "practice of medicine" as well as requirements and methods for licensure. They also define what constitutes unprofessional conduct in that particular state. While the laws vary from state to state, the more common items of unprofessional conduct include the following:

- Practicing medicine without a license
- Impaired ability to practice medicine due to addiction or mental illness
- Conviction of a felony
- Insufficient record keeping
- Allowing an unlicensed person to practice medicine
- Physical abuse of patients
- Prescribing drugs in excessive amounts

As we study law and ethics as they relate to medicine, we will frequently use court cases to illustrate points. For our purposes it is not necessary to memorize the specifics of a lawsuit, such as the legal citation, that has been decided in a court of law. But it is important to keep in mind that unless a decided case is overturned in an appeals court, it is considered to have established a **precedent.** This means that the decision of the case acts as a model for any future cases in which the facts are the same.

ETHICS

Ethics is the branch of philosophy related to morals, moral principles, and moral judgments. A more practical explanation from ethics experts tells us that ethical behavior is that which puts the common good above self interest. Ethics is concerned with the obligation of what we "should" or "ought to" do. **Morality** is the quality of being virtuous or practicing the right conduct. A person is said to be **amoral** if he or she is lacking or indifferent to moral standards. However, the terms *ethics* and *morality* are used interchangeably by many people. Ethics, as part of philosophy, uses reason and logic to analyze problems and find solutions. Ethics, in general, is concerned with the actions and practices that are directed at improving the welfare of people in a moral way. Thus, the study of ethics forces us to use reason and logic to answer difficult questions concerning life, death, and everything in between. In modern terms, we use words such as *right, wrong, good,* and *bad* when making ethical judgments. In other cases, people refer to issues or actions that are *just* and *unjust* or *fair* and *unfair.* **Medical ethics** concerns questions specifically related to the practice of medicine. This branch of ethics is based on principles regulating the behavior of healthcare professionals, including practitioners such as physicians, nurses, and other allied health professionals. It also applies to patients, relatives, and the community-at-large.

> ### MED TIP
> Ethics always involves people. This includes patients, caregivers, healthcare professionals, and the general public.

Ethics is meant to take the past into account, but also to look to the future and ask, "What should I do now?" Unfortunately, using moral views based only on those of parents and peers can lead to radical subjectivism that can make ethical discussion of issues such as euthanasia, abortion, or cloning difficult, if not impossible. Many of our beliefs are based on emotions—for example, we believe that something is wrong if we feel guilt when we do it. While most healthcare practitioners, other than physicians, will not be required to make life and death decisions about their patients, it is still important for everyone to develop his or her own personal value system. Whenever you are involved in an ethical dilemma, you must analyze actions and their consequences to all concerned parties. Law also does this by directing actions into "legal" and "illegal" human actions. Ethical issues are not so easily divided into two categories such as "right" and "wrong."

As we study ethics, we will also analyze various actions and their effects. When following a moral line of reasoning it is advisable to carefully take apart the issues, restate them in your own words, and offer an interpretation, and even a criticism, of them.

> ### MED TIP
> Remember that ethics always involves formal consideration of the interests of others in deciding how to act or behave. In fact, some philosophers believe that almost every decision to do anything is an ethical decision.

Theories of Ethics

Basic questions relating to the study of ethics have been the subject of much debate and analysis, particularly among philosophers. Various philosophers have defined ethics under several categories, such as utilitarianism, natural rights or rights-based, duty-based, justice-based, and virtue-based ethics. A division is often made between *teleological* and *deontological* theories in ethics. A teleological theory asserts that an action is right or wrong depending on whether it produces good or bad consequences. Utilitarianism is an example of this theory. Deontological ethical theory asserts that at least *some* actions are right or wrong and, thus, we have a duty or obligation to perform them or refrain from performing them, without consideration of the consequences. Duty-based ethics is an example of deontological theory. These ethical theories are the basis for many of our country's regulations, such as OSHA, and the norms of our society.

Utilitarianism

Utilitarianism is an ethical theory based on the principle of what is the greatest good for the greatest number of people. This ethical theory is concerned with the impact of actions, or final outcomes, on the welfare of society as a whole. In other words, the "rightness" or "wrongness" of an act is determined solely by its consequences. This view looks at what would satisfy the interests, wants, and needs of *most* people. Additionally, utilitarianism is a consequences-based ethical theory that follows the premise that the ends (consequences) justify the means (methods for achieving the ends). For example, in the case of limited financial resources, money would be spent in a way to benefit the greatest number of people. In this respect, utilitarianism is considered to be an efficient allocation of resources. In a professional context, a **cost/benefit analysis** justifies the means of achieving a goal. In other words, if the benefit (or well-being) of a decision outweighs the cost (financial or otherwise) of achieving a goal, then the means to obtain the goal would be justified. A problem arises when utilitarianism, or cost/benefit analysis, is used for making ethical decisions, because some people will inevitably "fall through the cracks." This could result in serious consequences if a person is denied treatment, and eventually suffers and/or dies because of this denial.

The nation's Medicare system, in which all persons over the age of 65 receive healthcare benefits, is one example of utilitarianism. Congress has limited amounts to allocate for medical coverage and uses those funds to cover the elderly and others, such as the disabled, under the government Medicare Act. However, not *all* people require the benefit. In the case of Medicare, for example, not all elderly persons need to have medical coverage provided for them by this act, because some are wealthy and can afford their own coverage. On the other hand, there are people with low incomes who are not yet 65, and are not **indigent** (impoverished) enough to qualify for Medicaid, but still require some type of medical insurance. Another example of utilitarianism occurs when there is a limited supply of donor organs. Under a utilitarianism approach, patients with the most immediate need (and who would benefit the most) would receive the organ. Using this approach for organ distribution, terminally ill or elderly persons with a limited lifespan would not be the first to receive a scarce resource such as a new heart. A weakness of the utilitarianism approach to moral reasoning is that it is impossible to quantify all the variables. Therefore, it can result in a biased allocation of resources, ignoring the rights of some vulnerable people such as the young, sick, handicapped, or elderly who lack representation or a voice.

Rights-Based Ethics

Rights-based ethics, or a natural rights ethical theory, places the primary emphasis on a person's individual rights. This ethical theory states that rights belong to all people purely by virtue of their being human. Under our rights-based democracy, all Americans have the right to freedom of speech. Employees have the right to due process, which entitles them to a fair hearing in the case of dismissal from their jobs. In the previous example of limited donor organs, using a rights-based ethical approach, every patient needing a donor organ would have the same right to receive the available organ.

The strength of rights-based ethics is a strong attempt to protect the individual from injury. Laws such as OSHA (Occupational Safety and Health Act) benefit society as a whole because everyone in the workplace is protected by this act. The downside to this approach is that there can be incidents of individualistic selfish behavior which is independent of the outcomes (consequences). For example, unions protect their membership while excluding the rights of the non-union members of society.

Duty-Based Ethics

Duty-based ethics focuses on performing one's duty to various people and institutions such as parents, employers, employees, and customers (patients). This line of moral reasoning follows the belief that our actions should be universal which means that everyone would act the same way with the same set of circumstances. For example, Americans have a duty to adhere to laws enforced by government authorities. Duties also arise from our own actions. Therefore, we have a duty to keep promises, not to lie, and to make reparations to those whom we have harmed. These reparations include compensation for any damage to another person. An example is the financial compensation a medical practitioner would make if he or she caused harm to a patient.

One of the problems encountered with this moral line of reasoning is the mandate to do things out of a sense of duty regardless of the consequences. In addition, we may hear conflicting opinions about what is our "duty" or responsibility in particular circumstances. If our employer asks us to do something that we are sure is wrong or unethical, we have a duty not to perform the action. However, this violates our duty to our employer. Most religions have statements that address one's duty as a member of that faith or religion. However, many people do not accept their faith's beliefs concerning issues such as birth control and working on the Sabbath, but do adhere to other doctrines of their religion. Many people claim that a sense of duty is not enough when dealing with ethical dilemmas. Rules do not always work. And people from different cultures may have a different sense of what "duty" means.

Justice-Based Ethics

Justice-based ethics is based on an important moral restraint called "the veil of ignorance." The philosopher John Rawls believed that all social contracts, such as who should receive a scarce organ donation, should be handled so that no one would know the gender, age, race, health, number of children, income, wealth, or any other arbitrary personal information about the recipient. This "veil of ignorance," meaning we would not *see* the recipients of our choices, would allow the decision-makers (such as Congress or medical experts) to be impartial in their decisions. The so-called "veil of ignorance" means that no one person is advantaged or disadvantaged. In effect, the "least well off" person would then have the same chance for scarce resources and justice as the more educated and wealthy. Rawls, who equated justice with fairness, assumed that people have a self-interest when forming social contracts such as who will receive medical care. The justice-based model of ethics infers that every citizen should have equal access to medical care. For example, children with genetic diseases which would require large financial resources deserve good care simply as a matter of justice. Proponents of justice-based ethics believe insurance premium rates and risk should be spread over all members of the nation such as in a federal single-payer system.

Opponents of this theory believe it is unfair for the healthy to subsidize the unhealthy. Furthermore, under the current gigantic healthcare system and media coverage it is impossible to have the "veil of ignorance" that is demanded by this ethical model.

Virtue-Based Ethics

A moral virtue is a character trait that is morally valued. The emphasis of **virtue-based ethics** is on persons and not necessarily on the decisions or principles that are involved. Most people agree that virtues are just good habits, such as fairness and honesty. Other examples of virtues and good character traits are integrity, trust, respect, empathy, generosity, truthfulness, and the ability to admit mistakes.

Virtue-based ethics, or seeking the "good life," is our legacy from the philosopher Aristotle. According to him, the goal of life, for which we all aim, is happiness. He believed that happiness is founded not solely on what we gain in life, but also on who we are. For example, the joy of being a medical professional cannot be present without having the traits or virtues that make one a good physician, nurse, medical assistant, technologist, or other healthcare professional. These virtues include perseverance, integrity, compassion, and trust. Aristotle's theory is considered inadequate by many because it does not take into account the consequences of an action, as in utilitarianism, or the rights of others, as in rights-based ethics. In addition, there are some who believe that people might take advantage of someone who is too trusting.

While each of these five ethical theories can have positive outcomes and are useful in certain circumstances, no one ethical theory or system is perfect.

Ethical standards that relate to the medical profession are set and defined by professional organizations such as the American Medical Association. All professional disciplines, such as nursing and medical assisting, have their own organizations and standards of guiding ethical codes of conduct. Codes of ethics are discussed more fully in Chapter 5.

In general, people believe an action is wrong or unethical if it

- Causes emotional or physical harm to someone else.
- Goes against one's deepest beliefs.
- Makes a person feel guilty or uncomfortable about a particular action.
- Breaks the law or traditions of their society.
- Violates the rights of another person.

No one ethical theory is perfect. The medical community and the healthcare professional use a combination of many theories to determine the correct action to take.

See Table 1.1 ■ for comparison of the advantages and disadvantages of the five ethical theories.

Principles or Values That Drive Ethical Behavior

Most people have established, throughout their lifetime, their own set of principles or values that drive their ethical behavior. Benjamin Franklin included in his list of virtues such things as cleanliness, silence, and industry. In today's world, we don't think of these things as virtues; they are assumed by many people to be a part of everyday life.

MED TIP
One should not perform an action which might threaten the dignity and welfare of another individual.

Theory	Strengths	Weaknesses
Utilitarianism The greatest good for the greatest number	1. Encourages efficiency and productivity 2. Consistent with profit maximization—getting the most value (benefit) for the least cost 3. Looks beyond the individual to assess impact of the decision on all who are affected	1. Virtually impossible to quantify all variables 2. Can result in biased allocations of resources, especially when some who are affected lack representation or voice 3. Can result in ignoring the rights of some people to achieve a utilitarian outcome
Rights-Based Ethics Individual's rights to be protected	1. Protects the individual from injury; consistent with rights to freedom and privacy	1. Can encourage individualist selfish behavior that, if misinterpreted, may result in anarchy
Duty-Based Ethics Based on absolute moral rules	1. Absolute rules or principles help us determine what is our duty toward others 2. People are not treated as a means to an end 3. A mandate for respect and impartiality	1. Hard to identify who should determine the rules and principles of moral behavior 2. Who determines what our duty is to one another
Justice-Based Ethics Fair distribution of benefits and burdens	1. A democratic approach 2. Based on a "veil of ignorance" 3. No one person is advantaged or disadvantaged	1. Some believe it is unfair for the healthy to subsidize the unhealthy
Virtue-Based Ethics Based on belief that we have a duty or responsibility to others	1. Based on premise that our actions are universal 2. Virtuous behavior includes perseverance, courage, integrity, compassion, humility, and justice	1. Concern that people can be taken advantage of if they are too complacent or trusting

TABLE 1.1

Strengths and Weaknesses of Five Ethical Theories

However, in today's fast-paced healthcare environment, it is important to slow down enough to consider some of the most respected virtues. Some of these virtues include beneficence, fidelity, gentleness, humility, justice, perseverance, responsibility, sanctity of life, tolerance, and work.

▶ Beneficence—The action of helping others and performing actions that would result in benefit to another person. It cautions all those working in the healthcare field to do no harm to anyone. In fact, when we prevent harmful actions from happening to our patients, we are using this virtue to its fullest extent (Figure 1.1 ■).

▶ **Fidelity**—Loyalty and faithfulness to others. Fidelity implies that we will perform our duty. We must use caution when practicing fidelity. A strict adherence to a sense of duty or loyalty to an employer does not mean that we must perform actions that are wrong or harmful to our patients.

▶ Gentleness—A mild, tenderhearted approach to other people. Gentleness goes beyond compassion since it can exist in the absence of a person's pain and suffering.

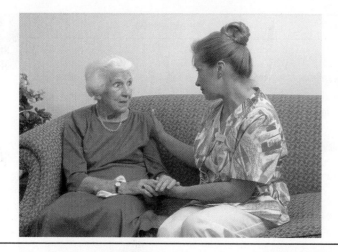

FIGURE 1.1
Beneficence: Helping Others

A gentle approach to patient care is considered by patients to be one of the most welcome virtues. Both men and women have the ability to demonstrate gentleness.

▶ Humility—Acquiring an unpretentious and humble manner. Humility is considered to be the opposite of vanity. It has been said, "honesty and humility are sisters." This means that to be truly humble, we must be entirely honest with ourselves. Humility requires that we recognize our own limits. Vanity and a sense of self-importance have no place in medicine. When mistakes are made, they must be reported so that corrections can take place. It takes a humble—and honest—person to admit mistakes.

▶ Justice—Fairness in all our actions with other people. It means that we must carefully analyze how to balance our behavior and be fair to all. Justice implies that the same rules will apply to everyone. This means that as healthcare workers we cannot demonstrate favoritism with our patients or our coworkers. The four cardinal virtues are justice, temperance, prudence, and courage. Of these four, only justice is considered to be an absolute good. To emphasize this point, the philosopher Immanuel Kant said, "If legal justice perishes, then it is no longer worthwhile for men to remain alive on this earth."

▶ Perseverance—Persisting with a task or idea even against obstacles. This virtue implies a steady determination to get the job done. For example, it takes perseverance to complete one's education. This is an outstanding virtue for a healthcare worker to have. It implies that one will finish the job even if it is difficult.

▶ Responsibility—A sense of accountability for one's actions. Responsibility implies dependability. A sense of responsibility can become weakened when one is faced with peer pressure. Medical professionals must be able to "answer" or be accountable for their actions. Taking responsibility is a sign of maturity.

▶ **Sanctity of life**—The sacredness of human life. All human beings must be protected. This means that we may have to become an advocate for people who cannot speak out for themselves, such as children and many elderly.

▶ **Tolerance**—A respect for those whose opinions, practices, race, religion, and nationality differ from our own. Tolerance requires a fair and objective attitude toward opinions and practices with which we may or may not agree.

▶ Work—An effort applied toward some end goal. Work, if performed well, is clearly a virtue that almost everyone enters into at one time or another. In its broadest sense, work is part of our everyday existence that includes activities such as studying, child rearing, home maintenance, gardening, hobbies, and religious activities. The work we do to earn a living can be performed with pride or can be performed poorly and grudgingly. The most satisfying work involves achieving a goal that we believe is worthwhile and worthy of our talent.

Interpersonal Ethics

The expectation of employees in the workplace is that they will be treated ethically with respect, integrity, honesty, fairness, empathy, sympathy, compassion, and loyalty. Professional healthcare employees are no different in their expectation of receiving such treatment.

MED TIP

Remember to treat each person, whether patient or coworker, the way you wish to be treated.

▶ Respect implies the ability to consider and honor another person's beliefs and opinions. This is a critical quality for a healthcare worker because patients come from a variety of racial, ethnic, and religious backgrounds. Coworkers' opinions must also be respected, even if contrary to one's own.

▶ **Integrity** is the unwavering adherence to one's principles. People with integrity are dedicated to maintaining high standards. For example, integrity means that healthcare professionals will wash their hands between each patient contact even when no one is looking. Dependability, such as being on time for work every day, is a key component of integrity. Integrity is so important that many professions include a statement regarding this quality in their code of ethics. For example, the Pharmacy Technician Code of Ethics states that this healthcare professional "supports and promotes honesty and integrity in the profession, which includes a duty to observe the law, maintain the highest moral and ethical conduct at all times, and uphold the ethical principles of the profession."

▶ Honesty is the quality of truthfulness, no matter what the situation. Healthcare professionals must have the ability to admit an error and then take corrective steps. Anyone who carries out orders for a physician has a duty to notify the physician of any error or discrepancy in those orders.

▶ Fairness is treating everyone the same. It implies an unbiased impartiality and a sense of justice. This is a particularly important characteristic for supervisors.

▶ **Empathy** is the ability to understand the feelings of others without actually experiencing their pain or distress. Acting in this caring way expresses sensitivity to patients' or fellow employees' feelings (Figure 1.2 ■).

▶ **Sympathy,** on the other hand, is feeling sorry for or pitying someone else. Most people, including patients, react better to empathetic listeners than to sympathetic ones.

▶ **Compassion** is the ability to have a gentle, caring attitude toward patients and fellow employees. Any illness, and in particular a terminal illness, can cause fear and loneliness in many patients. A compassionate healthcare professional can help to ease this fear.

▶ Loyalty is a sense of faithfulness or commitment to a person or persons. Employers expect loyalty from their employees. This loyalty should be granted unless the practice of one's employer is unethical or illegal. For example, it is never appropriate to recommend that a patient seek the services of another physician unless instructed to do so by the employer. By the same token, employees expect loyalty, or fair treatment, from their employer.

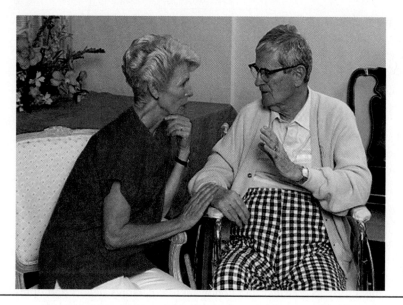

FIGURE 1.2
Empathy Draws a
Positive Response
from the Patient

MED TIP

Loyalty to one's employer does *not* mean hiding an error that has been committed by that employer or by a physician.

Additionally, there are specific issues that affect the workplace, such as privacy, due process, sexual harassment, and comparable worth.

▶ Privacy, or confidentiality, is the ability to safeguard another person's confidences or information. Violating patient confidentiality is both a legal and ethical issue that carries penalties. Employees have a right to expect the contents of their personnel records to be held in confidence by their employer. By the same token, it is inappropriate for employees to discuss the personal life of their physician/ employer.

▶ **Due process** is the entitlement of employees of the government and public companies to have certain procedures followed when they believe their rights are in jeopardy. The Fourteenth Amendment of the Constitution acts to prevent the state's deprivation or impairment of "any person's life, liberty, or property without due process of the law." The Fifth Amendment also restricts the federal government from depriving individuals of these rights without due process of the law. In a work environment, this means that employees of the government and public companies accused of an offense are entitled to a fair hearing in their defense. Due process is also a protection guaranteed to healthcare workers as it relates to their state certification, license, or registration to practice. To remove a person's license to practice his or her profession is the same as removing a person's livelihood. Thus, the removal of this documentation is not to be taken lightly. If there are allegations (accusations) made claiming that a healthcare worker, such as a medical technologist, nurse, or a physician, has committed malpractice, then their rights to defend themselves and due process must be protected. This means that they must receive a notice of the charges, an investigation of the allegations, and a hearing if enough evidence is found. If these allegations are proven to be false, then the individual must not be penalized.

▶ **Sexual harassment, or gender harassment,** is defined in the Equal Employment Opportunity Commission guidelines, which are part of Title VII of the Amended Civil Rights Act of 1964:

> Unwelcome sexual advances, requests for sexual favors, and other verbal or physical conduct of a sexual nature constitute sexual harassment when (1) submission to such conduct is made either explicitly or implicitly a term or condition of an individual's employment; (2) submission to or rejection of such conduct by an individual is used as the basis for employment decisions affecting such individual; or (3) such conduct has the purpose or effect of interfering with an individual's work performance or creating an intimidating, hostile, or offensive working environment.

MED TIP

Any type of gender harassment, whether male or female, is seen as one person exerting power over another.

Both males and females working in the healthcare field have reported sexual harassment.

▶ **Comparable worth,** also known as pay equity, is a theory that extends equal pay requirements to all persons who are doing equal work. The principle of fairness and justice dictates that work of equal value performed by men and women in the workplace should be rewarded with equal compensation. However, research demonstrates that there is a wage gap, with some estimates as high as 36 percent, due to the undervaluation of work performed by women. This results in injustice; equals are not treated equally. Because pay scales are the same for males and females in many of the healthcare professions, the situation is not as intense as it is in the business world. However, employers and supervisors who are involved in the hiring process must be committed to providing equal pay for equal work.

While it is important to reflect on the above concepts, many ethical topics relating to the medical field fall into categories of common sense. See Table 1.2 ■ for examples that might fall into the category of a "common sense" approach to ethics.

			TABLE 1.2
Avoid harming others	Keep promises and contracts	Be fair	
Respect the rights of others	Obey the law	Reinforce these imperatives in others	**Common Sense Approach to Ethics**
Do not lie or cheat	Help those in need		

MODELS FOR EXAMINING ETHICAL DILEMMAS

The decision-maker must always be objective when making ethical decisions. It is critical to examine all the facts of a given situation by gathering as much information or data as possible. Alternative solutions to the problem must be assessed if they are available. All sides of every issue should be studied before ethical decisions are made. The following are three decision-making models that can be helpful when resolving ethical issues: the three-step (Blanchard-Peale) ethics model, the seven-step decision model, and Dr. Bernard Lo's clinical model.

Three-Step Ethics Model

Kenneth Blanchard and Norman Vincent Peale advise the use of a three-step model when evaluating an ethical dilemma. The three steps are to ask yourself each of the following questions:

- Is it legal?
- Is it balanced?
- How does it make me feel?

1. *Is it legal?* When applying this three-step model, if the situation is clearly illegal, such as inflicting bodily harm on another, then the matter is also clearly unethical, and you do not even have to progress to the second question. However, if the action is not against the law, then you should ask yourself the second question.

2. *Is it balanced?* This question helps to determine if another person or group of people is negatively affected by the action. In other words, is there now an *imbalance* so that one person or group suffers or benefits more than another as a result of your action? For example, in the case of a scarce resource such as donor organs, does one group of people have greater access?

3. *How does it make me feel?* This final question refers to how the action will affect you emotionally. Would you be hesitant to explain your actions to a loved one? How would you feel if you saw your name in the paper associated with the action? Can you face yourself in the mirror?

If you can answer the first two questions with a strong "Yes" and the final question with a strong "Good," then the action is likely to be ethical.

For example, student cheating is clearly unethical. By using the three-step ethics model, we have an even clearer idea of why it is unethical to look at even one answer on another student's test. We ask the three questions:

1. *Is it legal?* Yes, as far as we know there is no law against cheating.

2. *Is it balanced?* No, it is not. This question is where the model really helps us. One group or person (in this case the cheater) does have an advantage over another group or person. In addition, the grades will be skewed for the entire class, because the person who cheated will receive a higher grade than what he or she earned.

3. *How does it make me feel?* Remember that we have to live with ourselves. The philosopher Thomas Aquinas said, "We become what we do," meaning that if we lie, we become a liar. Or in this case, if we cheat, we become a cheater.

MED TIP

The three-step ethics model is a quick way to check yourself when you are uncomfortable about an ethical decision. Use it often!

Analysis is the ability to carefully take apart issues, restate them in your own words, and offer an interpretation, and even criticism, of them. The following two models require careful analysis of the problem.

The Seven-Step Decision Model

I. *Determine the facts by asking the following questions.*

What do we need to know?

Who is involved in the situation?

Where does the ethical situation take place?

When does it occur?

II. *Define the precise ethical issue.*

For example, is it a matter of fairness, justice, morality, or individual rights?

III. *Identify the major principles, rules, and values.*

For example, is this a matter of integrity, quality, respect for others, or profit?

IV. *Specify the alternatives.*

List the major alternative courses of action, including those that represent some form of compromise. This may be a choice between simply doing or not doing something.

V. *Compare values and alternatives.*

Determine if there is one principle or value, or a combination of principles and values, that is so compelling that the proper alternative is clear.

VI. *Assess the consequences.*

Identify short-term, long-term, positive, and negative consequences for the major alternatives. The short-term gain or loss is often overridden when long-term consequences are considered. This step often reveals an unanticipated result of major importance.

VII. *Make a decision.*

The consequences are balanced against one's primary principles or values. Always double-check your decision.

The seven-step decision model forces us to closely examine the facts before we make an ethical decision. This model is helpful when making a decision that has many sub-decision questions to examine; for example, "Who should the physician treat first?," "Should I look at the exam paper of the person sitting next to me?," or even "What career choice should I make?" Obviously, some of these decisions require a quick response while others, such as selection of a career choice, require more time and research. This model can be used to examine all of the end-of-chapter cases in this textbook.

Dr. Bernard Lo's Clinical Model

Dr. Lo has developed a clinical model for decision-making to ensure that no important considerations relating to patient care are overlooked. He believes this approach can be used to help resolve important patient-care issues, such as when to proceed with life-sustaining interventions (for example, cardiopulmonary resuscitation [CPR] or kidney dialysis). His model also includes the patient's preferences and viewpoints.

I. *Gather information.*

If the patient is competent, what are his or her preferences for care?

If the patient lacks decision-making capacity, has he or she provided advance directives for care?

If the patient lacks decision-making capacity, who should act as surrogate?

What are the views of the healthcare team?

What other issues complicate the case?

II. *Clarify the ethical issues.*

What are the pertinent ethical issues?

Determine the ethical guidelines that people are using.

What are the reasons for and against the alternative plans of care?

III. *Resolve the dilemma.*

Meet with the healthcare team and with the patient or surrogate.

List the alternatives of care.

Negotiate a mutually acceptable decision.

Dr. Lo emphasizes that patients should play an active role in decisions. Everything should be done to ensure that the patient has been well informed by providing information in an easy-to-understand way. This model cautions the healthcare team to seek the patient's decision on advance directives. He requires that the entire healthcare team—including medical students, nurses, social workers, and all others who provide direct care for the patient—be involved in the decisions. These caregivers should voice any moral objections they have to the proposed care. Finally, the patient's best interests must always be protected. This model is more commonly used in a hospital or clinic setting.

MED TIP

When following a moral line of reasoning, it is always advisable to examine all of the facts rather than to predetermine what should be done.

WHAT ETHICS IS NOT

Ethics is not just about how you feel, the sincerity of your beliefs, or your emotions; nor is it only about religious viewpoints. Feelings, such as in the statement "I feel that capital punishment is wrong," are not sufficient when making an ethical decision. Others may feel that capital punishment is right in that it helps to deter crime. All people have feelings and beliefs. However, ethics must be grounded in reason and fact. For example, a statement such as "I feel that cheating is wrong" doesn't tell us why you believe it is wrong to cheat. A better statement reflecting ethics would be, "I think cheating is wrong because it gives one student an unfair advantage over another student."

The sincerity with which people hold their beliefs is also not an adequate reason when making an ethical decision. For example, Hitler sincerely believed that he was right in exterminating more than 6 million Jews. His sincerity did not make him right.

Emotional responses to ethical dilemmas are not sufficient either. Emotions may affect why people do certain things, such as the woman who kills her husband in a rage after discovering he had an affair. However, we should not let our emotions dictate how we make ethical decisions. We may have helplessly watched a loved one die a slow death from cancer, but our emotions should not cloud the issue of euthanasia and cause us to kill our ill patients.

Ethics is not just about religious beliefs. Many people associate ideas of right and wrong with their religious beliefs. While there is often an overlap between ethics and what a religion teaches as right and wrong, people can hold very strong ethical and moral beliefs without following any formal religion.

MED TIP

Our determination of what is ethical or moral can have serious consequences in human action.

BIOETHICS

Bioethics, also known as biomedical ethics, is one branch of applied, or practical, ethics. It refers to moral dilemmas and issues prevalent in today's society as a result of advances in medicine and medical research. The term *bio,* meaning life, combined with *ethics* relates to the moral conduct of right and wrong in life and death issues. Ethical problems of the biological sciences, including research on animals, all fall under the domain of bioethics. Some of the bioethical issues discussed in this text include the allocation of scarce resources such as transplant organs, beginning-of-life issues, cloning, harvesting embryos, concerns surrounding death and dying, experimentation and the use of human subjects, who owns the right to body cells, and dilemmas in the treatment of catastrophic disease.

Bioethics uses a form of moral analysis to assist in determining the obligations and responsibilities of unique issues relating to modern healthcare. Today's modern medical care requires that decision-makers carefully examine facts, identify the moral challenges, and then look carefully at all alternatives. There are basically four principles that can serve as guidelines when confronting bioethical dilemmas. These include the principles of autonomy, beneficence, nonmalfeasance, and justice.

The **principle of autonomy** means that people have the right to make decisions about their own life. The concept of "informed consent" is included in this principle. It means that patients must be informed and understand what they are told before they can provide consent for the treatment. They must be told what the treatment involves, the risks involved, the chance for success, and the alternatives.

The **principle of beneficence,** or the principle of doing good, means that we must not harm patients while we are trying to help them. This principle recognizes that medical science must do what is best for each individual patient. If there are risks involved, then the principle of autonomy must be invoked so that decisions are made in conjunction with patient's wishes.

The **principle of nonmalfeasance** is taken from the Latin maxim *Primum non nocere,* which means "First, do no harm." This is a warning to all members of the health-care profession. Nonmalfeasance completes the principle of beneficence because we are now asking the medical profession to not only do good for the patient, but also to do no harm in the process. In some cases the risks of a treatment may outweigh the benefits. For example, when a surgeon removes a pregnant woman's cancerous uterus to save her life, her unborn child will not live. The principle of nonmalfeasance causes the medical profession to stop and think before acting.

Finally, the **principle of justice** warns us that equals must be treated equally. The same treatments must be given to all patients whether they are rich, poor, educated, uneducated, able-bodied, or disabled.

These four bioethical principles are guidelines for physicians and healthcare professionals to use when patients are unable to provide their personal wishes. For example, there have been cases of "wrongful life" in which a fetus is delivered too soon before development is complete. These infants, if they survive, may have severe disabilities. Physicians may be requested by parents to "do nothing" to resuscitate or save their undeveloped child. Issues such as these weigh heavily upon the shoulders of all medical professionals. Having a set of guidelines, such as the above four principles, to follow has helped in some of the decision-making.

Bioethicists, specialists in the field of bioethics, give thought to ethical concerns that often examine the more abstract dimensions of ethical issues and dilemmas. For example, they might ask, "What are the social implications of surrogate motherhood?" Bioethicists are often authors, teachers, and researchers. This branch of ethics poses difficult, if not impossible, questions for the medical practitioner. Examples of some of the difficult ethical and bioethical situations that face the healthcare professional are listed under Points to Ponder at the end of this chapter.

THE ROLE OF ETHICS COMMITTEES

Hospitals, as well as other healthcare organizations and agencies, have active ethics committees that examine ethical issues relating to patient care. This type of oversight committee consists of a variety of members from many healthcare fields as well as other disciplines, including physicians, nurses, clergy, psychologists, ethicists, lawyers, healthcare administrators, and family and community members. The ethics committee can serve in an advisory capacity to patients, families, and staff for case review of difficult ethical issues, especially when there is a lack of agreement as to what is in the patient's best interests. They also develop and review health policies and guidelines regarding ethical issues such as organ transplantation. After examining the facts surrounding the ethical issue, the committee often determines a recommendation based on predetermined criteria. These criteria might include the severity of the patient's medical condition, the age of the patient, and the chance for ultimate recovery.

The ethics committee may examine issues such as when hospitalization or treatment needs to be discontinued for a patient. For example, a hospital ethics committee will assist in determining the best action to take for a terminally ill patient who is on a respirator. In some cases, the committee may be asked to examine if a patient received the appropriate care.

Ethics committees have tremendous power in today's healthcare environment. Patients are holding their doctors and hospitals to a high standard of care. While it is necessary for the committee meetings to be confidential in order to protect the patient's privacy, nevertheless, there should be a strong set of policies that govern how the meetings are conducted.

Unfortunately in some cases, members of an ethics committee will never see or talk to the patient whose life and care they are discussing. Mistakes can be made when a group of people makes a judgment without reviewing all the facts.

MED TIP

It has been suggested that ethics committees make an effort to have disabled people represented on their committee either as a member or as a resource person to represent the viewpoint of the handicapped patient. In some cases decisions are made based on committee members' own prejudice against living with a disability.

QUALITY ASSURANCE PROGRAMS

In addition to ethics committees, most hospitals and healthcare agencies have a quality assurance (QA) program. These programs were established in the early 1960s as a response to the increasing demand from the public for accountability in quality medical care. **Quality assurance** (QA) is gathering and evaluating information about the services provided, as well as the results achieved, and comparing this information with an accepted standard.

Quality assessment measures consist of formal, systematic evaluations of overall patient care. After the results of the evaluations are compared to standard results, then any deficiencies are noted and recommendations for improvements are made (Figure 1.3 ■). The types of issues that are reviewed by a QA committee are

- Patient complaints relating to confidentiality.
- Errors in dispensing medications.
- Errors in labeling of laboratory specimens.
- Adverse reactions to treatments and/or medications.
- Inability to obtain venous blood on the first attempt.
- Safety and monitoring practices for radiology and laboratory areas.
- Infection control.

MEDICAL ETIQUETTE

There are certain rules of **medical etiquette,** or standards of professional behavior, that physicians practice in their relationship and conduct with patients and other physicians. These are general points of behavior and are not generally considered to be medical ethics issues. For instance, physicians expect that their telephone calls to fellow physicians will be taken promptly and that they will be seen immediately when visiting a physician's office. This courtesy is extended to physicians because they are often consulting about patients with other physicians. However, ethical issues are present when one physician overlooks or "covers up" the medical deficiencies of another physician.

In addition, physicians should be referred to as "Doctor" unless they request to be called by their first name. The same courtesy is required for the patient. Many patients, especially the elderly, prefer to be addressed by their surname (with Ms., Miss, Mrs., or Mr.). Many nurses and other allied health professionals prefer to be

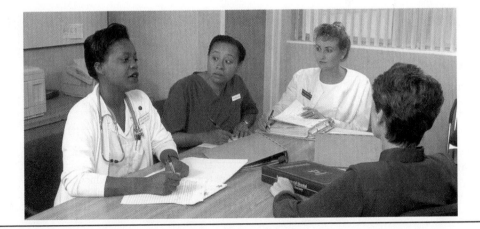

FIGURE 1.3
Quality Assurance (QA)
Committee Meeting

addressed in this manner also. There are allied health professionals who have decades of experience and do not wish to be addressed by either the patient or physician by their first name.

MED TIP

The outdated medical courtesy of physicians providing free medical care to their colleagues is not advisable. If their colleagues were to need further treatment, their insurance coverage may be in jeopardy because of the initial "free" care.

POINTS TO PONDER

1. Should an alcoholic patient, who may die of liver disease, be eligible for an organ transplant?

2. Should a suicidal patient be allowed to refuse a feeding tube?

3. Should prisoners be eligible to receive expensive medical therapies for illnesses?

4. Is assisting with suicide ever ethically justified?

5. Should medical personnel suggest other treatment modes or suggest the patient request a consultation with another physician?

6. Under what circumstances should you report a colleague or physician who is physically, psychologically, or pharmacologically impaired?

7. Is experimentation on human subjects ever justified?

8. When, if ever, should you disclose a patient's medical condition to the family?

9. Should parents be allowed to refuse medical treatment, such as chemotherapy, for their child?

10. If you are an employee in a medical office with access to medical records, should you protect your friend by telling him that you know that his partner has tested positive for AIDS?

These questions, and others like them, are addressed throughout this book.

DISCUSSION QUESTIONS

1. Discuss the difference between the terms *legal* and *moral*.

2. Give an example for each of the following: a medical ethics dilemma, a bioethics situation, and a medical–legal problem.

3. Determine if the ten questions under Points to Ponder are ethical or legal issues or both.

4. Describe five ethical situations that you may face in the profession you intend to follow.

REVIEW CHALLENGE

Short Answer Questions

1. Why do we study law, ethics, and bioethics?

_____

_____

2. What is the purpose of the Medical Practice Acts?

_____

_____

3. What are five theories of ethics?

_____

_____

_____

_____

_____

4. What are ten virtues that drive ethical behavior?

_____ _____ _____

_____ _____ _____

_____ _____ _____

_____

5. What are the three steps of the Blanchard-Peale Model?

   a. _____

   b. _____

   c. _____

6. What is bioethics?

   _____

   _____

7. What is the role of an ethics committee?

   _____

   _____

8. Discuss what's wrong with the following rationalizations for unethical behavior:

   a. "Everybody does it!" _____

   b. "It's not _really_ illegal." _____

   c. "No one will find out." _____

   d. "My employer will protect me." _____

   e. "It's not wrong to do it just this once." _____

Matching

Match the responses in column B with the correct term in column A.

Column A

_____ 1. medical etiquette
_____ 2. ethics
_____ 3. applied ethics
_____ 4. laws
_____ 5. medical ethics
_____ 6. beneficence
_____ 7. veil of ignorance
_____ 8. three-step ethics model
_____ 9. R/O
_____ 10. gut feeling

Column B

a. justice-based
b. decision based on emotion
c. binding rules determined by an authority
d. principle of doing good
e. standards of professional behavior
f. practical application of moral standards
g. rule out a diagnosis
h. moral conduct to regulate behavior of medical professionals
i. branch of philosophy
j. Kenneth Blanchard and Norman Vincent Peale's approach to ethics

Multiple Choice

Select the one best answer to the following statements.

1. A problem that occurs when using a duty-based approach to ethics is

   a. the primary emphasis on a person's individual rights.
   b. determining the greatest good for the greatest number of people.
   c. the conflicting opinions regarding what our responsibility is.
   d. remembering the three-step model approach to solving ethical dilemmas.
   e. understanding the difference between what is fair and unfair.

2. Moral issues that occur as a result of modern medical technology are covered under what specific discipline?

   a. law
   b. medicine
   c. philosophy
   d. bioethics
   e. none of the above

3. When trying to solve an ethical dilemma, it is necessary to

   a. do what everyone else is doing.
   b. use logic to determine the solution.
   c. do what we are told to do by others.
   d. base the decision on religious beliefs only.
   e. allow our emotions and feelings to guide us.

4. The three-step approach to solving ethical dilemmas is based on

   a. asking ourselves how our decision would make us feel if we had to explain our actions to a loved one.
   b. asking ourselves if the intended action is legal.
   c. asking ourselves if the intended action results in a balanced decision.
   d. a, b, and c.
   e. none of the above.

5. A utilitarian approach to solving ethical dilemmas might be used when

   a. allocating a limited supply of donor organs.
   b. trying to find a just decision in which everyone will benefit.
   c. finding a decision based on a sense of duty toward another person.
   d. making sure that no one will "fall through the cracks" and not receive access to care.
   e. none of the above.

6. An illegal act is almost always

   a. hidden.
   b. unethical.
   c. performed with the full knowledge of the healthcare worker.
   d. obvious.
   e. all of the above.

7. A practical application of ethics is

   a. philosophy.
   b. the law.
   c. illegal.
   d. applied ethics.
   e. b and d.

8. An employee who is entitled to a fair hearing in the case of a dismissal from a job is an example of

   a. duty-based ethics.
   b. utilitarianism.
   c. rights-based ethics.
   d. justice-based ethics.
   e. c and d.

9. Laws that affect the medical profession

   a. often overlap with ethics.
   b. have a binding force.
   c. are always fair to all persons.
   d. are determined by a governmental authority.
   e. a, b, and d.

10. Modern laws

   a. may allow some unethical acts such as lying on job applications.
   b. are interpreted by some people to require no ethical responsibility beyond what the law requires.
   c. are not used as a type of yardstick for group behavior.
   d. a and b only.
   e. a, b, and c.

DISCUSSION CASES

1. Analyze the following case using the five theories discussed in this chapter.
   It has become necessary to ration a vaccine for a contagious disease. There is only enough vaccine available to cover 75% of the U.S. population. It is necessary to determine an appropriate method for doing this.

   a. Utilitarianism: _____
   _____

   b. Rights-based ethics: _____
   _____

   c. Duty-based ethics: _____
   _____

   d. Justice-based ethics _____
   _____

   e. Virtue-based ethics: _____
   _____

2. Using the Three-step Ethics Model (Blanchard-Peale) analyze the following case:
   A student knows that two other students who sit next to each other in class are cheating on exams because they talk about it after class. Is this an ethical dilemma? What, if anything, should the student do?

   a. _____

   b. _____

   c. _____

3. *Your friend shows you some books he took from the bookstore without paying for them. When you question him about it, he says, "Sure I took them. But I'm no different from anybody else around here. That's how we all manage to get through school on limited funds. I'll be a better medical professional because of all the knowledge I gain from these books."*

   a. Do you agree or disagree with his rationalization? Why or why not?

   _____

   _____

   b. What do you say to your friend?

   _____

   _____

   c. Is the example in this case any different from taking home medical supplies or equipment from the workplace? Why or why not?

   _____

   _____

   d. What ethical principles discussed in this chapter helped you with your answer?

   _____

   _____

4. *Are there any groups of people (such as children) who should be "protected" based upon one of the ethical theories? If so, who are they and what is the ethical theory?*

   _____

   _____

PUT IT INTO PRACTICE

Talk to someone who is currently working in the medical field that you are working in or plan to enter. Ask him or her for a definition of medical ethics. Then compare it with the textbook definition. Does it match? Discuss with that person an ethical dilemma that he or she has faced and handled.

WEB HUNT

Search the Web site of the American Society of Law, Medicine, and Ethics (www.aslme.org). Check on **Instant Ethicist.** Read and summarize the entry for today.

CRITICAL THINKING EXERCISE

What would you do if, when you leave work at the end of the day, you notice an elderly woman in a wheelchair sitting in the reception area and you recall that you saw her sitting in that same spot when you came in to work in the morning?

BIBLIOGRAPHY

Boatright, J. 2005. *Ethics and the conduct of business*. New York: William Morrow.

Brincat, C., and V. Wike. 2000. *Morality and the professional life.* Upper Saddle River, NJ: Prentice Hall.

Espejo, R. ed. 2003. *Biomedical ethics*. New York: Greenhaven Press.

Jervis, R. 2010. "Katrina case alleges negligence." *USA Today*, Jan. 11, p.1A.

Levine, C. 2004. *Taking sides*. New York: McGraw Hill.

Lo, B. 1995. *Resolving ethical dilemmas: A guide for clinicians.* New York: Lippincott Williams & Wilkins.

Mappes, T., and D. DeGrazia. 2005. *Biomedical ethics*. New York: McGraw Hill.

Munson, R. 2004. *Raising the dead*. New York: Oxford University Press.

Nossiter, A. 2007. "Grand jury won't indict doctor in hurricane deaths." *New York Times*, July 25, A10.

Skipp, C., and A. Campo-Flores. 2006. "What the doctor did." *Newsweek*, July 31, 49.

Valinoti, A. 2009. "Exam-Room Rules: What's in a Name?" *New York Times*, December 15, p. D5.

The Legal System

2

Learning Objectives

1. Define the glossary terms.
2. Discuss why an understanding of the legal profession is necessary for the healthcare professional.
3. Describe the sources of law.
4. Describe the steps for a bill to become a law.
5. Discuss the difference between civil law and criminal law, explaining the areas covered by each.
6. List six intentional torts and give examples of each.
7. List examples of criminal actions that relate to the healthcare worker.
8. Discuss the difference between a felony and a misdemeanor.
9. Describe the types of courts in the legal system.
10. Explain the trial process.
11. Discuss why an expert witness might be used during a lawsuit.

Key Terms

Administrative law	Criminal case	Litigation
Assault	Criminal laws	Misdemeanors
Battery	Defamation of character	Plaintiff
Beyond a reasonable doubt	Defendant	Pleadings
Breach	Deposition	Preponderance of evidence
Breach of contract	Discovery	Prosecutor
Case law	Embezzlement	Regulations
Checks and balances	Expert witness	Slander
Civil law	Expressed contract	*Stare decisis*
Class action lawsuit	Felony	Statutes
Closing argument	Fraudulent	Subpoena
Common law	Implied contract	Subpoena *duces tecum*
Competent	Indictment	Summary judgment
Consideration	Intentional torts	Tort
Constitutional law	Jurisdiction	Unintentional torts
Contract law	Libel	Waive

THE CASE OF JACOB AND THE DISEASED LEG

Jacob is an outstanding quarterback on his high school football team who has been offered a college scholarship when he graduates. Unfortunately, Jacob was injured during a late summer practice just before his senior year. He suffered a compound fracture of the fibula bone in his lower leg. Since the fracture broke through his skin, he required a surgical repair to align or set the bone and close the skin. Dr. M., an orthopedic surgeon, kept Jacob in the hospital for three days and ordered intravenous antibiotics to be administered. When he was discharged from the hospital, Jacob was told to come in for an office visit once a week for six weeks.

At six weeks Jacob's parents took him into the surgeon's office for his cast removal, and except for a slightly inflamed and draining area around his stitches, Jacob's broken bone seemed to be healing. After his cast was removed, Jacob was told to wait for a few minutes while the surgeon went across the hall to check on another patient. Dr. M. removed his gloves, washed his hands in Jacob's exam room, and then went across the hall to examine another patient, Sarah K. The doors between the exam rooms were left open and Jacob's parents could see and hear Dr. M. examine Sarah's infected leg. They could tell that Dr. M. did not replace his gloves. He told Sarah that he was glad to see that her osteomyelitis (a serious bone infection) was almost better and he told her to come back in another week. Dr. M. then came back into Jacob's room, still without gloves, and examined Jacob's leg more carefully. He was concerned about the inflammation around the incision site and told the parents to keep the area clean and dry. He wrote Jacob a prescription for an oral antibiotic and said he could start to put a little weight on his leg. When Jacob came back the following week, his leg was grossly infected with a large abscess. Jacob had to have further surgery to drain the abscess. The pathology report of tissue specimens from Jacob's leg determined that he had developed osteomyelitis. This infection took several months to heal. The delay in his recovery meant that Jacob was unable to play football that fall and lost his chance at a college scholarship. Jacob's parents asked Dr. M. to provide them with the results of the tissue test. They then sued Dr. M. for negligence.

1. What obvious mistake did Dr. M. make?

2. Did Jacob or his parents contribute in any way to his condition?

3. What could all of the involved parties have done to prevent this situation from occurring?

Healthcare professionals must have a good understanding of the legal system for a variety of reasons. The advanced state of medical technology creates new legal, ethical, moral, and financial problems for the consumer and the healthcare practitioner. Today's healthcare consumer demands more of a partnership with the physician and the rest of the healthcare team. Patients have become more aware of their legal rights. Court cases and decisions have had a greater impact than ever on the way healthcare professionals practice business in the medical field. It's important to remember that while laws do protect an individual's rights, they are made for the protection of society as a whole. Laws tell us how we must conduct ourselves during interactions with other people as well as in business transactions, such as in providing healthcare services.

Introduction

MED TIP

Every effort should be made to provide a quality of care for patients that will not only help them recover their health but will also avoid lawsuits.

THE LEGAL SYSTEM

To understand the American legal system, it is important to first understand the two fundamental principles on which the U.S. system of government was founded—federalism and checks and balances. A federal form of government is one in which power is divided between a central government and smaller regional governments. The Constitution of the United States, which was drafted in Philadelphia in 1787, established a federal form of government, giving a limited and enumerated power to the central government (i.e., the federal government). All powers that have not been specifically delegated to the federal government by the Constitution are retained by the states.

The U.S. legal system has one federal legal system and fifty separate and unique state systems. For example, the federal government administers the U.S. Tax Court and the U.S. Bankruptcy Court. The state governments administer such courts as traffic and small claims courts. State governments also administer medical licensing acts. The majority of criminal cases originate in state courts. Most states have at least three court levels: trial, appellate, and supreme. The jurisdiction of a particular court refers to the subject matter of a particular case, territory the case occurred in, or people that a court has lawful authority over. An appellate court has the authority to review a decision made by a lower court, such as the trial court.

The court system is only one part of the government, however. In establishing a federal government, the U.S. Constitution separated the government's power into three branches: legislative, executive, and judicial. Each branch complements the others but does not take on the power of the other branches. The separation between the three branches created a system of **checks and balances** and was designed by the framers of the Constitution so that no one branch could have more power than another branch. See Figure 2.1 ■ for an illustration of the branches of the U.S. government.

The legislative branch, referred to as Congress, is the lawmaking body. It is composed of members of the Senate and House of Representatives and is responsible for passing legislation into law. The executive branch (consisting of the President of the United States, his or her cabinet, and various advisers) administers and enforces the law. The judicial branch (consisting of judges and the federal courts, including the Supreme Court) interprets the laws. Congress has the power to make laws, but the President has the power to veto these laws, although Congress can then override the veto with a two-thirds majority vote. The President can appoint all federal and Supreme Court judges, but Congress must confirm

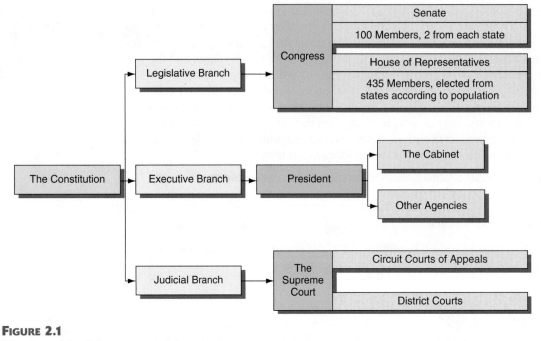

FIGURE 2.1
Branches of the U.S. Government

appointments. The judicial branch can review legislation and interpret the laws passed by Congress and the President, but the President must enforce the law. Congress can, in many instances, pass new laws to replace laws that are deemed unconstitutional by a judicial decision. See Figure 2.2 ■ for an illustration of the separation of powers.

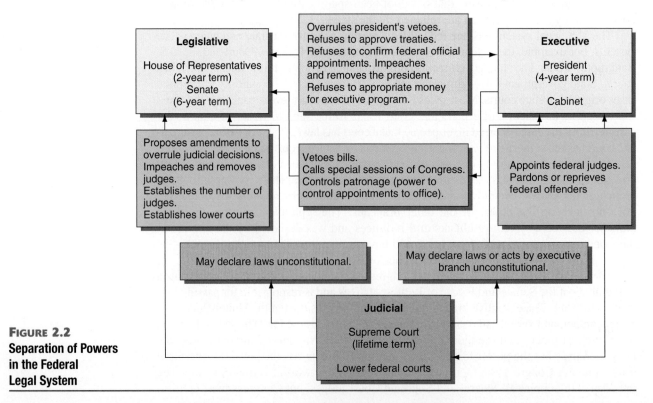

FIGURE 2.2
**Separation of Powers
in the Federal
Legal System**

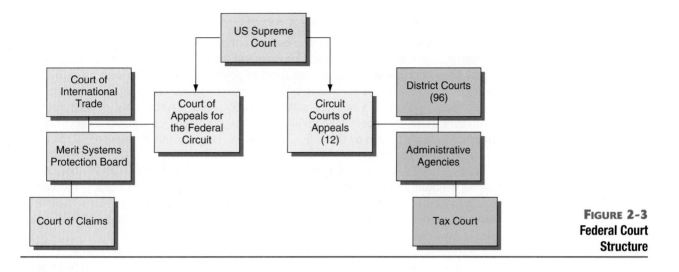

FIGURE 2-3
**Federal Court
Structure**

The states all have their own constitutions, which in many respects mirror the U.S. Constitution. The state constitutions likewise establish legislative, executive, and judicial branches within each state. See Figure 2.3 ■ for an illustration of the federal court system.

MED TIP

Federal law is administered the same in all states. However, individual states may vary on how they interpret and implement laws relegated to the states. Therefore, interpretation of legal acts for allied health professionals varies greatly from state to state.

SOURCES OF LAW

All laws—those enforceable rules prescribed by a government authority—must come from somewhere. Let's say that you are pulled over and given a ticket for driving 70 miles an hour, when the speed limit is only 55. You obviously broke a law. But where did that law come from? Did someone just walk down the highway and put up signs saying how fast he or she thought you should drive? Of course not. The speed limit, like all other laws, originated from a government body authorized to establish rules. These rules fall into four different categories: constitutional, statutory, regulatory, and common (or case) law.

Constitutional Law

Constitutional law consists of both the U.S. Constitution and the constitutions of the individual states. This is the country's highest judicial authority (since 1787). The U.S. Constitution sets up the government, defines the government's power to act, and sets limits on the government's power (i.e., individual rights such as the right to free speech). It takes precedence over all state laws and the state constitutions.

It is important to realize that the Constitution only addresses the relationship between individuals and their government; it does not apply to the relationship between private entities, whether they are individuals or businesses.

Statutory and Regulatory Law

Statutes are laws passed by legislative bodies, either Congress or a state legislature. This is called statutory or legislative law. Congress and the state legislatures have the authority to pass laws because in setting up our form of government, the Constitution authorized the legislature to make laws. Statutory law consists of ever-changing rules and regulations created by the U.S. Congress, state legislators, local governments, or constitutional lawmakers. These statutes are the inviolable rights, privileges, or immunities secured and protected for each citizen by the U.S. Constitution. They include written codes, bills, and acts (also called regulations).

Legislatures sometimes authorize agencies to make laws. The legislature does this by passing a statute, called enabling legislation. This statute creates an agency and authorizes it to pass laws regarding specific issues. For instance, the Food and Drug Administration is a federal agency that can pass rules governing the sale of food and drugs. The rules or laws made by agencies are called **regulations.**

Statutes begin as bills submitted by legislators at the state or federal level. The first step is taken when the bill is introduced in either of the two legislative houses: Senate or House of Representatives. If the bill does not "die" (fails to be acted upon) in one of the houses, it then goes to a committee for discussion and consideration. (Note that 85 percent of all bills die before they reach a committee.) The committee studies the bill and may hold a hearing to gain more facts about the bill. This first committee issues a report, including a recommendation to either pass or fail the bill. The bill then goes back to the house (Senate or House of Representatives) in which it originated, where a discussion and vote takes place. After the bill passes in one house, it becomes an act. The act is then sent back to the other house, where it goes through the same steps as it did as a bill. The act can always be amended by the second house, which results in its being returned to the originating house for a discussion and vote on the amendment.

If the second house passes the act, then the heads of each house—Speaker of the House of Representatives and the President Pro Tem of the Senate (the Vice President of the United States, in the case of a Federal act)—sign it. The act is then sent to the chief executive, who is, in the case of a federal act, the President, and for a state act, the governor. The act becomes a law if it is signed by the chief executive or if it is not vetoed within ten days. If vetoed, the bill goes back for an override vote. A presidential veto can be overridden by a two-thirds majority of both houses of Congress. After this complicated process, the act is referred to as a public law or statute.

MED TIP

A public law is designated by the initials P.L., the five or six digits that follow indicates the Congress that passed the law (the first 2 or 3 digits), and which piece of legislation the law was in that Congress. For example, a new law is issued with a public law number, such as PL 94-104, which indicates that it was the 94th Congress that passed the law (the first two or three digits) and the 104th piece of legislation in that Congress.

Laws that are passed by city governments are called municipal ordinances. Federal laws have precedence over state laws; state laws have precedence over city or municipal laws. In other words, a state or city may make laws and regulations more stringent than the federal law, but cannot make laws less stringent.

Common Law (or Case Law)

The final source of law is common law. Unlike the laws established by legislative bodies (statutory laws), common law is made by judges when they apply previous court decisions to current cases. This means it is based on the judicial interpretation of previous laws, leading to a common understanding of how a law should be interpreted. Thus, **common law,** as established from a court decision, may explain or interpret the other sources of law. Since common law evolves on a case-by-case basis, it is also called **case law.** For instance, a case may explain what the constitution, a statute, or a regulation means. In addition to interpreting the other sources of law, common law defines other legal rights and obligations. For example, a doctor's obligation to use reasonable care in treating a patient (i.e., not to commit medical malpractice) is a legal obligation created from actual court decisions.

Common law, or case law based on decisions made by judges, was originally established by English courts in the twelfth century and brought to America by the early colonists. The only state that doesn't follow common law is the state of Louisiana, which bases its law on early French law. Common law is based on precedent, the ruling in an early case that is then applied to subsequent cases when the facts are the same. Each time common, or judge-made, law is applied, it must be reviewed by the court to determine if it is still justified and relevant or has not been overturned by existing laws. As a result of this constant review of common law, many laws have been changed (or updated) over the years. The ultimate arbiter, or interpreter, of common law is the state supreme court or, if the law involves a federal question, the U.S. Supreme Court. The legal principle of *stare decisis,* or "let the decision stand," comes to us from the precedence of basing decisions on similar past case decisions.

MED TIP

Taken literally, *stare decisis* means to abide by, or adhere to, decided cases.

Many old case decisions, such as the ones described in the case law example, still influence today's medical practitioner.

EXAMPLE OF CASE LAW

In the 1616 case of *Weaver v. Ward,* Weaver sued Ward after Ward's musket accidentally fired during a military exercise, wounding Weaver. Weaver won, and Ward had to pay damages for Weaver's injury. The court concluded that Weaver did not have to show that Ward intended to injure him. Even though the injury was an accident, Ward was still liable (*Weaver v. Ward,* 80 Eng. Rep. 284, 1616). In *Lambert v. Bessey,* decided in 1681, the court stated, "In all civil acts the law doth not so much regard the intent of the actor, as the loss and damage of the party suffering" (*Lambert v. Bessey,* 83 Eng. Rep. 220, 1681). Cases such as these established the precedent that the person who hurt another person by unavoidable accident or self-defense was required to make good the damage inflicted.

Even though the facts of these cases are antiquated, we can still see their relevance when a patient suffers an injury while undergoing medical treatment. In the late nineteenth century, the courts recognized that there should be liability for a pure accident. Therefore, a person (defendant) may be liable for an injury to another person (plaintiff), even if the defendant did not intend to hurt the plaintiff.

CLASSIFICATION OF LAWS

Laws are classified as private and public. Private (or civil) laws can be divided into six categories: tort, contract, property, inheritance, family, and corporate law. Only tort and contract law are discussed here, since they most often affect the medical professional. Public law can be divided into four categories: criminal, administrative, constitutional, and international law. This chapter discusses criminal and administrative law.

Civil (Private) Law

Civil law concerns relationships either between individuals or between individuals and the government. It involves all the law that is not criminal law, although the same conduct may violate criminal and civil law. For instance, murder is a crime that the government prosecutes in order to punish the defendant by inflicting a prison term or even death, while the surviving family members can sue the person in a civil suit for wrongful death and receive compensation for their loss. Civil law cases generally carry a monetary damage or award as compensation for harm or injury. An individual can sue another person, a business, or the government. Some civil law cases include divorce, child custody, auto accidents, slander, libel, and trespassing.

In a civil law case there must be a **preponderance of evidence** in order to receive a determination of guilty. This means that it is more likely than not that the incident did occur.

Civil law includes tort law and contract law. Tort law covers private or civil wrongful acts that result in harm to another person or that person's property. A tort can result in money damages having to be paid. **Contract law** includes enforceable promises and agreements between two or more persons to do, or not do, a particular action. Healthcare employees are most frequently involved in cases of civil law, in particular, tort and contract law. Most medical malpractice lawsuits fall within the category of the civil law of torts.

MED TIP

In many cases, civil law matters are handled and settled outside of the courtroom.

Tort Law

A **tort** is a civil injury, or wrongful act, that is committed against another person or property, resulting in harm, and is compensated by money damages. To sue for a tort, a patient must have suffered a mental or physical injury that was caused by the physician or the physician's employee. A tort case is tried before either a judge or a jury. In certain cases in which a jury trial has been waived, a "bench trial" may take place in which the trial is held before a judge sitting without a jury. Torts can be either intentional or unintentional, and the patient may recover monetary damages. In order to recover damages there must be "fault" on the part of the defendant.

MED TIP

Under tort law, if a wrongful act has been committed against another person and there is no harm done, then there is no tort. However, in medical practice, every wrongful act or error must be reported, since patients may experience harm sometime later than when the tort occurs. For instance, if a woman in the first trimester (first three months) of her pregnancy has an x-ray procedure, the fetus may not demonstrate any harmful effects until several months later at birth.

Intentional Torts   Intentional torts occur when a person has been intentionally or deliberately injured by another. Intentional torts include assault, battery, false imprisonment, defamation of character, fraud, and invasion of privacy. Table 2.1 ■ provides a description and example of each.

Assault   No healthcare professional would knowingly perform a tort against a patient or any other person. However, even a trained professional can make a mistake if he or she is not aware of what constitutes a "wrongful act" under these torts. For example, for a tort of **assault,** it is sufficient for the patient to just fear that he or she will be hurt or has an "imminent apprehension of bodily harm." So, if a healthcare professional threatens a patient by saying, "If you don't lie still, we will have to hold you down," and the patient believes this will cause him or her injury or harm, this is considered a tort of assault. Shaking of one's fist in a patient's face in a threatening manner can also be considered assault.

Battery   The tort of **battery** requires bodily harm or unlawful touching (touching without the consent of the patient) and not just the fear of harm. No procedure, including drawing blood for a laboratory test, can be performed without the patient's knowledge and consent. When a patient offers an arm or rolls up a sleeve for the phlebotomist, this constitutes a form of consent (implied) for the procedure. When a surgeon has a patient sign an informed consent for a specific surgical procedure, then it is considered battery if he or she does anything to the patient that is not listed on the informed consent form. (This does not include emergency life-saving procedures such as CPR.) For example, if, during surgery for a hysterectomy (removal of the uterus), a surgeon notes that the patient's appendix is inflamed, he or she cannot remove that appendix unless this procedure was stated on the consent form. The surgeon would have to complete the surgery for the hysterectomy and then, after the patient is awake, discuss the need for surgical removal of the appendix. Often assault and battery occur together.

Other examples of battery include hitting a patient or forcing competent patients to do anything against their wishes, such as having therapy or getting out of bed.

Tort	Description	Example	TABLE 2.1
Assault	The *threat of* bodily harm to another. There does not have to be actual touching (battery) for an assault to take place.	Threatening to harm a patient or to perform a procedure without the informed consent (permission) of the patient.	**Intentional Torts**
Battery	Actual bodily harm to another person without permission. This is also referred to as unlawful touching or touching without consent.	Performing surgery or a procedure without the informed consent (permission) of the patient.	
False imprisonment	A violation of the personal liberty of another person through unlawful restraint.	Refusing to allow a competent patient to leave an office, hospital, or medical facility when he or she requests to leave.	
Defamation of character	Damage caused to a person's reputation through spoken or written word.	Making a negative statement about another physician's ability.	
Fraud	Deceitful practice that deprives another person of his or her rights.	Promising a miracle cure.	
Invasion of privacy	The unauthorized publicity of information about a patient.	Allowing personal information, such as test results for HIV, to become public without the patient's permission.	

False Imprisonment False imprisonment in healthcare occurs when a medical professional, or a person hired by that professional, takes an action to confine a patient. There have been cases in which patients were not allowed to leave a room or building when they wished, and had no reasonable means of escape resulting in a tort of false imprisonment in which the patient (plaintiff) won the case. This occurred in a Texas case in which the patient, who was assessed as being competent, was detained against his will from leaving a nursing home (*Big Town Nursing Home v. Newman,* 461 S.W.2d195, Tex. Civ. App. 1970).

A more common situation occurs when a patient wishes to leave a hospital against medical orders. In this case, the patient is asked to sign a statement that says he or she is leaving against the advice of the physician. There have also been a few cases of false imprisonment, resulting from hospitals trying to hold patients until their bills were paid (*Williams v. Summit Psychiatric Ctrs.,* 363 S.E.2d 794, Ga. App. 1987). However, no such cases have been reported in the last few years because hospitals now understand that this practice is unacceptable.

Defamation of Character Making false and/or malicious statements about another person constitutes **defamation of character** if the person can prove damages. Defamation can be in two forms: slander or libel. According to *Black's Law Dictionary,* **slander** (oral defamation) is speaking false and malicious words concerning another person that brings injury to his or her reputation. There are four recognized exceptions that require no proof of actual harm to a person's reputation in order to recover damages for slander: accusing a person of a crime; accusing someone of a "loathsome" disease, such as a venereal disease; using words against a person's business or profession; and calling a woman unchaste. **Libel** is, in general, any publication in print, writing, pictures, or signs that injures the reputation of another person. Physicians and nurses are protected against an accusation of libel when complying with a law to report venereal disease or cases of abuse. See Chapter 7, Public Duties of the Physician.

Fraud **Fraudulent** practices consist of attempts to deceive another person. For example, making a statement to a cancer patient that "Dr. Williams is a miracle worker; she'll have you feeling better in no time." is a false promise, since there are too many variables when dealing with cancer. However, a more common type of medical fraud consists of false billing practices, especially relating to Medicare and Medicaid.

Physicians are prohibited from accepting kickbacks, or payments of any kind, for the referral of Medicare and Medicaid patients under the Medicare-Medicaid Antifraud and Abuse Amendments. In some cases, physicians have received kickbacks from medical technology companies for using their products on patients. This is considered a criminal offense under the antifraud law and could result in a large penalty and even imprisonment.

Embezzlement, a form of fraud, is the illegal appropriation of property, usually money, by a person entrusted with its possession. It can occur in a physician's or dentist's office when a trusted office manager has total control over the office finances. To embezzle means to willfully take another person's rightly owned property or funds. For control purposes, more than one person should receive payments, issue receipts for payments, audit the accounts, and deposit the money.

Invasion of Privacy An invasion of privacy can occur at any time during a patient's treatment, even after the patient has granted permission to allow publicity. For example, in the case of allowing photographs or videotapes to be taken, the patient may cancel the permission at any time. In *Estate of Berthiaume v. Pratt,* an invasion of privacy case was tried after a patient with cancer of the larynx died. The deceased patient had allowed his physician to take several photographs that were to be used for the medical record but not for publication. A few hours before the hospitalized patient died, the surgeon and a nurse attempted to take more photographs in spite of the patient's indication he did not want this done and his wife's protests. The wife sued the surgeon for assault, since he had moved the patient's head during the photo taking, as well as invasion of privacy. An appeals court found in favor of the plaintiff and stated that taking photographs in spite of the patient's protests was an invasion of his legal rights to privacy (*Estate of Berthiaume v. Pratt,* 365 QA.2d 792, Me. 1976).

The famous Supreme Court case in 1973, *Roe v. Wade,* gave strength to the argument that a woman had a right to privacy over matters that related to her body, which included pregnancy (*Roe v. Wade,* 410 U.S. 113, 1973).

Unintentional Torts   **Unintentional torts,** such as negligence, occur, for example, when the patient is injured as a result of the healthcare professional's not exercising the ordinary standard of care. The term *standard of care* means that the professional must exercise the type of care that a "reasonable" person would use in a similar circumstance.

Morrison v. MacNamara illustrates the standard of care issue. In this case, MacNamara, a technician, took a urethral smear from the patient, Morrison, while the patient was standing. Morrison fainted, hit his head, and permanently lost his sense of smell and taste. An expert witness from Michigan testified that the national standard of care for taking a urethral smear requires the patient to sit or lie down. Thus, the court found in favor of the patient (*Morrison v. MacNamara,* 407 A.2d 555, D.C. 1979).

Standard of care is discussed more fully in Chapter 3.

An unintentional tort exists when a person had no intent of bringing about an injury to the patient. Healthcare professionals can be sued for a variety of situations, but most lawsuits relate to the unintentional tort of negligence.

Negligence is the failure or omission to perform professional duties to an accepted standard of care, such as a "reasonable person" would do. In other words, negligence occurs when a person's actions fall below a certain level of care. Negligence can involve doing something carelessly or failing to do something that should have been done. It can also involve doing something reckless such as performing a procedure without adequate training. Physicians and other healthcare professionals usually do not knowingly indulge in acts that are negligent. Malpractice, which is misconduct or demonstration of an unreasonable lack of skill, relates to a professional skill such as medicine or the law. Malpractice is a particular type of negligence that can be thought of as "professional negligence." While anyone can be accused of being negligent, only professionals can be sued for malpractice. Examples of professionals who are sued for malpractice include physicians, nurses, lawyers, accountants, pharmacists, and physical therapists.

Negligence and malpractice are similar in that both relate to wrongdoing. In medical malpractice, negligence is considered the predominant theory of liability. You can only be sued for malpractice if you are negligent in something done within your professional capacity. The topics of negligence and malpractice are discussed further in Chapter 6.

See Table 2.2 ■ for some actions that are considered unintentional or negligent torts.

	TABLE 2.2
▶ Altering or tampering with a medical record ▶ Failure to adequately assess or monitor a patient's condition ▶ Failure to maintain a safe environment ▶ Failure to dispense the correct medication ▶ Failure to document in a timely manner ▶ Failure to follow policies and procedures	**Unintentional or Negligent Torts**

> **MED TIP**
>
> Remember that it is easier to prevent negligence than it is to defend it.

Contract Law

Contract law addresses a **breach,** or neglect, of a legally binding agreement between two parties. The agreement or contract may relate to insurance, sales, business, real estate, or services such as healthcare.

> **MED TIP**
>
> Breach of contract refers to the failure, without legal excuse, to perform any promise or to carry out any of the terms of a contract.

A contract consists of a voluntary agreement that two parties enter into with the intent of benefiting each other. Something of value, which is termed **consideration,** is part of the agreement. In the medical profession, the consideration might be the performance of an appendectomy for a specific fee. An agreement would take place between the two parties that would include the offer ("I will perform the appendectomy") and the acceptance of the offer ("I will allow you to perform the appendectomy"). Therefore, a surgeon who has consent to perform a hysterectomy on a patient may not perform an appendectomy at the same time unless there is consent from the patient for both procedures.

In order for the contract to be valid (legal), both parties must be **competent.** The concerned party (patient) must be mentally competent and not under the influence of drugs or alcohol at the time the contract is entered into.

Types of Contracts   A contract can be either expressed or implied. An **expressed contract** is an agreement that clearly states all the terms. It can be entered into orally or in writing.

> **MED TIP**
>
> Most contracts are enforceable, even if oral.

Each state identifies certain types of contracts that must be in writing. The sale of property, mortgages, and deeds is required to be in writing by most state statutes.

There are state statutes and federal laws that relate to the medical profession. For example, if a third party agrees to pay a patient's bill, a contract must be placed in writing and signed by the third party. A copy of this document should be kept in the patient's chart or file. If physicians agree to allow their patients to pay bills in four or more installments, the interest (if any) must be stated in writing (Truth in Lending Act of 1969, discussed in Chapter 8).

A signed permit to receive a vaccine would be an example of an expressed or written contract in a medical situation.

An **implied contract** is one in which the agreement is shown through inference by signs, inaction, or silence. For example, when a patient explains his or her symptoms to the physician, and the physician then examines the patient and prescribes treatment, a contract exists, even though it was not clearly stated, and both parties must follow through on the implied agreement. This can cause problems for both parties if there is not a clear understanding of the implied contract. For example, a New York court found an implied contract to pay for medical services existed when a physician listened to a patient describe his symptoms over the telephone (*O'Neill v. Montefiore Hosp.,* 202 N.Y.S.2d, 436, App. Div. 1960). An implied contract can exist when a patient brought into an emergency department needs immediate treatment.

Termination of the Contract   A **breach of contract** occurs when either party fails to comply with the terms of the agreement. For example, if a physician refuses to perform a medical procedure he or she had agreed to perform, the physician has breached the contract. If a patient does not pay an agreed-upon fee, then the patient breached the contract with the physician.

The termination of a contract between patient and physician generally occurs when the treatment has ended and the fee has been paid. However, issues may arise that cause premature termination of a contract. It should be noted that both physicians and patients have the right to terminate the contractual agreement. A breach of contract occurs when one of the parties that entered into the contract does not keep his or her promise as, for example, when a patient refuses to pay a bill. A physician may be liable for breach of contract if he or she has promised to cure a patient and then failed to do so. The breach of contract can occur even if there were no negligence on the part of the physician.

When terminating a contract, physicians should be careful that they are not charged with abandonment of the patient. To protect against an abandonment charge, any letter from the physician to the patient should indicate the date his or her services will be terminated. A copy of this letter to the patient should be placed in the patient's record. In addition, there should be a notation in the patient's chart that a notification of termination letter was sent. See Chapter 5 for a complete discussion of abandonment. Some of the reasons for premature termination of a medical contract are

- failure to follow instructions.
- missed appointments.
- failure to pay for service.
- the patient states (orally or in writing) that he or she is seeking the care of another physician (for example, the patient's insurance may have changed and the physician may not be covered by the new insurance, or the patient may move).

Class Action Lawsuit

A **class action lawsuit** can be filed by one or more people on behalf of a larger group of people who are all affected by the same situation. For example, class action lawsuits are commonly filed in product liability or pharmaceutical cases in which a large number of people are negatively affected by the same product, such as cigarettes. In March 2000, a group of women in Florida filed a class action lawsuit against a group of physicians who failed to get informed consent before subjecting the women to random medical experimentation. See Figure 2.4 ■ for the components of civil law.

Public Law (Criminal Law and Administrative Law)

Criminal laws are made to protect the public as a whole from the harmful acts of others. The purpose of criminal law is to define socially intolerable conduct that is punishable by law. No citizen of the United States can bring a criminal lawsuit against another person, since these are offenses against society as a whole. A criminal act is one in which a person or institution commits an illegal act or a failure to act. Criminal law requires evidence **beyond a reasonable doubt,** which is evidence with an almost absolute certainty that a person did commit a crime. In a state crime, the local prosecutor in the District Attorney's office will bring about a criminal action against the accused person. In a federal crime, it will be the Federal Prosecutor who brings about this action.

In a **criminal case,** the government (the state in most cases) brings the suit against a person or group of people accused of committing a crime, resulting in a fine, imprisonment, or both if the defendant is found guilty. Federal criminal offenses include illegal actions that cross state lines—kidnapping, treason, or other actions that affect national security. Crimes involving the borders of the United States (for example, illegal transport of drugs and any illegal act against a federally regulated business, such as a bank) are also federal criminal offenses.

Criminal acts fall into two categories: felony and misdemeanor. A **felony** carries a punishment of death or imprisonment in a state or federal prison for more than one year. These serious crimes include murder, rape, sodomy, robbery, larceny, arson, burglary, tax evasion, and practicing medicine without a license. **Misdemeanors** are less serious

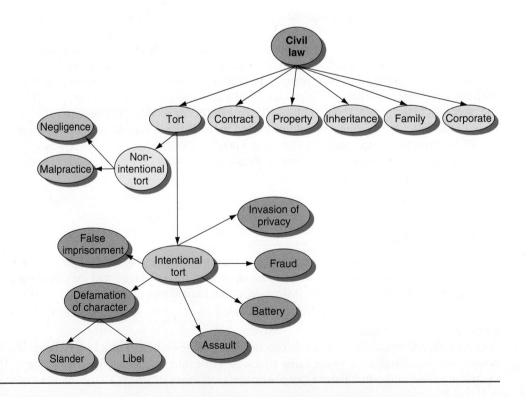

FIGURE 2.4
Components of Civil Law
(Courtesy of Amy Wilson, BS, RT(R), RDMS, RVT)

offenses. They include traffic violations, disturbing the peace, and minor theft. A misdemeanor carries a punishment of fines or imprisonment in jail for up to a year. See Figure 2.5 ■ for an illustration of the felony case process, and Figure 2.6 ■ for an illustration of the misdemeanor case process.

A physician's license may be revoked by the state licensing board if he or she is convicted of a crime. Criminal cases in the healthcare field have included revocation of a license for violating narcotics laws, sexual misconduct, income tax evasion, counterfeiting, and murder.

Administrative Law

Administrative law, a branch of public law, covers regulations that are set by government agencies. In the healthcare field, federal and state agencies, under authorization from Congress or state legislatures, have created a multitude of rules and regulations. Violations of these regulations may constitute criminal or civil violations. However, in most cases, they are civil law violations. Examples that are covered under administrative law include licensing boards for physicians and nurses, Workmen's Compensation

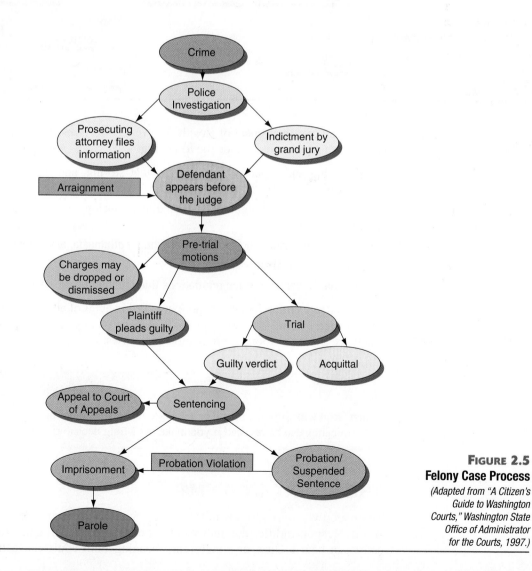

FIGURE 2.5
Felony Case Process
(Adapted from "A Citizen's Guide to Washington Courts," Washington State Office of Administrator for the Courts, 1997.)

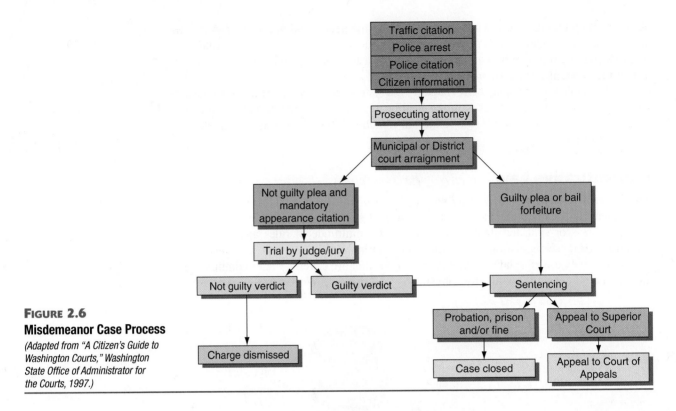

FIGURE 2.6
Misdemeanor Case Process
(Adapted from "A Citizen's Guide to Washington Courts," Washington State Office of Administrator for the Courts, 1997.)

Boards, and the Department of Health and Human Services. These wide-ranging health-care related regulations include the following:

▶ Licensing and supervision of prescribing, storing, and dispensing controlled substances

▶ Health department regulations, including reporting requirements of certain communicable diseases

▶ Regulations against homicide, infanticide, euthanasia, assault, and battery

▶ Regulations against fraud

▶ Internal Revenue Service regulations that are healthcare related.

Healthcare professionals are more involved in areas of administrative law than in any other source of law. The penalties for violations of this category of law include fines, sanctions, and revocation or termination of licenses.

MED TIP

When faced with difficult ethical or legal dilemmas, remember that your hard-earned license or certification can be revoked if you make the wrong decision.

THE COURT SYSTEMS

There are two court systems in the United States: state and federal. Each system has specific responsibilities that may be either exclusive, meaning that only that particular court can hear a case, or concurrent, meaning both courts have the power to hear the case. Which court hears the case depends on the plaintiff's choice, provided both courts have jurisdiction to hear the case. For a criminal case, this depends on the type of crime and where the criminal action occurred. For example, a bank robbery that took place in Alabama will usually be tried by a federal court in that state. In a civil case, the type of court used depends on where the incident occurred and the type of lawsuit.

Types of Courts

The federal court system has **jurisdiction,** or power to hear a case, when one of the following conditions is present:

▶ The dispute relates to a federal law or the U.S. Constitution.

▶ The U.S. government is one of the parties involved in the dispute.

▶ Different states' citizens are involved in the dispute and the case involves over $75,000.

▶ Citizens of another country are involved in a dispute with a U.S. citizen and the case involves over $75,000.

▶ The actual dispute occurred in international waters.

If the case does not involve one of these situations, it must be tried in state court. However, even if one of these situations exists, the case may still be heard in state court unless Congress has prohibited state courts from hearing the case, such as with a kidnapping that takes place across state lines. Cases involving a federal crime, bankruptcy law, and patent law must be heard in federal court. Cases involving divorce, child custody, and probate must be heard in state court.

The court system is divided into three levels. The levels for the federal court system are district (or municipal), court of appeals (or circuit courts), and the U.S. Supreme Court. A case is tried at the lowest level court first. If that court's decision is appealed, or challenged, then the next higher court may examine the decision.

The state courts, from lower to higher, are divided into district or municipal trial courts, state court of appeals, and the state's highest court for final appeals. The lower state courts hear cases such as small claims and traffic violations.

Physicians may have to take a patient who has a delinquent account to small claims court. Physicians may authorize their office manager, bookkeeper, or other office assistant to appear in court for the hearing. The clerk of small claims court can provide information on the requirements and procedures relating to this type of lawsuit.

Probate court, or estate court, handles cases involving estates of the deceased. A physician may have to contact the county court recorder for information about filing a claim for payment from the estate of a deceased patient.

MED TIP

It is always advisable to seek payment for all medical services that have been provided to dying or deceased patients. Failure to seek payment may be thought of as an indication of guilt or negligence over a patient's treatment or death.

THE TRIAL PROCESS

In a trial, the judicial process is designed to determine certain facts by hearing evidence, determine which facts are relevant, apply relevant principles of law, and then pass a judgment. A grand jury hearing is the first step in some cases.

The Grand Jury

The federal government and many states use the grand jury process. A grand jury, usually consisting of from twelve to twenty-three private citizens, hears evidence about a criminal case in order to determine if the case has enough merit to be heard in court. Thus, a grand jury can serve as a filter to prevent cases from being heard when there is insufficient evidence. The grand jury hearings are held in private, and the **defendant,** the person being sued in a court of law, may or may not appear to speak before the grand jury. The defendant can be a physician, a nurse, the healthcare facility (employer), and/or other healthcare providers. The grand jury can ask to see documents relating to the investigation and speak with witnesses. After hearing all the evidence and deliberating among themselves, the grand jury votes on whether they should move the **indictment,** a written legal charge against the defendant, to a trial court.

The Procedure

When two parties are unable to solve a dispute by themselves, it may result in **litigation,** a dispute or lawsuit that is tried in court. A physician may be the **plaintiff,** the person bringing an action into litigation, or the defendant. A plaintiff can be a patient, the patient's family, or anyone else who has a right to be compensated under the law due to the injury the patient (plaintiff) has received. A **prosecutor** brings a criminal lawsuit on behalf of the government. Not all lawsuits end up in court. In many situations, attorneys for both sides work out a settlement, or agreement, between the parties, so there is no need for a trial. This is called settling out of court.

If the parties are unable to settle the dispute, a trial may be held. A court case can be tried before a judge only or before a judge and jury of the defendant's peers. Both parties (defendant and plaintiff) in the case may **waive,** or give up their right, to a jury trial or request a jury trial.

If a jury is requested, then six to twelve people are selected from a large pool of potential jurors. The jurors are most commonly summoned from a list of residents of a particular region, registered voters, or driver's license holders. The judge and attorneys for both sides of the case (plaintiff and defendant) question the potential jurors to find an impartial jury. Once the final selection of jurors is made, the case is ready to begin.

A trial begins with opening statements made by the attorneys for each side of the case that describe the facts they will attempt to prove during the case. The plaintiff's attorney then questions the first witness. A witness is generally someone who has knowledge of the circumstances of the case and can testify, under oath, as to what happened. This witness can then be cross-examined (asked questions) by the defendant's attorney. After all of the plaintiff's witnesses have been examined and cross-examined, the defendant's attorney (defense counsel) presents witnesses for the defense side of the case. The plaintiff's attorney then has an opportunity to cross-examine the defense witnesses. When this portion of the case has been completed, and once any additional witnesses are called and cross-examined, both sides "rest their case," which means that all the evidence and witnesses have been examined.

MED TIP

The U.S. legal system is based on the premise that all persons are innocent until proven guilty. Because the plaintiff is claiming that the defendant violated a law, the *burden of proof* is placed upon the plaintiff to prove that the defendant is liable.

Subpoena

Discovery is the legal process by which facts are discovered before a trial begins. A court of law may need to subpoena a person or records. A **subpoena** is a written command from the court for a person or documents to appear in court. In some cases, a **deposition** can be taken, meaning that the person's statement is recorded with witnesses present, and the person may not be required to appear in court. The deposition is submitted by an attorney during the court case. A **subpoena** *duces tecum,* a Latin phrase meaning "under penalty, take with you," is a court order requiring a witness to appear in court and to bring certain records or other material to a trial or deposition. There is a penalty for failure to appear, or present documents, if subpoenaed by the court. A person or documents may also be produced in court on a voluntary basis, thus not requiring a subpoena. (Subpoena *duces tecum* is explained more fully in Chapter 9.)

A subpoena must be sent by registered mail or hand-delivered (served) to the person who is being requested to appear in court, that is, the person who is named on the subpoena. Unless requested to do so, an assistant cannot accept a subpoena on behalf of a physician without his or her knowledge; otherwise, the subpoena is considered "not served." The physician may delegate the responsibility to an assistant to accept a subpoena on his or her behalf, but this practice is not encouraged. If there are any questions, it is always a good idea to consult with an attorney if you are served a subpoena. A failure to appear in court, or produce materials, as asked in the subpoena is considered to be a "contempt of court" and carries a serious penalty.

Summary Judgment

A request may be made by an attorney on either side for a summary judgment to take place in a civil lawsuit. A **summary judgment** is a decision made by the court (judge) in response to a motion that declares there is no necessity for a trial since there is no dispute as to the material fact. Any person who is involved in a civil action can request, through their attorney, a summary judgment by the judge if he or she believes there is no issue of law involved in the case. When the evidence supporting the position of one of the parties involved in the lawsuit is very clear from the onset, there may be no need for a trial to take place. It is a procedural device that can assist in bringing a controversy to quick closure without a trial. Summary judgment can result in a win for one side of the case and is based on **pleadings** (formal written statements) alone.

Closing Arguments

Attorneys for both the plaintiff and the defendant then present summaries of the evidence or summaries of their case, called **closing arguments.** In a jury trial, the judge instructs the jury on the areas of law that affect the case. The jury is then excused and taken to another room so they can deliberate, examine the evidence presented, and come to a conclusion, or verdict. If the trial has been conducted in front of a judge without a jury, then the judge makes a decision based on the evidence presented and the law. In a civil case, if the judge or jury finds in favor of the plaintiff, then the defendant is typically ordered to pay the plaintiff a monetary award. In a criminal case, if the defendant is found guilty, the judge sentences the defendant with a fine and/or a prison sentence. In some cases, if the state statutes allow it, the death penalty may be applied. If the defendant wins in either a civil or criminal case, the case is over unless an appeal is made. See Figure 2.7 ■ for an illustration of a civil trial procedure.

A plaintiff or defendant may appeal the decision to a higher court. Ultimately, a case can be appealed to the highest court, either in the state or, in a federal case, the U.S. Supreme Court.

MED TIP

A judgment of not guilty, or not liable as in a malpractice case, does not mean that the defendant did not commit the crime or perform the misconduct. It only means that, based on the evidence presented, the plaintiff failed to prove it to a jury.

Standards of Proof

When deciding a case in a court of law, there are several different levels of proof that are required depending on how serious society considers the crime to be. In a civil case, the court will generally look at a "preponderance of evidence." This is evidence that, as a whole, shows that the fact sought to be proved is more probably true than not. This means that the burden of proof in a civil case will place greater weight on evidence that is more credible and convincing. This does not mean that the cases will be decided on a greater number of witnesses, but rather on a greater weight of all the evidence.

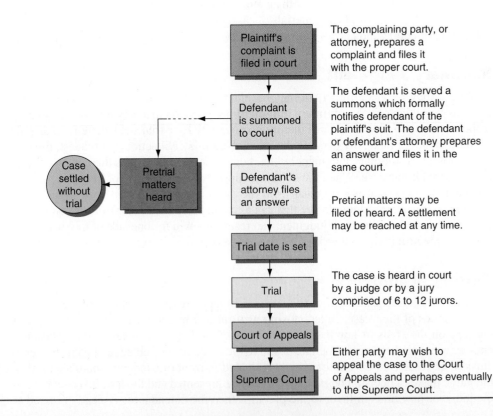

FIGURE 2.7
The Procedure for a Civil Trial
(Adapted from "A Citizen's Guide to Washington Courts," Washington State Office of Administrator for the Courts, 1997.)

In juvenile abuse cases, the court tends to use "clear and convincing evidence." This means that there is a reasonable certainty of the truth. "Clear and convincing evidence" or proof, requires more than a "preponderance of evidence" or proof, as in a civil case, and less than proof "beyond a reasonable doubt" as in a criminal case. In criminal trials, a judge or jury must find the defendant guilty "beyond a reasonable doubt," which means that the facts when proven must establish guilt.

Expert Witness

An **expert witness** is a person called as a witness in a case where the subject matter is beyond the general knowledge of most people in the court or on the jury. In healthcare related cases, this person, usually a medical professional, has special knowledge or experience not only about the facts of a case but also about the professional conclusions that are drawn from the facts. The testimony of the expert witness should assist the jury or judge in evaluating the facts in a particular case. In a medical malpractice suit, an expert witness often is called to testify as to what the standard of care for a patient is in a similar circumstance and locality. An expert witness in a medical malpractice suit involving a physician is generally a physician. In cases involving nurses, an expert witness is often a nurse.

Expert witnesses, who are generally paid a fee, may use visual aids such as charts, photos, x-rays, models, and diagrams. They do not testify about the actual facts of the case, but clarify points of knowledge that may not be readily understood by all present. Physicians and nurses often serve as expert witnesses to describe the standard of care in a community when another physician or nurse is being sued for negligence. For example, an expert witness on the topic of DNA may be called to testify in a paternity case.

Testifying in Court

If you are called to testify in court, remember the following:

- Always tell the truth.
- Be professional. People are judged by their appearance as well as by their behavior in court. An attorney can offer further advice on this.
- Remain calm, dignified, and serious at all times. The opposing attorney may try to make the witness nervous by asking difficult questions.
- Do not answer a question you do not understand. Simply ask the attorney to repeat the question or state, "I don't understand the question."
- Just present the facts surrounding the case. Do not give any information that is not requested. Do not insert your opinion. "The patient was shouting" is stating a fact; "He was angry" is your opinion.
- Do not memorize your testimony ahead of time. You will generally be allowed to take some notes with you to refresh your memory concerning such things as dates.

MED TIP

Keep in mind that a lawsuit can take years to come to closure. The mean age for a lawsuit from beginning to settlement is three to five years. Every necessary step should be taken to avoid a lawsuit in the first place.

Appellate Court System

The U.S. legal system at both the state and federal levels has a built-in appeals process for decisions that need to be reviewed. If the losing party in a lawsuit believes that the case was handled improperly or unfairly, it can "appeal" to a higher court of law to have the decision corrected or changed in its favor. The appellate court, or higher court, reviews the written transcripts of the original trial. This court will examine the evidence to determine if, in its opinion, the ruling was correct and fair. The appellate court does not retry the case but acts as a reviewing court. After reading the transcripts from the case, the judge affirms the original decision, reverses it, or modifies it.

POINTS TO PONDER

1. Why do I have to know how a bill becomes a law?
2. Why is common law important?
3. How can I avoid a lawsuit?
4. Can I restrain a person against his or her will if I know it is for his or her own good?
5. Can I be sued if I make a statement to a patient about a mistake a physician has made?
6. What should I do if I see a physician or another healthcare employee make an error?
7. Can I be sued if I unintentionally leave a patient record with a diagnosis of AIDS within sight of another patient?
8. What do I do if I am subpoenaed?

DISCUSSION QUESTIONS

1. Discuss the significance of common laws for the healthcare professional.
2. Explain what is meant by the statement, "It is easier to prevent negligence than it is to defend it."
3. Differentiate between common law and statutory law.
4. Explain what the numbering system in public law means.
5. What is meant by *burden of proof?*
6. What is a subpoena and who can accept it?

REVIEW CHALLENGE

Short Answer Questions

1. How can embezzlement be prevented?

_____

_____

2. What is the difference between libel and slander?

_____

_____

3. What are some of the reasons for termination of a medical contract?

_____

_____

4. What is an expert witness and why might one be used during a lawsuit?

_____

_____

5. What is the difference between a felony and a misdemeanor? Give an example of each.

_____

_____

6. What is a subpoena *duces tecum?*

_____

_____

7. What is a class action lawsuit? Give an example of one.

_____

_____

8. What is the role of the appellate court within the court system?

_____

_____

_____

Matching

Match the responses in column B with the correct term in column A.

Column A

_____ 1. breach
_____ 2. deposition
_____ 3. plaintiff
_____ 4. defendant
_____ 5. felony
_____ 6. misdemeanor
_____ 7. waive
_____ 8. tort
_____ 9. subpoena
_____ 10. precedent

Column B

a. order for a person or documents to appear in court
b. person who is being sued
c. give up the right to something
d. law that covers harm to another person
e. earlier ruling applied to present case
f. failure
g. person who sues another party
h. less serious crime such as a traffic violation
i. oral testimony to be used in court
j. serious crime such as practicing medicine without a license

Multiple Choice

Select the one best answer to the following statements.

1. Sources of law include all of the following except
   a. regulatory law.
   b. executive law.
   c. statutory law.
   d. common law.
   e. constitutional law.

2. Subpoena *duces tecum* means
   a. "let the master answer."
   b. "under penalty, take with you."
   c. "let the decision stand."
   d. "the thing speaks for itself."
   e. "the thing has been decided."

3. *Stare decisis* means
   a. "let the master answer."
   b. "under penalty, take with you."
   c. statutory law has been invoked.
   d. constitutional law has been invoked.
   e. "let the decision stand."

4. Administrative law covers all of the following except
   a. health department regulations.
   b. licensing of prescription drugs.
   c. Internal Revenue Service regulations.
   d. fraud.
   e. all of the above are covered under administrative law.

5. The person who brings the action into litigation is called a(n)
   a. attorney.
   b. plaintiff.
   c. defendant.
   d. judge.
   e. juror.

6. A court order that requires a witness to appear in court with certain records is called a
   a. deposition.
   b. discovery.
   c. subpoena *duces tecum.*
   d. *res judicata.*
   e. waiver.

7. The common law of the past that is based on a decision made by judges is called
   a. civil law.
   b. constitutional law.
   c. case law.
   d. criminal law.
   e. statutory law.

8. The threat of doing bodily harm to another person—
stating, for example, "If you won't allow us to continue
this procedure, we will have to tie your hands."—is

   a. assault.
   b. battery.
   c. fraud.
   d. invasion of privacy.
   e. all of the above.

9. Standard of care refers to the care that

   a. a reasonable person would use.
   b. is ordinary care.
   c. a prudent person would use.
   d. healthcare professionals in all specialties must practice.
   e. all of the above.

10. Removing one's clothing in order to allow the physician
to perform a physical examination is a(n)

   a. invasion of privacy.
   b. defamation of character.
   c. implied contract.
   d. abandonment.
   e. none of the above is correct.

DISCUSSION CASES

1. Analyze *"The case of Jacob and the Diseased Leg"* (found at the beginning of the chapter) using the
Three-step Ethics Model (Blanchard-Peale).

   a. _____
   _____

   b. _____
   _____

   c. _____
   _____

2. Using Figure 2.7, explain the procedure for a civil trial.

   _____
   _____
   _____
   _____

3. *Adam Green is an orderly in the Midwest Nursing Home. His supervisor, Nora Malone, has asked
him to supervise the dining room while twenty residents eat their evening meal. Bill Heckler is an
80-year old resident who is very alert and ambulatory. He tells Adam that he doesn't like the meal
that's being served, and he wants to leave the dining room and go back to his own room. Adam is
quite busy, as he has to watch the behavior of several patients who are confused. He's concerned
that patients might choke on their food or otherwise harm themselves. Adam becomes impatient
with Bill and tells him that he cannot leave the room until everyone is finished eating. Adam then
locks the dining room door. Bill complains to the nursing home administrator that he was unlawfully
detained. He then hires an attorney, who brings forth a charge of false imprisonment.*

   a. Was Adam's action justified?

   _____
   _____

   b. In your opinion, was this a case of false imprisonment?

   _____
   _____

c. What could Adam have done to defuse the situation?

_____

_____

d. Do the nursing home administrator and Nora Malone have any legal responsibility for Adam's action?

_____

_____

PUT IT INTO PRACTICE

Give an example of a violation of each of the six torts mentioned in this chapter (assault, battery, false imprisonment, defamation of character, fraud, and invasion of privacy) as it might affect your particular area of medical specialization.

WEB HUNT

Search the website of the National Institutes of Health (www.nih.gov). What types of information and service does this site offer?

CRITICAL THINKING EXERCISE

What would you pick if you had a choice between having a legal system that never punishes an innocent person but often lets the guilty go free, or a system that sometimes punishes the innocent but never frees the guilty?

BIBLIOGRAPHY

Aiken, T. 2002. _Legal and ethical issues in health occupations._ Philadelphia: Saunders.

Beaman, N., and L. Fleming-McPhillips. 2007. _Comprehensive medical assisting._ Upper Saddle River, NJ: Prentice Hall.

Black, H. 2009. _Black's law dictionary,_ 8th ed. St. Paul, MN: West Publishing.

Hall, M., and M. Bobinski. 2003. _Healthcare law and ethics in a nutshell._ St. Paul, MN: West Publishing.

McWay, D. 2003. _Legal aspects of healthcare information._ New York: Delmar.

Posgar, G., and N. Santucci. 2005. _Legal and ethical issues for health professionals._ Sudbury, MA: Jones and Bartlett.

Schmallager, F. 2007. _Criminal justice today._ Upper Saddle River, NJ: Pearson/Prentice Hall.

Taber's cyclopedic medical dictionary. 2009, 21st ed. Philadelphia: F.A. Davis Company.

Importance of the Legal System for the Physician and the Healthcare Professional

Learning Objectives

1. Define all glossary terms.
2. List the four basic characteristics of state medical practice acts.
3. Describe the three methods by which a state grants a license to practice medicine.
4. Discuss conduct that may result in a physician's loss of license to practice medicine.
5. Identify the difference between licensure and certification.
6. Discuss what the term *standard of care* means for the physician and what it means for someone in your profession.
7. Describe the importance of the discovery rule as it relates to the statute of limitations.
8. Discuss the importance of the phrase *respondeat superior* as it relates to the physician.

Key Terms

Accreditation

Bonding

Confidentiality

Discovery rule

Endorsement

Good Samaritan laws

Guardian ad litem

Incident report

Joint Commission on Accreditation of Healthcare Organizations (JCAHO)

Prudent person rule

Reciprocity

Respondeat superior

Revoke

Risk management

Scope of practice

Standard of care

Statute of limitations

Tolling

THE CASE OF LATOYA AND THE PHYSICAL THERAPY PATIENT

Latoya is in training to become a physical therapist. Dr. B., the head of the Physical Therapy Department, has told her that she helps the patients too much. Many times he has said, "You can't go home with the patients. They must learn to care for themselves." Nearing the end of her program, Latoya is doing very well in all her studies, but she fears that Dr. B. will not give her a good performance evaluation unless she can better prepare the patients for independence.

One of her patients, a 72-year-old-woman, recovering from a stroke, is adamant in her refusal to walk with either a walker or a cane. She insists on remaining in her wheelchair because she is afraid of falling. Latoya is sympathetic toward this patient's fears. She remembers seeing a patient fall during a physical therapy session resulting in a fractured vertebra (bone) in her spine. The woman was, subsequently, bedridden for several weeks while she recovered. In addition, a statement that Latoya heard in one of her classes, *primum non nocere* meaning "first of all, do no harm," has always influenced her behavior. Latoya is very reluctant to force her patient to do something she doesn't want to do.

1. How can Latoya balance the benefits and harm of encouraging her patients to do something they do not want to do?

2. In your opinion, is Dr. B. placing too much pressure on a student?

3. Is this a legal or ethical problem, or both?

4. Who should Latoya talk to about her dilemma?

Even though only a small portion of malpractice suits actually end up in court, it is still important that all healthcare professionals realize how the law impacts the physician's practice. The physician has a responsibility to respect the conditions of licensure. Healthcare employees must understand their obligations to their physician/employer and to the patients they serve.

MEDICAL PRACTICE ACTS

Each state has statutes that govern the practice of medicine in that state. These are called medical practice acts and are meant to protect the health and safety of the general public. The acts were originally established in a limited number of states to protect the general public from quackery, or persons practicing medicine without a legitimate education and training. Each state legislature establishes a state medical board that has the authority to control the licensing of physicians. While some slight differences exist from state to state, in general these practice acts define who must be licensed to perform certain procedures. These acts also specify the requirements for licensure; the duties of the licensed physician; grounds on which the license may be revoked, or taken away; and reports that must be made to the government or other appropriate agencies. Medical practice acts also define the penalties for practicing without a license. These state acts seek to protect patients from harm caused by persons who are not qualified to practice medicine. Therefore, each state licensing board has the authority to grant a medical license to qualified individuals as well as to revoke or take away that license for cause, and to fine, reprimand, and censure the physician (Figure 3.1 ■).

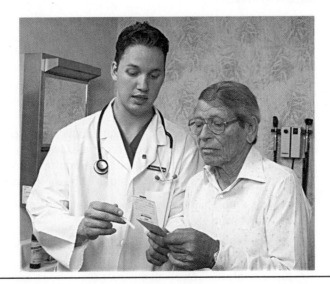

FIGURE 3.1
Fundamentals of Human Resource Management

MED TIP

Every state has a state board set up to handle issues relating to physician registration. The title for these boards varies from state to state (for example, State Board of Registration or State Board of Medical Examiners). However, the functions are similar for all state boards.

State licensing boards receive complaints about physicians from a variety of sources: patients; other physicians; employees, including hospital employees; the media; and insurance companies. The board has the authority to investigate each complaint, but cannot prosecute the physician. However, the board may access records that relate to each incident, including patient hospital records, individual physician medical records, and insurance reimbursement records. The board may declare the name of the physician but is obligated to keep a patient's name confidential.

A physician who moves to another state must obtain a license to practice in that state also. The physician may be required to pass another state's medical examination, or the physician may receive reciprocity or endorsement from the state.

While medical practice acts vary from state to state, they generally

▶ provide for the establishment of a medical examining board, also called a State Board of Registration or State Board of Examiners, that has authority to license physicians.

▶ establish the baseline for the practice of medicine in that state.

▶ determine the prerequisites for licensure.

▶ forbid the practice of medicine without a license.

▶ specify the conditions for license renewal, suspension, and revocation.

LICENSURE OF THE PHYSICIAN

The board of examiners in each state may grant licensure through examination, endorsement, or reciprocity.

Examination

Each state offers its own examination for licensure. Some states also accept or endorse the National Board of Medical Examiners (NBME) licensing examination, usually taken before the end of medical school, for licensure. Within the United States, the official medical licensing exam is the Federal Licensing Examination (FLEX). The license is issued to those who pass the examination, graduate from an accredited school, and complete an internship. Successful completion of these criteria entitles one to set up private practice as a general practitioner.

The U.S. Medical Licensing Examination (USMLE), which was introduced in 1992, is a single licensing examination for graduates from accredited medical schools that allows them to practice medicine. In addition to successfully passing the examination (written and oral), the applicant is required by most states to

▶ provide proof that he or she has completed the professional education as required by his or her state.

▶ provide proof of the successful completion of an approved internship/residency program.

▶ provide information about any past convictions, and history of drug or alcohol abuse.

▶ have obtained an age of majority, generally 21 years old.

▶ be of good moral character.

▶ be a U.S. citizen or have evidence of filing a declaration of intent to become a citizen. (Some states have dropped this requirement.)

▶ be a resident of that state.

Endorsement

Endorsement means an approval or sanction. A state may grant a license by endorsement to applicants who have successfully passed the NBME exam. In fact, most physicians in the United States are licensed by endorsement. Any medical school graduate who is not licensed by endorsement is required to pass the state board examination. Graduates of foreign medical schools must fulfill the same requirements as U.S. graduates. Licensure by endorsement is considered for acceptance or denial on a case-by-case basis. In some cases, a physician trained in a particular country or foreign school may not be able to obtain a license to practice in the United States without attending a U.S. medical school.

Reciprocity

Physicians must satisfy the licensure requirements of any and all states in which they practice. In some cases, the state to which the physician applies for a license will accept the state licensing requirements of the state from which the physician already holds a license. In that case, the physician will not have to take another examination. This practice of cooperation by which a state grants a license to practice medicine to a physician already licensed in another state is known as **reciprocity.** Reciprocity is automatic if a reciprocity agreement exists between the states where the current license is held and licensure is being sought and if the requirements of the agreement are satisfied. For instance, some states require a physician to be licensed for a certain number of years before qualifying for reciprocity.

Registration

It is necessary for physicians to maintain their license by periodic re-registration or renewal either annually or biannually. In addition to paying a fee to renew their license, physicians are generally required to complete 75 hours of continuing medical education (CME) units in a three-year period to assure that they remain current in their field of practice. While state requirements differ for renewal of a medical license, they generally include (1) attending approved workshops, courses, and seminars; (2) completing self-instruction modules; (3) teaching other health professionals; and (4) reading a variety of approved medical literature.

There are a few exceptions to the requirement of having a valid state license to practice medicine within that state. These include

▶ A physician employed by a federal medical facility, such as a Public Health Service wellness center or a Veterans Administration (VA) hospital. However, the physician does have to be licensed to practice medicine, but it doesn't have to be in the state where the facility is located.

▶ An out-of-state physician who is providing emergency medical care.

▶ A physician who is waiting to become a qualified resident in a state in order to obtain a license.

▶ A research physician who does not practice patient-based medicine.

▶ Military physicians at military hospitals.

Generally, physicians in different states may consult with each other without being licensed in each other's state.

Revocation and Suspension of Licensure

A state may **revoke** a physician's license for cases of severe misconduct, including unprofessional conduct, commission of a crime, or personal incapacity to perform one's duties. Unprofessional conduct involves behavior that fails to meet the ethical standards of the profession, such as inappropriate use of drugs or alcohol, gross immorality, or falsifying records. Crimes may include Medicare/Medicaid fraud, rape, murder, larceny, and narcotics convictions. Personal incapacity often relates to a physical or mental incapacity that prevents the physician from performing professional duties. Professional incompetence, such as malpractice or negligence, can also result in revocation of a medical license.

The physician's state licensing board oversees the suspension or revocation of a license. The board will provide the physician with sufficient notice of any charges and then perform a thorough investigation of the charges. In some states, the licensing board can temporarily suspend a physician's license to practice if a potentially dangerous situation exists, such as drug impairment or criminal charges. The physician is always accorded due process of the law, which includes a written description of the claim and a hearing before the state medical examiners. The physician can then appeal the board's decision.

Practicing Medicine Without a License

No physician wishes to have a license expire for failure to renew or have their license revoked for inappropriate behavior. A physician cannot legally practice medicine without this license.

MED TIP

Remember that if a physician continues to practice medicine without renewal of his or her license, under the law it is considered practicing medicine without a license.

Accreditation

Accreditation is a voluntary process in which an agency is requested to officially review healthcare institutions such as hospitals, nursing homes, and educational programs to determine competence. This is accomplished by sending in an objective third party, such as the **Joint Commission on Accreditation of Healthcare Organizations (JCAHO),** to examine the policies and procedures of the organization being accredited. The accreditation process can be rigorous and generally requires an onsite examination of the program under review. The institution or program must demonstrate that it maintains high standards of care, as set by the reviewing body, for patients and education of its participants. Accreditation of healthcare agencies and institutions became especially important with the advent of Medicare. The federal government stopped surveying hospitals providing care for Medicare patients and allowed JCAHO to perform this function. If an institution loses its accreditation, it also loses the ability to provide for Medicare patients.

JCAHO, established in 1952, accredits such organizations as: all types of hospitals, including psychiatric, long-term care facilities; managed care organizations such as HMOs; visiting nurse associations (VNA); and clinical laboratories. JCAHO emphasizes the use of qualitative standards and looks for compliance with outcome measures such as those found in quality assurance (QA) programs (see Chapter 1 for QA programs.) A JCAHO survey team visits the organization for an onsite inspection every three years. Upon successful completion of the accreditation process, an institution may display signage that it is accredited by JCAHO.

Another organization that provides accreditation for the healthcare profession is the Commission on Accreditation of Allied Health Education Programs (CAAHEP). CAAHEP provides accreditation for programs such as medical assisting, emergency medical technicians (EMTs), physician assistants and respiratory therapists. Many other allied health professions also have accreditation programs . . .

STANDARD OF CARE

Standard of care refers to the ordinary skill and care that all medical practitioners such as physicians, nurses, physician assistants, medical assistants, and phlebotomists must use, as determined by their state license or certification and that a "reasonable" person would use in a similar circumstance. This level of expertise is that which is commonly used by other practitioners in the same medical specialty when caring for patients.

> ### MED TIP
>
> The term *reasonable* is a broad, flexible word to make sure the decision is based on the facts of a particular situation rather than on abstract legal principles. It can mean fair, rational, or moderate. Reasonable care has been defined as "that degree of care a person of ordinary prudence (the so-called reasonable person or reasonable healthcare professional) would exercise in similar circumstances.

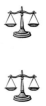

The standard of care for particular professions has changed somewhat over the years. For instance, in a Louisiana case, the court concluded that because doctors and nurses are both members of the medical profession, they should both be held to the same high standard of professional competence (*Norton v. Argonaut Ins. Co.,* 144 So.2d 249, La. App. 1962). However, in a later case, the court recognized that "situations could arise in which a doctor would be considered negligent in his performance of some task where he failed to act to the best of his ability as a physician, while a nurse, performing the same task in the same manner, could be acting to the best of her ability as a nurse." (*Thompson v. Brent,* 245 So.2d 751, La. App. 1971).

While physicians are not obligated to treat everyone (except in the case of an emergency), once a physician accepts a patient for treatment, he or she has entered into the physician–patient relationship (contract) and must provide a certain standard of care (see Figure 3.2 ■). This means that the physician must provide the same knowledge, care, and

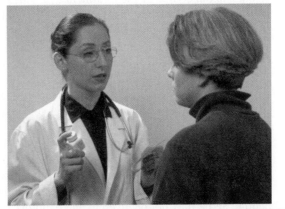

FIGURE 3.2
Standard of Care
Applies to
All Healthcare
Professionals.

skill that a similarly trained physician would provide under the same circumstances. The law does not require the physician to use extraordinary skill, only reasonable, ordinary care and skill. The physician is expected to perform the same acts that a "reasonable and prudent" physician would perform. This standard also requires that a physician not perform any acts that a "reasonable and prudent" physician would not.

Physicians are expected to exhaust all the resources available to them when treating patients and not expose patients to undue risk. If they violate this standard of care, they could be liable for negligence.

The Prudent Person Rule

The **prudent person rule,** also called the "reasonable person standard," means that a healthcare professional, usually a physician, must provide information to a patient that a reasonable, prudent person would want before he or she makes a decision about treatment or refusal of treatment. In general, a reasonable, prudent person would want to know the following.

- The diagnosis.
- The risks and potential consequences of the treatment, excluding any remote or improbable outcomes; this information should include the success and failure rates of the physician and/or institution.
- The expected benefits of the treatment or procedure.
- Potential alternative treatments.
- The prognosis if no treatment is received.
- That an acceptable standard of care is followed.
- The costs, including the amount of expected pain.

In general, the physician discusses these issues with the patient; however, ancillary healthcare professionals may be present during these conversations. The patient should always be treated in terms of what a "reasonable, prudent person" would want. Unfortunately, not all patients are provided the same courtesy.

CONFIDENTIALITY

Confidentiality refers to keeping private all information about a person (patient) and not disclosing it to a third party without the patient's written consent. The duty of medical confidentiality is an ancient one. The Hippocratic Oath states, "What I may see or hear in or outside the course of the treatment . . . which on no account may be spread abroad, I will keep to myself, holding such things shameful to speak about." This duty seeks to respect the patient's privacy, and it also recognizes that if the physician does not keep information confidential, patients may be discouraged from revealing useful diagnostic information to their physician.

According to the Medical Patients Rights Act, a law passed by Congress, all patients have the right to have their personal privacy respected and their medical records handled with confidentiality. Information such as test results, patient histories, and even the fact that the person is a patient, cannot be passed on to another person without the patient's consent. No information can be given over the telephone without the patient's permission. No patient records can be given to another person or physician without the patient's written permission, unless the court has subpoenaed it.

In short, any information that is given to a physician by a patient is considered confidential, and it may not be given to an unauthorized person unless specifically required by the law. Information should be communicated only on a need-to-know basis. (See Chapter 10 for a more detailed discussion of confidentiality and the Health Insurance Portability and Accountability Act of 1996, or HIPAA.)

MED TIP

Be especially careful about discussing anything relating to a patient within earshot of others. A comment such as, "Did Ms. Jones come in for her pregnancy test?" can result in a breach-of-confidentiality lawsuit against the physician. Remember: "Walls have ears."

STATUTE OF LIMITATIONS

The **statute of limitations** refers to the period of time that a patient has to file a lawsuit. The court will generally not hear a case that is filed after the time limit has run out. This time limit varies from state to state, but typically is one to three years. The only exception is that there is no statute of limitations for murder and some other criminal cases. One of the purposes of the statutes is to prevent potential plaintiffs from "sitting on their rights" while the memories surrounding the controversy grow dim or witnesses die or move away. In addition, the statutes allow potential defendants to go on with their lives without worry about a lawsuit that could be filed relating to some long-ago occurrence.

The statute of limitations, or the time period, however, does not always start "running" at the time of treatment. It begins when the problem is discovered or should have been discovered, which may be some time after the actual treatment. This is known as the **discovery rule.** In *Teeters v. Currey,* the plaintiff sued her doctor, alleging that as a result of Dr. Currey's negligence in performing surgery to sterilize Teeters, she gave birth to a premature child with severe complications several years later. Teeters brought an action for malpractice, and Currey pleaded the statute of limitations. The court found in favor of the defendant, Currey. However, Teeters successfully appealed and the case was remanded back to the lower court. The court adopted the "discovery doctrine" under which the statute does not begin to run until the injury is, or should have been, discovered (*Teeters v. Currey,* 518 S.W.2d 512, Tenn. 1974).

In some cases, the statute of limitations is *tolled,* or stops running. **Tolling,** or running, of the statute of limitations means that time has not expired, even if it is past the usual two-to-three year time frame, such as two-to-three years after reaching the age of majority for a child. For instance, most states say that the statute of limitations does not begin to run until the injured person reaches age 18. So, when a minor is injured, the minor may sue years after learning of the injury. While generally the court will appoint a *guardian ad litem,* an adult to act in the court on behalf of a child in litigation, the child does not have to sue through the *guardian ad litem.* The child may wait until he or she reaches adulthood before suing an obstetrician and his or her healthcare assistants 18 years (plus the statute of limitations period, which varies slightly in each state) after a birth injury has occurred, assuming the parents hadn't already sued.

MED TIP

The statute of limitations is a state law that varies by state.

GOOD SAMARITAN LAWS

Good Samaritan laws are state laws that help to protect from liability healthcare professionals and ordinary citizens who provide care to a victim of an accident or other emergency. The emergency aid covered under this law must be given at the scene of the accident or emergency. These laws exist in most states to encourage such aid. However, with the possible exception of Vermont, there is no *legal* duty to assist a stranger in a time of distress. But the law does state that those who do volunteer must exercise reasonable care and skill in rendering such aid. This law protects those professionals who do offer aid, outside of their work environment, in good faith, without gross negligence. "Good faith" is an abstract quality that is best defined as being faithful to one's duty or obligation. It is an honest belief that a person can provide aid to an emergency victim with no intention to defraud that victim. Under this law, the emergency care must be provided without an expectation of payment.

The protection under this law does have its limits, which can vary from state to state. If an emergency provider performed an action that was grossly negligent and acted in a way that a reasonable person would know would harm the victim, then the law's protection would be withdrawn and a lawsuit could then take place. This can be difficult to determine, however. For example, an elderly person, with brittle bones, who receives chest compressions during cardiopulmonary resuscitation (CPR) might accidentally receive fractured ribs, which puncture his or her lungs. A reasonable person would also have provided CPR in the same manner with the same result. In this case the emergency care would be covered under the Good Samaritan law even though the victim received an injury to her lungs.

Some states have provided additional protection under this law. For example, the Ohio Good Samaritan law extends protection to emergency medical technicians (EMTs) during ambulance runs. Since these laws vary from state to state, it is vital that every healthcare professional knows and understands the Good Samaritan laws in his or her own state.

Someone responding in an emergency situation is only required to act within the limits of acquired skill and training. For example, a nursing assistant would not be expected, or advised, to perform advanced emergency treatment that is considered within the scope and practice of a physician or nurse.

Even though trained healthcare professionals are generally not under a legal obligation to offer aid to an emergency victim, some believe they do have an ethical obligation. Their personal ethics set the guidelines for care provided in emergency situations. The statute of limitations does apply when filing a case under this law, with the time period starting to run when the injury occurs or is identified by the victim.

MED TIP

The Good Samaritan laws do not protect physicians or their employees from liability while practicing their profession in their work environment. The laws are meant to encourage medical professionals to assist with emergencies outside of the work setting. Always check on the coverage of the Good Samaritan Law in your own state.

RESPONDEAT SUPERIOR

Respondeat superior is a Latin phrase meaning, "let the master answer." Under the principle of *respondeat superior,* an employer is liable for acts of the employee within the scope of employment. What this means for physicians is that they are liable for negligent actions of the employees working for them even though the employer's conduct may be without fault. The employee's wrongful action must be within the scope of their employment. This means that the employer has assumed the right to control the employee's performance of duties (see Figure 3.3 ■).

MED TIP

Even though the doctrine of *respondeat superior* mainly refers to the employer, in all states both the physician and the employee may be liable.

In effect, when a physician delegates certain duties to staff employees—nurses, physician assistants, and medical assistants—the ultimate liability for the correct performance of those duties rests with the physician. For example, in the case of *Thompson v. Brent,* a medical assistant removed a cast from Thompson's arm with an electrically powered saw, known as a Stryker saw. While sawing through the cast, the medical assistant cut the plaintiff's arm, causing a scar almost the length of the cast and the width of the saw blade. The court held that even though the medical assistant was negligent in the use of the saw, the physician was liable for the assistant's actions under the doctrine of *respondeat superior* (*Thompson v. Brent,* 245 So.2d 751, La. Ct. App. 1971).

In similar cases, the courts have consistently found both the employer *and* the healthcare employee negligent. In the case of *Goff v. Doctors General Hospital,* the court held that the nurses who attended a mother, and who knew that she was bleeding excessively, were negligent in failing to report the circumstances so that prompt measures could be taken to safeguard her life (*Goff v. Doctors General Hospital,* 333 P.2d 29, Cal. Ct. App. 1958).

In some cases the hospital may also incur liability under this doctrine. The most well-known case in which a nurse failed to bring the condition of the patient to the doctor's attention was *Darling v. Charleston Community Memorial Hospital.* This case involved a minor patient who sued a hospital and a physician for allegedly negligent medical and hospital treatment, which resulted in the amputation of the patient's right leg below his knee. On November 5, 1960, the 18-year-old plaintiff broke his leg while playing football. At the hospital emergency room, his leg was set and placed in a cast, and he was hospitalized. He complained of great pain in his toes, which became swollen, dark, and eventually cold and insensitive. Over the next few days, the physician relieved the pressure in the cast by

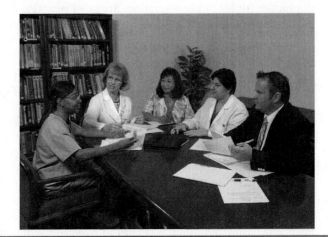

FIGURE 3.3
Physician Working with the Rest of the Healthcare Team.

"notching" the cast and cutting it three inches above the foot. On November 8, the physician split both sides of the cast, cutting the patient's leg as the cast was removed. Blood and seepage were observed coming from the leg as the cast was removed. The plaintiff was eventually transferred to another hospital on November 19 under the care of a specialist. After several attempts to save the plaintiff's leg, it was finally amputated eight inches below the knee. The plaintiff's attorney argued that it was the duty of the nurses to check the circulation of the leg frequently and the duty of the hospital to have, at the bedside, a staff of trained nurses who could recognize gangrene of the leg and bring it to the attention of the medical staff. If the physician failed to act, it was the duty of the nurse to then advise hospital authorities so that medical action could be taken. In this famous case, the court found liability existed on the part of all three: the physician, the hospital, and the nurse (*Darling v. Charleston Community Mem. Hosp.,* 211 N.E. 2d 253, 1965).

Employee's Duty to Carry Out Orders

Healthcare employees have a duty to interpret and carry out the orders of their employer/physician. They are expected to know basic information concerning procedures and drugs that may be used. The nurse or other healthcare professional has a duty to clarify the physician's orders when they are ambiguous or erroneous. If the procedure or drug appears to be dangerous for the patient, the healthcare professional has a duty to decline to carry out the orders and should immediately notify the physician. In the case of *Cline v. Lund,* a hospital was held liable for the death of a patient because a nurse failed to check the patient's vital signs every 30 minutes as ordered by the physician. The nurse also failed to notify the physician when the patient's condition became life threatening (*Cline v. Lund,* 31 Cal. App.3d 755, 1973).

> ### MED TIP
>
> Healthcare workers have a duty to be assertive and question those orders that they believe are erroneous or appear to be harmful to the patient. They also have a duty to refuse to carry out orders that violate their own practice acts.

Scope of Practice

Every employee in a medical setting must clearly understand and work within the scope of practice for his or her discipline. **Scope of practice** refers to the activities a healthcare professional is allowed to perform as indicated in their licensure, certification, and/or training. This means that a nurse can legally, through licensure, provide care and treatment to patients that a medical assistant is not licensed or certified to perform. For example, in some states a nurse may be permitted to renew medical prescriptions, with the physician's knowledge and authority, to a pharmacy over the telephone. A medical assistant is not licensed to do this. A trained and certified medical assistant can draw a sample of blood from a patient and perform certain tests on the sample, such as a blood count. However, a nurse's aide is typically not qualified or certified to perform these procedures.

It is imperative that employees understand and practice within the guidelines of their profession. However, the physician/employer also has a responsibility to instruct members of the healthcare team to perform activities that are within their respective scope of practice.

In addition, a physician/employer must clearly designate a chain of command for the healthcare team, assigning a person to oversee the functions of the healthcare team. In some cases, the physician assumes this duty. However, a nurse manager may also be designated for this role. In some medical offices, medical assistants can assume this function due to the intensive administrative portion of their training. Each employee must understand the chain of command so that when a question occurs regarding patient treatment or procedure, there is a clear route for obtaining the correct answer. A clear chain of command provides a "failsafe" mechanism so that no employees are left to make decisions that they are unqualified to make.

MED TIP

All employees must understand that there are limits to their authority when it comes to healthcare decisions. The ultimate decision always rests with the physician, provided it does not violate their professional practice.

Employer's Duty to Employees

Physicians/employers have a responsibility to provide a safe environment for their employees and staff. However, accidents and unforeseen incidents do happen while performing work-related tasks, such as theft, fires, auto accidents, and injuries from falls. Most physicians have liability insurance to cover any injuries or thefts occurring on the owner's grounds and within the buildings. They may also bond employees who handle money. **Bonding** is a special type of insurance made with a bonding company that covers employees who handle financial statements, records, and cash. If the employee embezzles (steals) money from the physician/employer, the physician can then recover the loss up to the amount of the bond.

Some physicians also carry liability insurance to cover the employee who has an automobile accident while conducting work-related business, such as making a bank deposit, for the employer.

Just as employers have a duty to provide a safe work environment, the employee has a duty to the employer to maintain this safe environment. Healthcare workers are, by the very nature of their work, surrounded with equipment and drugs that could be dangerous if misused. For example, employees must use caution when handling electrical equipment with multiple cords. Yanking an electrical cord out of the wall instead of gently pulling it out at the wall socket can result in an electric spark to occur. Even a simple act such as wiping up a spill on the floor can cause an injury if a "Wet Floor" sign is not posted. Most physicians' offices and all hospitals have a multitude of medications, including narcotics, that must be kept locked at all times.

In addition, it is an employee's duty to refrain from discussing their employer's personal life with patients and coworkers.

RISK MANAGEMENT

Risk management is a practice used to control or minimize the incidence of problem behavior that might result in injury to patients and employees, and ultimately to liability for the physician/employer. A key factor in risk management is to identify problem behaviors and practices in an organization such as a hospital or medical office. A plan of action is then put into practice to eliminate these problem behaviors. Risk management factors include environmental issues such as wet floors, improper grounding of electrical equipment, and poor security. Risk factors that affect employees include poor record keeping, improper storage of drugs and needles, improper follow-up for patient care, and abandonment of patients. Corrective actions for these factors are often addressed in updated policies and procedures books and employee handbooks. Many offices and hospitals employ risk managers whose sole job is to oversee the practices and behaviors that might harm patients and even result in malpractice suits (see Figure 3.4 ■).

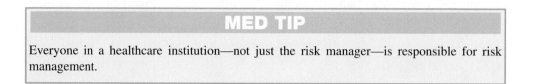

MED TIP

Everyone in a healthcare institution—not just the risk manager—is responsible for risk management.

Incident Report

One means of documenting problem areas within a hospital or other medical facility is the **incident report.** This report, using a form developed by the individual facility, should be completed whenever there is an unusual occurrence such as a fall, error in medication dispensing, needle sticks, fire, or a patient or employee complaint. An incident report can be completed by anyone who observed or or became aware of an unusual occurrence or incident such as an employee, manager, or physician. The purpose of the report is to document exactly what happened, when it happened, and what was done about the incident. The goal of using an incident report immediately after the situation happened is to accurately recall what happened as well as to prevent another incident.

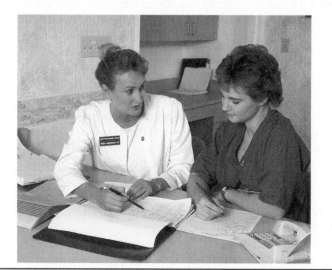

FIGURE 3.4
**Everyone Must
Participate in Risk
Management.**

POINTS TO PONDER

1. If a patient who suffers from cirrhosis tells me in confidence that she has started drinking again, what should I do?

2. Does *respondeat superior* mean that I am fully protected from a lawsuit? Why or why not?

3. Does the Medical Practice Act in my state allow a registered nurse to prescribe birth control pills for patients? Why or why not?

4. Is it really beneficial for me to become a licensed or certified member of my profession? Why or why not?

5. Am I expected to maintain the same standard of care for patients that my physician/employer is held to?

6. Am I protected by Good Samaritan laws if I perform CPR on a patient in a hospital emergency room waiting area and the patient dies?

7. Am I protected from a lawsuit if I have reported a medical emergency to my supervisor that I did not believe I was capable of handling?

8. If an injury occurred four years ago, am I protected from a lawsuit if the statute of limitations is two years in my state?

DISCUSSION QUESTIONS

1. A patient collapses on the floor in your department (office) and you must administer CPR. If the patient is injured when you administer CPR, are you protected from a malpractice suit under the Good Samaritan laws?

2. Describe the process Dr. Williams might use to become licensed to practice medicine when she moves from Chicago to New York.

3. Describe what *reasonable and prudent* means as it relates to standard of care.

REVIEW CHALLENGE

Short Answer Questions

1. What are some of the duties that an employee has to his or her employer as discussed in this chapter?

_____

_____

2. Does the doctrine of *respondeat superior* always protect the employee? Explain why or why not.

_____

_____

3. When does the "discovery rule" begin to "run?"

_____

_____

4. What is the purpose of the JCAHO?

_____

_____

5. Explain the difference between endorsement and reciprocity for licensure.

_____

_____

6. What does "standard of care" mean and why is it important?

_____

_____

7. Explain the "prudent person rule" as it relates to the patient.

_____

_____

8. Who or what determines the length of time for the statute of limitations?

_____

_____

Matching

Match the responses in column B with the correct term in column A.

Column A

_____ **1.** endorsement
_____ **2.** *guardian ad litem*
_____ **3.** revoked
_____ **4.** *respondeat superior*
_____ **5.** statute of limitations
_____ **6.** discovery rule
_____ **7.** reciprocity
_____ **8.** standard of care
_____ **9.** Good Samaritan law
_____ **10.** nonrenewal of license

Column B

a. begins at the time the injury is noticed or should have been noticed
b. ordinary skill that medical practitioners use
c. "let the master answer"
d. court-appointed representative
e. law to protect the healthcare professional
f. period of time that a patient has to file a lawsuit
g. sanction
h. medical license taken away
i. practicing medicine without a license
j. one state granting a license to a physician in another state

Multiple Choice

Select the one best answer to the following statements.

1. According to the Medical Patients Rights Act, patient information
   a. may be given over the telephone without the patient's consent.
   b. must be communicated on a need-to-know basis.
   c. can always be given out to another physician.
   d. other than test results, cannot be given out to a relative.
   e. can never be given out to a third party.

2. The term for a court-appointed person to represent a minor or unborn child in litigation is
   a. *respondeat superior.*
   b. advanced directive.
   c. *guardian ad litem.*
   d. durable power of attorney.
   e. living will.

3. Standard of care refers to
   a. ordinary skill.
   b. type of care given to patients by other practitioners in the same locality.
   c. only the care given by the physician.
   d. a, b, and c.
   e. a and b only.

4. The statute of limitations varies somewhat from state to state but is typically
   a. ten years.
   b. five years.
   c. one to three years.
   d. there is no limitation.
   e. none of the above.

5. *Respondeat superior* means that
   a. a healthcare employee can act independently of the employer.
   b. the healthcare employee is never found negligent by the courts.

c. the employer is liable for the actions of the employee.
d. healthcare employees have a duty to carry out the orders of their employers without question.
e. all of the above.

6. A process by which a physician in one state is granted a license to practice medicine in another state is
   a. endorsement.
   b. reciprocity.
   c. statute of limitations.
   d. revocation.
   e. suspension.

7. Patients' rights to have their personal privacy respected and their medical records handled with confidentiality is covered in the
   a. statute of limitations.
   b. rule of discovery.
   c. FLEX act.
   d. Medical Patients Rights Act.
   e. Good Samaritan Laws.

8. The prudent person rule refers to
   a. the needs of a medical assistant.
   b. the information that a reasonable patient would need.
   c. the type of employee that a physician would wish to hire in his or her office.
   d. the credentials for a malpractice attorney.
   e. none of the above is correct.

9. When a physician places an ambiguous order, the healthcare professional
   a. has a duty to carry out the order.
   b. can decline to carry out the order.
   c. should immediately notify the physician.
   d. b and c only.
   e. none of the above is correct.

10. Both physicians and employees are

a. liable in a lawsuit.

b. have the same responsibility to protect patient's confidentiality.

c. operate under a standard of care.

d. must be trained to perform a procedure before attempting it.

e. all of the above.

DISCUSSION CASES

1. Analyze the case at the beginning of this chapter, The Case of Latoya and the Physical Therapy Patient, by answering the following questions:

a. How can Latoya balance the benefits and harm of encouraging her patients to do something they do not want to do?

_____

_____

b. In your opinion, is Dr. B. placing too much pressure on a student?

_____

_____

c. Who should Latoya talk to about her dilemma?

_____

_____

d. Is this a legal or ethical problem, or both?

_____

_____

2. You are a phlebotomist drawing a specimen of blood on Emma Helm, who says she doesn't like having blood drawn. In fact, she tells you that the sight of blood makes her "queasy." You attempt to make her feel relaxed by quietly talking to her as you help her onto a chair in the hospital laboratory. While you are taking her blood specimen, she faints and hits her head against the side of a cabinet.

a. Are you liable for Emma's injury? Why or why not?

_____

_____

b. If you are not liable, do you know who is?

_____

_____

c. Is Emma Helm at fault for her accident? Why or why not?

_____

_____

d. What might you do to prevent this type of injury from happening?

_____

_____

3. *Jessica, a registered nurse (RN), and her husband were finally leaving on their vacation trip. They pull up to a red light as it is about to change to green. They watch in horror as a large truck, moving fast down a hill, is unable to stop before crashing into a van carrying a mother and her child. The van is thrown into the air and lands in a small park. Jessica runs over to offer aid. She finds a semi-conscious woman in the driver's seat and an unconscious 4-year-old boy in the back seat strapped in his car seat. The mother asks Jessica if Christopher is alright before she slips into unconsciousness. Christopher is unconscious and not breathing, with his head down and chin touching his chest. He has a gash bleeding on the side of his head caused by his tricycle flying over the backseat during the crash.*

   A truck driver, who had also stopped to give help, yells in the window at Jessica, "Don't move him!" Jessica knows that she has to get Christopher's breathing started. Even though the truck driver is still yelling at her not to move the boy, she gently lifts his head up off his chest. Christopher, still unconscious, starts breathing immediately. Jessica stops the bleeding on his head by applying pressure using a clean handkerchief from her husband. Emergency help arrives ten minutes later.

   a. In your opinion, even though Jessica knew that, in most cases, an injured victim should not be moved, did she do the right thing by moving Christopher's chin up so he could breathe?

   _____

   _____

   b. Was Jessica covered by the Good Samaritan Act or was she held to a higher standard because she had a nursing license?

   _____

   _____

   c. Would Jessica have been covered by the Good Samaritan Act if Christopher had not started breathing when she moved his head and he had suffered a further injury from the movement?

   _____

   _____

   d. Was Jessica, an RN, legally required to stop and provide aid? Was she ethically obligated to stop and provide aid?

   _____

   _____

   e. In your opinion, is it always a good idea to stop and give assistance at an accident site before medical help arrives?

   _____

   _____

PUT IT INTO PRACTICE

Search the newspapers in your area for an article relating to medical malpractice or medical ethics issues. Discuss whether the standard of care was violated in the situation discussed in the newspaper.

WEB HUNT

Using a search engine, find out about the Good Samaritan laws in your state.

CRITICAL THINKING EXERCISE

What would you do if you were just certified in CPR last week and a large woman collapsed in front of you on a very crowded bus? Her color is very dusky and she does not appear to be breathing. No one on the bus does anything. You are worried that you will do something wrong and might even hurt her with the chest compressions. Besides—everyone will be looking at you.

BIBLIOGRAPHY

American Medical Association. 2008–2009. *Code of medical ethics: Current opinions on ethics and judicial affairs.* Chicago: American Medical Association.

Badasch, S., and D. Chesebro. 2004. *Introduction to health occupations.* Upper Saddle River, NJ: Prentice Hall.

Beaman, N., and L. Fleming-McPhillips. 2007. *Comprehensive medical assisting.* Upper Saddle River, NJ: Pearson/Prentice Hall.

Black, H. 2009. *Black's law dictionary.* 8th edition. St. Paul, MN: West Publishing.

Stanfield, P. 2002. *Introduction to the health professions.* Boston: Jones & Bartlett.

Taber's cyclopedic medical dictionary. 2009. 21st edition. Philadelphia: F. A. Davis.

Today's Healthcare Environment

4

Learning Objectives

1. Define all glossary terms.
2. Describe today's healthcare environment.
3. Discuss the similarities and differences among HMOs, PPOs, and EPOs.
4. Describe five types of medical practice.
5. Discuss the term *diplomat* as it relates to medical specialty boards.
6. Identify three categories of licensed nurses and describe their educational requirements.
7. Describe five categories of certified healthcare professionals.
8. Describe the diagnostic related group (DRG) system of classification.
9. State the differences between Medicare and Medicaid.

Key Terms

Associate practice
Capitation rate
Certification
Conscience clause
Copayment
Corporation
Diagnostic related groups (DRGs)
Exclusive provider organization (EPO)
Fee splitting
Fixed-payment plan
Franchise

Franchisee
Gatekeeper
Group practice
Health Care Quality Improvement Act
Health maintenance organization (HMO)
Indigent
Licensure
Managed care organization (MCO)
Medicaid
Medicare

National Practitioner Data Bank (NPDB)
Partnership
Per diem
Preferred provider organization (PPO)
Primary care physician (PCP)
Prospective payment system
Registration
Sole proprietorship
Solo practice
Third-party payers

THE CASE OF MARION AND THE PACEMAKER

Marion is a 92-year-old patient who weighs 78 pounds. She has had poor eating habits for at least twenty years and refused all attempts by her two daughters to improve her nutrition. In addition, Marion had been a heavy smoker all her life and suffered frequent respiratory problems. During the past two years she has become quite forgetful, has suffered a broken hip as a result of a fall out of bed, and has been treated for pneumonia. Her daughters, who have their own family responsibilities and cannot bring their mother to live with them, have found an excellent nursing home near them. In spite of Marion's protests, she enters the nursing home. However, she quickly adjusts to her new home and likes the care and the attention that she receives.

During her third week in the nursing home, Marion develops a cough, high temperature, and respiratory problems. She is hospitalized with a diagnosis of pneumonia. Marion immediately becomes disoriented and attempts to remove her intravenous and oxygen tubing. Because she tried to climb out of bed, her daughters must remain at her side. The attending physician tells the daughters that in addition to treatment for pneumonia, Marion will also need to have a pacemaker inserted to regulate her heartbeat. Marion would then be unable to return to the nursing home, as the facility is not equipped to care for someone recovering from surgery.

One of Marion's daughters has been granted a medical power of attorney for her mother. Before Marion became confused, she clearly explained to her daughters her wishes not to receive extraordinary measures to prolong her life. She also signed a living will indicating her wishes. After thoughtful discussions with other family members, Marion's daughters tell the physician that they do not want to put their confused mother through the surgical procedure. They state that they want to spare her the pain of recovery from a surgical procedure because she is quite confused and elderly. Further, they are concerned that their mother will not survive an anesthetic and surgical procedure in her frail condition.

The physician seems to be understanding of this decision. He says that he will place into Marion's chart their request not to have the pacemaker inserted. However, the floor nurses take the daughters aside on several occasions to tell them that this is not a dangerous procedure and that they need to sign a permit for surgery. In fact, the nurses make the daughters feel that they are not acting in their mother's best interests by not signing the surgical permit. Marion returns to the nursing home without a pacemaker. She lives another four years without any cardiac problems.

1. Were the nurses carrying out their responsibility as licensed healthcare professionals or were they overstepping their role?

2. Were Marion's daughters acting in the best interests of their mother because they knew that if she had the surgery she could not return to the nursing home where she was receiving good care?

3. What should happen when a physician agrees with the family members and the nursing staff does not?

Today's healthcare professionals are immersed in an ever-changing environment. The advent of managed care, a variety of medical practice arrangements, and a multitude of healthcare specialty areas have resulted in the continual need to understand healthcare law. Unfortunately, due to the rise in the number of malpractice suits, many physicians are protecting themselves by ordering multiple testing procedures, some of which might not be needed. In addition, many patients no longer want older, more conservative approaches to testing and diagnosis—and these newer tests are more expensive.

As demonstrated in the above case, all healthcare professionals need to pay attention to the wishes of their patients. And in circumstances where the patient has given family members or others authority to make a healthcare decision on their behalf, healthcare professionals must respect the patient's wishes. They also should use care not to place their own opinions ahead of the decisions made by physicans and other healthcare professionals in consultation with the patient. However, an ethical dilemma arises when the healthcare professional's moral and religious beliefs conflict with their role in healthcare. There are no easy, or perfect, answers to these dilemmas.

TODAY'S HEALTHCARE ENVIRONMENT

Healthcare has undergone major changes since 1965 when Medicare and Medicaid became law. The growth rate of the older adult population and the remarkable technological discoveries and applications, such as heart and kidney transplants and mobile mammogram units, are just a few of the developments that have caused a rapid expansion of the healthcare system. In addition, insurance companies, managed care plans—such as **health maintenance organizations (HMOs),** which stress preventive care and patient education—and government legislation have significantly impacted the way healthcare is delivered.

Currently, about $3 billion a day is spent on healthcare in the United States. However, this does not mean that all Americans are receiving good care, or even any care. We, as a nation, are far from the top in life expectancy at birth. Traditionally, the emphasis in healthcare has been on quality. However, with rising healthcare costs, many U.S. citizens are concerned about the cost of services and access to medical care. Another critical issue is the crisis in health insurance coverage as many Americans do not have adequate medical insurance.

Health insurance includes all forms of insurance against financial loss resulting from illness or injury. Private health insurance is more than a $200 billion business annually. The most common type of health insurance covers hospital care. Relatively new types of insurance are the fixed-payment plans. These are offered by organizations that operate their own healthcare facilities or that have made arrangements with a hospital or healthcare provider within a city or region. The **fixed-payment plan** offers subscribers (members) complete medical care in return for a fixed monthly fee. HMOs, for example, base their operations on fixed prepayment plans.

Insurance companies and other **third-party payers,** such as HMOs, recognize that persons who are well covered by medical insurance have no incentive to economize. Insurers, however, want to keep their costs for reimbursement as low as possible. Physicians want to order more tests to avoid malpractice suits. Patients want adequate tests and complete care. Keeping these differing viewpoints in mind, who then decides on the allocation of the health resources?

Managed Care

Managed care is a method for restructuring the healthcare system, including delivery of a broad range of services, financing of care, and purchasing. Managed care provides incentives to keep costs of healthcare down by using an administrative structure to manage the enrolled population of patients. The managed care movement is known for its goal of offering medical care at lower costs and decreasing the amount of unnecessary medical procedures. Managed care provides a mechanism for a **gatekeeper,** such as the insurance company, to approve all nonemergency services, hospitalizations, or tests before they can be provided. A **primary care physician (PCP)** also acts in a gatekeeper capacity, because he or she is responsible for the patient's medical care and any referrals to other physicians or services. Physicians used to receive a fee for each service, procedure, test, or surgery they provided, called the fee-for-service (FFS) method of payment. In addition, patients could select any physician or specialist to treat them.

MED TIP

One of the fundamental principles of managed care is "managed choice." Patients have a choice about their medical care but only within certain parameters that are determined by the managed care organizations (MCOs).

Managed care organizations (MCOs) pay for and manage the medical care a patient receives. One of the means an MCO uses to manage costs is to shift some of the financial risk back onto the physician and hospitals—when the costs go up their income from the MCO goes down. This mechanism poses many ethical dilemmas. MCOs offer a variety of financial incentives, including bonuses to physicians for reducing the number of tests, treatments, and referrals to hospitals and specialists. These incentives can create a conflict of interest for physicians.

The offer of financial inducements to physicians who order fewer tests and hospitalizations for their patients is a widely discussed concern. Many fear that physicians may withhold services from patients in order to increase their own profits. Some of the reasons for these concerns are that MCOs attempt to limit the

- Choice of physician.
- Treatments a physician can order.
- Number and type of diagnostic tests that can be ordered.
- Number of days a patient can stay in the hospital for a particular diagnosis.
- Choice of hospitals.
- Drugs a physician can prescribe.
- Referrals to specialists.
- Choice of specialists.
- Ordering of a second opinion for diagnosis and treatment.

The managed care movement—with the implementation of health maintenance organizations (HMOs), preferred provider organizations (PPOs), and exclusive provider organizations (EPOs)—sought to bring healthcare costs under control by monitoring healthcare and hospital usage.

1. **Health Maintenance Organization (HMO)**—a type of managed care plan in which a range of healthcare services are made available to plan members for a predetermined fee (the *capitation rate*) per member, by a limited group of providers (such as physicians and hospitals). HMOs use a physician as the primary care

physician (PCP) to manage and control the enrolled patient's medical care. This capitation rate replaced the former "fee-for-service" rate which was considered to be more costly. In addition, the HMO places the PCP at some financial risk if there are excessive medical expenses in conjunction with the patient's medical care.

2. **Preferred Provider Organization (PPO)**—a plan in which the patient uses a medical provider (physician or hospital) who is under contract with the insurer for an agreed fee in order to receive **copayment** (usually $10 to $20) from the insured. PPOs differ from HMOs in two main areas: (a) A PPO is a fee-for-service program not based on a prepayment or a fixed monthly fee paid to the healthcare provider for providing patient services (capitation rate) as with an HMO—physicians and hospitals designated as PPOs are reimbursed for each medical service they provide; and (b) PPO members are not restricted to certain designated physicians or hospitals.

3. **Exclusive Provider Organization (EPO)**—a new managed care concept that is a combination of HMO and PPO concepts. In an EPO, the selection of providers (such as physicians and hospitals) is limited to a defined group, but the providers are paid on a modified fee-for-service (FFS) basis. Unlike a PPO, there is no insurance reimbursement if nonemergency service is provided by a non–EPO provider.

Federal Assistance Programs

Medicare

Medicare is the federal program that provides healthcare coverage for three groups of people: persons age 65 and over; disabled persons who are entitled to Social Security benefits or Railroad Retirement benefits; and end-stage renal disease victims who qualify, regardless of age. It was established under Title XVIII of the Social Security Act as part of the Social Security Amendments of 1965. Medicare was designed as a traditional third-party private insurance that emphasized free choice of healthcare. The accounting details were handled by private insurance companies, usually Blue Cross and Blue Shield. Medicare expenditures quickly rose beyond the initial projections. In addition, traditional Medicare reimbursement became very complex in both the administration and review process. This led to several problems, including a long delay for physicians and hospitals to receive reimbursement for providing services (see Figure 4.1 ■).

As a result of the rising costs of the Medicare program, a rationing of healthcare under Medicare has occurred. For example, the first $500 of the hospital care costs may have to be paid by the recipients once during each benefit period as a deductible; there is a cutoff of reimbursement of care beyond sixty days; and long-term care is not fully reimbursed. These cost-saving devices result in a fixed allocation of healthcare services for many elderly who will not use a hospital or nursing home facility because they cannot afford the deductible payment. In addition, most Medicare recipients who can afford to also pay for supplemental insurance to cover those costs not covered under Medicare.

Medicare patients have a right to appeal care that may be denied under existing Medicare rules and regulations. As a result of a court case, new rules by the Department of Health and Human Services for HMOs went into effect in August 1997. In the case of *Grijalva v. Shalala* (Donna Shalala was secretary of the department when the suit was filed), an Arizona court found that a 71-year-old Medicare patient, whose healthcare coverage was refused by her HMO, was denied the right to appeal when her request for home healthcare was refused by her HMO. The judge ruled that the Department of Health and Human Services, which oversees Medicare, was at fault for failing to force HMOs to follow federal law that mandates allowing appeals when there are denials for treatment. Under the current rules, a Medicare patient in an HMO may appeal when there are denials for treatment (*Grijalva v. Shalala*, 946 F. Supp. 747, Ariz. 1996).

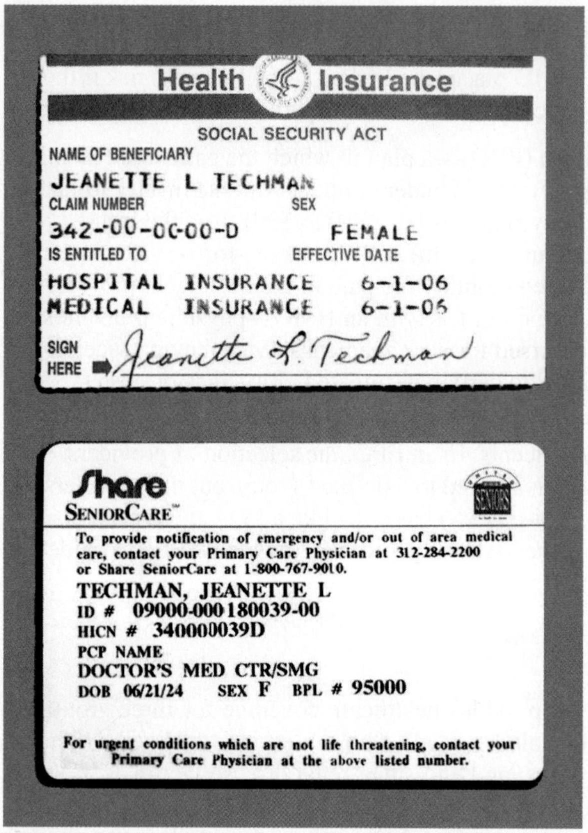

FIGURE 4.1
Medicare and Supplemental Private Insurance Cards

Diagnostic Related Groups (DRGs)

Another method of rationing healthcare was implemented in 1983, when Medicare instituted a hospital payment system—**diagnostic related groups (DRGs)**—that classifies each Medicare patient by illness. DRGs, now used for all patients, are designations which categorizes diagnoses and treatments into groups that are used to identify reimbursement conditions. There are currently nearly 1000 illness categories of medical conditions under the DRG system.

Hospitals receive a preset sum for treatment of an illness category, regardless of the actual number of "bed days" of care used by the patient. This method of payment provides a further incentive to keep costs down. However, it has also discouraged the treatment of severely ill patients due to the high costs associated with their care. In addition, patients are often discharged before they are ready to take care of themselves. This has resulted in hospital readmissions and, in some cases, death from embolisms (blood clots) that could have been prevented if the patient had remained under hospital supervision a few days longer.

Medicaid

Medicaid is a federal program implemented by the individual states, with the federal government paying 57.3 percent of Medicaid expenditures. Enacted at the same time as Medicare, it provides financial assistance to states for insuring certain categories of the poor and **indigent** (a person without funds). There is a growing concern that these two programs operate at cross purposes, as they serve some of the same beneficiaries, and that better coordination of the two programs is needed. Cases of abuse and fraud are reported within both programs. For example, there are cases of physicians and others employed in the healthcare field submitting bills for reimbursement under these two programs for patients they have never treated.

Rationing also takes place in the Medicaid program. For instance, several state Medicaid programs have resisted funding procedures such as liver transplants. The state of Oregon voted to abolish Medicaid funding for liver transplants and instead fund intensive prenatal screening programs. Voters apparently believed that the millions spent to save a few lives with liver transplants are better spent on effective prenatal screening that would help to prevent premature births and thus save more lives.

Individual states enact their own legislation to direct the way funds such as Medicaid are spent. Ethical dilemmas surface as patients on Medicaid find they have little or no access to funds within their own state. For example, while this does unfortunately happen, hospitals have gotten themselves into trouble for discharging a patient too early. Hospitals have been found guilty for negligently discharging patients because adequate discharge planning was not implemented.

Medicaid patients in long-term-care facilities are required under the law to use their own excess income to help to pay for their care. This means that they must use their own income before Medicaid will assist them. This has proved to be a burden for married couples, because it may impoverish the spouse as well as the patient. Some states have enacted laws in which the spouse may separate his or her financial resources from the patient's. In other words, the total amount of resources is divided in half so as not to leave the patient's spouse without a home or other resources. Some states offer nursing homes a **per diem,** or daily rate, payment for a patient's care. Other states may use a **prospective payment system** in which the payment amount or reimbursement for care is known in advance.

Ethical Considerations of Managed Care

Managed care, including Medicare and Medicaid, has many flaws. Because the basis for a managed care approach is an economic one of cost containment, those who know how to use the system will fare better than the poor and less educated. The wealthy patient may receive better care than the poor patient. For example, the wealthy Medicare patient may be able to carry a supplemental health insurance policy to cover the items, such as prescription drugs and long-term care, which are not fully covered under Medicare. Other ethical considerations and questions concerning managed care include the following:

- Some physicians will not accept patients who are on Medicare. They are concerned that the reimbursement is not sufficient to treat patients who may require a great deal of care as they age.
- Many believe it is difficult, if not impossible, to provide a decent minimum standard of care or treatment to everyone under the managed care concept.
- Are all the families and patients who agree to a managed care contract at the closest clinic fully informed of the consequences of trying to obtain healthcare elsewhere?
- Is a bait-and-switch approach being used by the MCO in which the patient is lured into joining a managed care plan only to realize that only minimal services are provided in such areas as rehabilitation or long-term care?
- Are the patient's interests being sacrificed to the bottom line? In other words, does a profit for the MCO become more important than the patient?
- Do the wealthy have better access to care and treatment?

Medicare and Medicaid laws prohibit physicians referring their patients to any service, such as physical therapy or dialysis centers, in which they may have a financial ownership or interest. In addition, physicians must be cautious that their patient charges do not violate Medicare's fee-for-service reimbursement rule.

Managed care poses the question of how to maximize the services available to the maximum number of people. This ideal equity approach would bring access to healthcare for all at an appropriate level. This would result in a relationship between access, cost, and quality of care. However, changing any one of these three elements (access, cost, and quality of care) impacts on the other two areas. For example, if we provide more access to care without increasing the cost, then quality will be negatively affected. If there is a proposal to increase quality and access to care, then there will be an increase in cost. In the current healthcare system, the public perception is that managed care has sacrificed quality and access for cost.

In spite of the potential problems with managed care, it is not an inherently unethical system of healthcare. Under this system, monitoring and control of the excessive use of testing and surgical procedures have improved. In addition, a reputable MCO can provide better preventive programs and healthcare screening for early detection of disease. It can also reduce the unnecessary testing, treatments, and hospitalizations that were present under the old fee-for-service (FFS) system.

Health Care Quality Improvement Act (HCQIA) of 1986

Congress passed the **Health Care Quality Improvement Act** in response to a growing concern about medical malpractice. The act provides for peer review of physicians by other physicians and healthcare professionals. The act also provides protection from lawsuits (liability) that whistleblowers may face when they report issues of potential malpractice. The main purpose of this act is to improve the quality of medical care. The act also sets up a **National Practitioner Data Bank (NPDB)** which assists with the peer review of physicians. The NPDB collects information about physicians' medical malpractice losses and settlements, investigations into licensure, and other damaging professional conduct. The NPDB has become a resource for organizations, such as state licensing boards, that require information about the qualification of doctors and dentists, in particular. This data bank information has become a necessary requirement when physicians are seeking medical staff hospital privileges. The data bank does not disclose this information to the general public.

TYPES OF MEDICAL PRACTICE

In the early part of the twentieth century, the main form of medical practice was the solo practice set up by a family practitioner within a designated town or geographic area. Over the years, the practice of medicine and the legal environment have changed. Few physicians make house calls any longer. However, patients now expect to be able to reach their physicians on a 24-hour basis.

MED TIP

The increase in the number of patients who have initiated malpractice lawsuits has necessitated not only increased insurance coverage costs for physicians and patients, but different methods of practice.

Other forms of medical practice have become popular, including some that meet patient needs for around-the-clock coverage and some that provide the opportunity for a group of physicians to share insurance premium costs, staff, and facilities investments.

Solo Practice

In **solo practice,** a physician practices alone. This is a common type of practice for dentists. However, physicians generally enter into agreements with other physicians to provide coverage for each other's patients and to share office expenses. Physicians are becoming increasingly reluctant to enter into solo practice because of the large burden of debt they incurred during their medical training and the high cost of operating an independent office.

A type of solo practice called **sole proprietorship** is one in which a physician may employ other physicians and pay them a salary. However, the sole proprietor of the medical practice is still responsible for making all the administrative decisions. The physician–owner pays all expenses and retains all assets.

The advantages of this type of practice include being able to retain all of the profits and to make the major decisions concerning policies and staffing. However, in a sole proprietorship, the owner is responsible and liable for the actions of all the employees. In addition, the physician may have to work long hours to provide his or her patients with the care they need. It is often difficult to find the correct balance of qualified physicians to help out during vacations and illnesses of the solo practitioner. This form of practice is diminishing rapidly due to increasing expenses and the lack of another physician to share the patient load.

Partnership

A **partnership** is a legal agreement to share in the business operation of a medical practice. A partnership may exist between two or more physicians. In this legal arrangement, each partner becomes responsible for the actions of all the other partners. This responsibility includes debts and legal actions unless otherwise stipulated in the partnership agreement. It is always advisable to have partnership agreements in writing. A document or "certificate of doing business as partners" is registered in the local county clerk's office.

The advantages of a partnership include greater earning power than a physician just working alone can realize. There are also other physicians in a partnership to carry any burden of patient care, liability, overhead expenses, or capital requirements to improve the office facility. The disadvantages often relate to personality conflicts. In addition, all the partners in the group must share in the liabilities even if only a few of the members are responsible for incurring them (see Figure 4.2 ■).

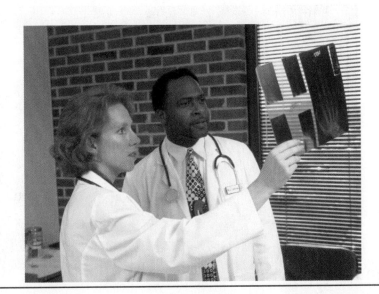

FIGURE 4.2
Physicians in Partnership

Associate Practice

The **associate practice** is a legal agreement in which physicians agree to share a facility and staff but not the profits and losses. They do not generally share responsibility for the legal actions of each other, as in a partnership. The legal contract of agreement stipulates the responsibilities of each party. The physicians act as if their practice is a sole proprietorship.

The legal arrangement of an associate practice must be carefully described and discussed with patients. Patients may mistakenly believe that there is a shared responsibility by all the physicians in the practice. This can lead to legal difficulties if one physician is accused of committing malpractice.

> **MED TIP**
>
> To avoid the appearance that a partnership exists when one does not, physicians must be sure the signage on their offices, their letterhead and other stationery, and the manner in which the staff answers the telephone is not misleading.

Group Practice

A **group practice** consists of three or more physicians who share the same facility (office or clinic) and practice medicine together. This is a legal form of practice in which the physicians share all expenses and income, personnel, equipment, and records. A physician may be a member of a group practice as a partner or as an employee. Some areas of medicine frequently found in group practice are anesthesiology, rehabilitation, obstetrics, radiology, and pathology. In some cases, physicians who practice in a single specialty area such as radiology join together in group practice. The membership of a group practice can be quite large, and thus it may be a difficult setting to work in for those who prefer to work alone. In some cases, the income level may not be as high as in a more limited type of partnership due to the large number of physicians creating the expenses (see Figure 4.3 ■).

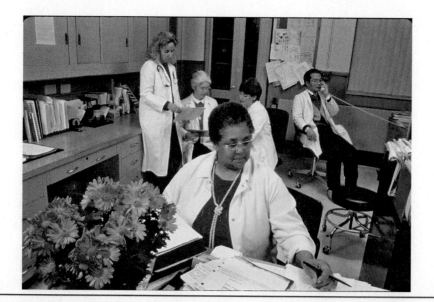

FIGURE 4.3
Group Practice

A group practice can be designated as a health maintenance organization (HMO) or as an independent practice association (IPA). Group practices have grown rapidly during the last decade, and large groups of more than one hundred doctors are not uncommon. A large group practice often forms a legal professional corporation.

Professional Corporations

During the 1960s, state legislatures passed laws (statutes) allowing professionals—for example, physicians and lawyers—to incorporate. A **corporation** is managed by a board of directors. There are legal and financial benefits to incorporating the practice.

Professional corporation members are known as shareholders. Some of the benefits that can be offered to employees of a corporation include medical expense reimbursement, profit sharing, pension plans, and disability insurance. These fringe benefits may not always be taxable to the employee and are generally tax deductible to the employer. While a corporation can be sued, the individual assets of the members cannot be touched (as they can in a solo practice). In some cases, a physician in solo practice will take legal steps to incorporate in order to provide some protection of assets. A corporation will remain until it is dissolved. Other forms of practice, such as the sole proprietorship, stop with the death of the owner. Today, most medical practices are corporations. Table 4.1 ■ describes the types of medical practice along with the advantages and disadvantages of each.

MED TIP

Physicians are moving away from solo practice and forming partnerships or corporations to better serve patient needs, share the costs of insurance, and, in the case of corporations, provide legal protection.

Type of Practice	Advantages	Disadvantages
Solo practice (only one physician)	Physician retains independence; simplicity of organization; physician retains all assets	Difficulty raising capital, sole responsibility for liability and management functions; inadequate coverage of patients' needs; practice may die with the owner
Sole proprietorship	Physician retains all assets; autonomy; hires other physicians to provide assistance	Pays all expenses; responsible for all liability
Partnership	Legal responsibility is shared among partners; work, assets, and income are shared	Partners may have personality differences; all partners are liable for actions of the other partners
Associate practice	Work is shared	Legal responsibility is not shared by all members
Group practice	All expenses and income are shared; all equipment and facilities are shared	Income may not be as great as when a physician practices alone; possible personality clashes among members
Single specialty	Expenses and staff are shared	Possible competition among specialists within the group
Corporation	Protection from loss of individual assets; many fringe benefits offered; corporation will remain until it is dissolved	Income may not be as great as in other forms of practice

TABLE 4.1

Types of Medical Practices

> ## MED TIP
>
> Remember that in all forms of practice, the physician is responsible for the actions of his or her employees.

THE ETHICS OF FEE SPLITTING

Fee splitting occurs when one physician offers to pay another physician for the referral of patients. Fee splitting has long been considered unethical and is a basis for professional discipline. The payment of a referral fee is also considered a felony in states such as Alaska, New Mexico, Vermont, and California. However, the most prohibitive statements against accepting a fee for referrals are at the federal level. The Medicare and Medicaid programs both contain antifraud and abuse provisions. These provisions declare that anyone who receives or pays any money, directly or indirectly, for the referral of a patient for service under Medicare or Medicaid is guilty of a felony punishable by five years' imprisonment, a $25,000 fine, or both.

Fee splitting is not the same as referrals to a hospital **franchise,** such as a pharmacy or radiology department. In this case, the holder of the franchise, or the **franchisee,** may legally pay the hospital in proportion to the amount of business received from hospital patients.

It is not necessarily considered fee splitting if the franchisee is paying an amount equal to expenses incurred. For instance, in a California case, a court held that a radiologist's payment of two-thirds of his receipts to a hospital did not constitute fee splitting because the evidence showed that fees paid to the hospital were equal to expenses incurred by the hospital to furnish the diagnostic center (*Blank v. Palo Alto-Stanford Ctr.,* 44 Cal. Rptr. 572, Cal. Ct. App. 1965).

MEDICAL SPECIALTY BOARDS

Of the 9 million people employed in the healthcare system, there are approximately 600,000 physicians, 35,000 doctors of osteopathy, and 150,000 dentists. Of the 600,000 physicians, only 150,000 practice primary patient care: family medicine, internal medicine, obstetrics, and pediatrics. The majority of physicians work in specialty fields such as anesthesiology, psychiatry, or a surgical specialty. Many physicians now work at salaried staff positions in hospitals, as members of group practices, for a corporate-sponsored medical care firm, or for community clinics.

> ## MED TIP
>
> It's important that the physician's support staff, including nurses, physician assistants, certified medical assistants, and technicians, understand the different medical specialty categories because they are often the ones who respond to patients' questions regarding these specialties.

Currently, twenty-three specialty boards are covered by the American Board of Medical Specialists. Included among these specialties are the American Board of Allergy and Immunology, American Board of Anesthesiology, American Board of Emergency Medicine, American Board of Internal Medicine, American Board of Surgery, and American Board of Urology. The specialty boards seek to improve the quality of medical care and treatment by encouraging physicians to further their education and training. The board evaluates the qualifications of candidates who apply and pass an examination. The physicians who pass the board review become certified as diplomats. As board-certified physicians, they may be addressed as either diplomats or fellows, a designation they can use after their name—for instance, Paul Smith, M.D., Diplomat of the American Board of Pediatrics.

Due to the dramatic advances in medicine over the past two decades, there continues to be an interest in specialization among physicians. Transplant surgery, including liver, kidney, lungs, and pancreas, has expanded the need for medical and surgical specialties. A description of some of the more common medical and surgical specialties is found in Table 4.2 ■.

Medical Specialty	Description
Adolescent medicine	Treats patients from puberty to maturity (ages 11 to 21)
Allergy and immunology	Treats abnormal responses or acquired hypersensitivity to substances with medical methods such as testing and desensitization
Anesthesiology	Administration of both local and general drugs to induce a complete or partial loss of feeling (anesthesia) during a surgical procedure
Cardiology	Treats cardiovascular disease (of the heart and blood vessels)
Dermatology	Treats injuries, growths, and infections to the skin, hair, and nails
Emergency medicine	Trained in emergency medicine with the ability and skills to quickly recognize, prioritize (triage), and treat acute injuries, trauma, and illnesses
Family practice	Treats the entire family regardless of age and gender
Geriatric medicine	Focuses on the care of diseases and disorders of the elderly
Hematology	Study of blood and blood-forming tissues
Infection control	Focuses on the prevention of infectious disease by maintaining medical asepsis, practicing good hygiene, and promoting immunizations
Internal medicine	Treats adults who have medical problems
Neurology	Treats the nonsurgical patient who has a disorder or disease of the nervous system
Nephrology	Specializes in pathology of the kidney, including diseases and disorders
Nuclear medicine	Specializes in the use of radioactive substances for the diagnosis and treatment of diseases such as cancer
Obstetrics and gynecology	Obstetrics treats the female through prenatal care, labor, delivery, and the postpartum period; gynecology provides medical and surgical treatment of diseases and disorders of the female reproductive system
Oncology	The study of benign tumors and cancer-related tumors
Ophthalmology	Treats disorders of the eye
Orthopedics	Specializes in the prevention and correction of disorders of the musculoskeletal system
Otorhinolaryngology (ENT)	Specializes in medical and surgical treatment of the ear (otology), nose (rhinology), and throat (laryngology)
Pathology	Specializes in diagnosing abnormal changes in tissues that are removed during surgery or an autopsy
Pediatrics	Specializes in the care and development of children
Physical medicine/ rehabilitative medicine	Treats patients after they have suffered an injury or disability
Preventive medicine	Focuses treatment on the prevention of both physical and mental illness or disability
Psychiatry	Specializes in the diagnosis and treatment of patients with mental, behavioral, or emotional disorders
Radiology	Specializes in the study of tissue and organs based on x-ray visualization

TABLE 4.2

Medical and Surgical Specialties

TABLE 4.2	Medical Specialty	Description
Medical and Surgical Specialties (*continued*)	Rheumatology	Treats disorders and diseases characterized by inflammation of the joints, such as arthritis
	Surgery	Corrects illness, trauma, and deformities using an operative procedure
	Surgical Specialty	**Description**
	Cardiovascular	Surgically treats the heart and blood vessels
	Colorectal	Surgically treats the lower intestinal tract (colon and rectum)
	Cosmetic/plastic surgery	Surgically reconstructs underlying tissues
	Hand	Surgically treats defects, traumas, and disorders of the hand
	Neurosurgery (CNS)	Surgically intervenes for diseases and disorders of the central nervous system
	Orthopedic	Surgically treats musculoskeletal injuries and disorders, congenital deformities, and spinal curvatures
	Oral (periodontics/orthodontics)	Treats disorders of the jaws and teeth by means of incision and surgery as well as tooth extraction; treats malocclusion (misalignment) of teeth
	Thoracic	Surgically treats disorders and diseases of the chest

American College of Surgeons

The American College of Surgeons also confers a fellowship degree upon applicants who have completed additional training and submitted documentation of 50 surgical cases during the previous three years. A successful candidate becomes a Fellow of the American College of Surgeons (FACS).

American College of Physicians

The American College of Physicians offers a similar fellowship and entitles the applicant to become a Fellow of the American College of Physicians (FACP) in a nonsurgical area.

The designation doctor (Dr.) is the proper way of addressing—verbally or in writing—someone who holds a doctoral degree of any kind. In the medical field, the title of doctor indicates that a person is qualified to practice medicine within the limits of the degree received; in other fields, the title means that a person has attained the highest educational degree in that field. Several designations for doctor are listed in Table 4.3 ■.

MED TIP

The term doctor comes from the Latin word *docere,* meaning "to teach."

TABLE 4.3	Designations	Abbreviations
Designations and Abbreviations for Doctors	Doctor of Chiropractic	D.C.
	Doctor of Dental Medicine	D.M.D.
	Doctor of Dental Surgery	D.D.S.
	Doctor of Medicine	M.D.
	Doctor of Optometry	O.D.
	Doctor of Osteopathy	D.O.
	Doctor of Philosophy	Ph.D.
	Doctor of Podiatric Medicine	D.P.M.

ALLIED HEALTH PROFESSIONALS

A physician works with a variety of trained personnel, depending on the area of special-ization. Healthcare professionals are also called allied healthcare practitioners. There are specific requirements for healthcare professionals, including licensure, certification, and registration as well as a means of establishing competency. In addition, programs for edu-cating healthcare professionals may seek accreditation such as through the Joint Com-mission on Accreditation of Healthcare Organizations (JCAHO). (See more about the JCAHO in Chapter 3.)

Licensure, generally issued at the state level, is a mandatory credentialing process that allows an individual to legally perform certain skills. As dictated by law, there is usually a requirement to pass certain tests and exhibit the ability to perform certain skills. For example, nurses and pharmacists must graduate from an accredited educational program and pass a national examination that shows competency in their chosen medical field. Licensed personnel, including registered nurses, nurse practi-tioners, licensed practical nurses, and pharmacists are licensed in the state in which they practice. Licensed medical professionals can place their license in jeopardy, or even lose their license to practice their profession, if they abuse drugs or alcohol, steal from their employer or patients, lie about their education and training, or commit a criminal act.

Certification is a voluntary credentialing process usually offered by a private profes-sional organization, such as a school, college, or other accreditation body. Certification indicates that the allied health professional has met the standards set by the certification entity. The individual programs will have requirements to adequately perform certain skills. Certified, but not licensed, personnel include physician assistants or registered/cer-tified medical assistants, certified medical transcriptionists, laboratory technicians, and ultrasound technologists.

The American Association of Medical Assistants (AAMA), founded in 1956, is a key association in the field of medical assisting. This organization is responsible for the medical assistants' certification process. Certification indicates that a candidate has met the standards of the AAMA by achieving a satisfactory test result. A certificate, or legal document, is issued to a person who has successfully passed the examination (see Figure 4.4 ■).

Registration indicates that a person whose name is listed on an official record or register has met certain requirements in their particular profession. The registry list of names can then be accessed by healthcare providers to determine if a potential employee has met certain requirements. For example, registered nurses' names are listed in the reg-istry of the state in which they hold a license. The American Medical Technologists (AMT) association provides oversight for the registration and testing of medical assis-tants, medical technologists, and phlebotomists. This association, in cooperation with the AMT Institute for Education (AMTIE) has developed a continuing education (CE) pro-gram and recording system.

The AMT, a nonprofit certifying body, provides a Registered Medical Assistant (RMA) certification for medical assistants who meet the eligibility requirements and who can prove their competency to perform entry-level skills through written examination. The RMA is awarded to candidates who pass the AMT certification examination.

Nonphysician health professionals also cannot practice medicine outside of their own licensure and expertise. If one acts outside the area of his or her competency and the patient is injured as a result, that healthcare practitioner is liable for malpractice or, in other terms, medical negligence. In this situation, the healthcare practitioner could be fined and/or lose his or her license. For example, it is against the law for a licensed practical nurse (LPN) or medical assistant to prescribe medications: this function lies

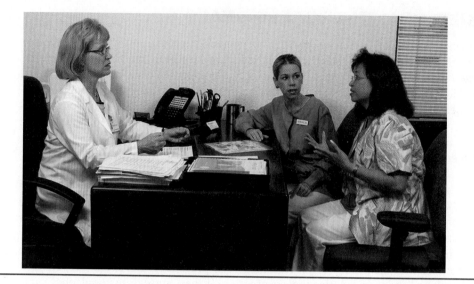

FIGURE 4.4
Health Professionals Working Together

only within the domain of a physician, nurse practitioner, or physician assistant. A phlebotomist is not licensed to discuss the results of a patient's laboratory tests with the patient: only the physician is licensed to interpret and discuss this information with the patient.

MED TIP

Physicians and their staff who assist with hiring personnel have a responsibility to check the licensure and certification of all employees. For example, patients expect that when they see the initials R.N. after an employee's name that the person is trained and licensed as a registered nurse.

Accreditation agencies for allied health educational programs include the Commission on Accreditation of Allied Health Education Programs (CAAHEP) and the Accrediting Bureau of Health Education Schools (ABHES). This accreditation, which is voluntary, requires that the educational facilities maintain particular standards which usually include an internship. (See Table 4.4 ■ for a description of healthcare occupations.)

TABLE 4.4	Occupation	Description
Healthcare Professions	Certified Medical Assistant (CMA)	Duties are grouped into two categories: administrative and clinical. Works in a variety of healthcare settings including physicians' offices and clinics. Must graduate from an accredited program and pass a national certification exam.
	Certified Medical Transcriptionist (CMT)	Types dictation recorded by a physician or surgeon. Must pass a certification exam. Works in medical records departments in hospitals and other healthcare facilities.
	Certified Professional Coder (CPC)	Evaluates medical orders using the Health Care Procedure System (HCPCS) used for billing purposes.

Occupation	Description
Dental Assistant	Works under the supervision of a dentist to prepare the patient for treatment, take dental x-rays, and hand instruments to the dentist.
Dental Hygienist	Works directly with the dental patient to clean teeth, take x-rays, and discuss results of the patient's dental exam with the dentist.
Electrocardiograph Technologist	Operates electrocardiograph (EKG/ECG) machines to record and study the electrical activity of the heart.
Emergency Medical Technician (EMT/paramedic)	Provides emergency care and transports injured patients to a medical facility. Works for ambulance service or a hospital (see Figure 4.5) ■.
Laboratory or Medical Technologist (MT)	Performs laboratory analysis, directs the work of laboratory personnel, and maintains quality assurance standards for all equipment. Also referred to as clinical laboratory scientist.
Licensed Practical Nurse (LPN)	Performs some, but not all, of the same tasks as the registered nurse. Must graduate from a recognized one-year program and become licensed by the National Federation of Licensed Practical Nurses. Works under the supervision of physicians and registered nurses.
Medical Records Technician (ART)	Skilled in health information technology; maintains medical records in healthcare institutions and medical practices. Successfully completes the Accredited Record Technician examination.
Nurse Practitioner (NP)	A registered nurse who has additional training in a specialty area such as obstetrics, gerontology, or community health. This nurse usually holds a master's degree.
Occupational Therapist (OT)	Provides treatment to people who are physically, mentally, developmentally, or emotionally disabled in the area of personal care skills; goal of OT is to restore the patient's ability to manage activities of daily living.
Pharmacist	A licensed professional who orders, maintains, prepares, and distributes prescription medications.
Pharmacy Technician	Prepares and dispenses patient medications (see Figure 4.6) ■.
Phlebotomist	Draws blood from patients; certification is required in some states.
Physical Therapist (PT)	Provides exercise and treatment of diseases and disabilities of the bones, joints, and nerves through massage, therapeutic exercises, heat and cold treatments, and other means.
Physician Assistant (PA)	Assists the physician in the primary care of the patient. Requires additional education similar to a master's level program; must work or have an internship experience and pass an accreditation exam. Works under the supervision of a physician.
Registered Nurse (RN)	A professional caregiver who has successfully completed a national licensure exam known as the National Council Licensure Examination (NCLEX).
Respiratory Therapist (RT)	Evaluates, treats, and cares for patients who have breathing abnormalities.
Social worker	Provides services and programs to meet the special needs of the ill, physically and mentally challenged, and older adults.
Surgical Technician	Trained in operating room procedures and assists the surgeon during invasive surgical procedures.
Ultrasound Technologist (ARRT)	Uses inaudible sound waves to outline shapes of tissues and organs.
X-ray Technologist (radiologic technologist)	Uses radiologic technology such as nuclear medicine and radiation.

TABLE 4.4

Healthcare Professions (*continued*)

Patients often refer to anyone wearing a white laboratory coat as "doctor" or a white uniform as "nurse." Always correct patients and tell them exactly what your position is. If you are a student, be sure to wear an identifying badge so that you will not be asked to perform an action outside of your scope of practice.

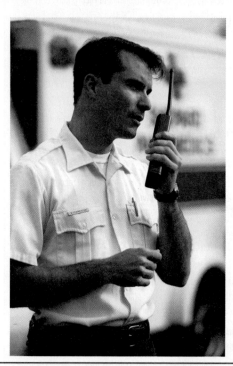

FIGURE 4.5
Emergency Medical Technician

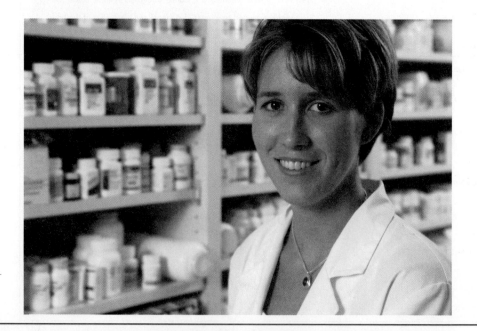

FIGURE 4.6
Pharmacy Technician

Conscience Clause

Because many employees in a variety of healthcare settings have religious or moral objections to assisting with certain procedures, such as sterilization and abortion, several states have enacted legislation called a **conscience clause.** These clauses state that hospitals may choose not to perform sterilization procedures and that physicians and hospital personnel cannot be required to participate in such procedures or be discriminated against for refusing to participate. In 1979, a Montana nurse-anesthetist was awarded payment (damages) from a hospital that violated the Montana conscience clause. The hospital had fired her for refusing to participate in a tubal ligation (*Swanson v. St. John's Lutheran Hosp.*, 579 P.2d 702, Mont. 1979).

On the other hand, there have been situations in which employees do not wish to leave their work setting even though they are morally unable to assist with sterilization or abortion procedures. In one New Jersey case, a court held that a hospital could transfer a nurse from the maternity ward to the medical-surgical staff because the nurse refused to assist in sterilization or abortion procedures. The court ruled that the transfer was not illegal because the nurse did not lose her seniority and it did not alter her pay (*Jeczalik v. Valley Hosp.*, 434 A.2d 90, N.J. 1981).

There are numerous examples of healthcare providers and patients clashing over the right to refuse to give treatment if it violates a person's beliefs. This conflict stimulates bitter debate over religious freedom versus patients' rights. Patients claim their rights are being ignored. Healthcare workers claim they are victims of religious discrimination when they are discharged or fired for refusing to provide service or care to patients. For example, a Chicago ambulance driver refused to transport a woman who was having an abortion, a Texas pharmacist refused to fill a prescription for a rape victim who was seeking the morning-after pill, and a California fertility clinic refused to give assistance to a gay woman who was requesting artificial insemination. Some respiratory therapists have objected to removing terminally ill patients from ventilators; gynecologists have declined to prescribe birth control pills; and some anesthesiologists have refused to provide anesthetics in sterilization procedures or to participate in executions.

Patient advocates claim that there is a long tradition in medicine that medical professionals have an ethical, as well as a professional, responsibility to place the patient's needs first. Believers in a "right of conscience" or the "conscience clause" in medicine believe that U.S. citizens should not be forced to violate their moral and religious values. This debate is not new. After the 1973 *Roe v. Wade* decision allowing abortion, several states passed laws to protect doctors and nurses who did not want to participate in performing an abortion. Oregon's law in 1994 to legalize physician-assisted suicide allows doctors and nurses to decline to participate.

Many such conflicts are quietly and informally handled. In some cases an employee will seek a position elsewhere; in others, a coworker will step in to assist with a procedure, usually without the patient's even knowing of the change. The ethical dilemma facing both patients and healthcare workers becomes critical during an emergency. This is especially difficult in poor or rural areas where there are few options for care. There is currently no perfect solution, legal or otherwise, to this problem.

POINTS TO PONDER

1. What impact will managed care have upon your career as an allied health professional?

2. What type of practice does your physician/employer have? If it is not a solo practice, what are the other specialties involved in the practice?

3. What are the advantages of forming a corporation?

4. Why is it important to include the medical specialty and initials indicating a particular degree or license after one's name?

5. What should you say if a patient refers to you as "doctor" or "nurse" even though your degree is in another discipline?

6. How should healthcare plans balance the interests of all the enrolled patients with the interests of a patient who has special medical needs and extraordinary expenses?

7. In the interest of maintaining a successful practice, should a physician refuse to provide care for patients who are uninsured or minimally insured?

8. Consider the question of ethics that arises when we ask ourselves if we are reducing unnecessary tests, as the HMOs and others believe we should, or if we are limiting tests for patients who really need them.

DISCUSSION QUESTIONS

1. Discuss your role as a medical professional in relation to the physician and other healthcare providers.

2. Discuss the impact that managed care is likely to have on your career in healthcare.

3. What can be done to ensure that MCOs provide ethical care for all patients?

4. Discuss "managed choice" as described in this chapter. Is there a choice?

REVIEW CHALLENGE

Short Answer Questions

1. What are the differences between Medicare and Medicaid?

   _____

   _____

2. What are the advantages and disadvantages of a group medical practice for a physician?

   _____

   _____

3. What are some of the areas that might be limited to patients under an MCO?

   _____

   _____

4. Explain the titles for the following abbreviations.

   D.P.M. _____ O.D. _____

   D.O. _____ D.M.D. _____

   M.D. _____ D.C. _____

5. Explain the titles for the following abbreviations.

   NP _____ CMT _____

   CMA _____ RT _____

   PT _____ ARRT _____

   PA _____ ART _____

6. Explain the differences between licensure, certification, and registration.

   _____

   _____

7. What is the purpose of a conscience clause?

   _____

   _____

8. What is the National Practitioner Data Bank (NPDB)?

   _____

   _____

9. Explain the difference between a per diem payment system and a prospective payment system.

   _____

   _____

Matching

Match the responses in column B with the correct term in column A.

Column A

_____ **1.** HMO
_____ **2.** EPO
_____ **3.** PPO
_____ **4.** solo practice
_____ **5.** associate practice
_____ **6.** sole proprietorship
_____ **7.** corporation
_____ **8.** third-party payer
_____ **9.** Medicaid
_____ **10.** Medicare

Column B

a. preferred provider organization
b. physicians agree to share expenses of a facility
c. health maintenance organization
d. managed by a board of directors
e. financial assistance for the elderly
f. exclusive provider organization
g. one physician may employ others
h. financial assistance for the indigent
i. physician practices alone
j. insurance company

Multiple Choice

Select the one best answer to the following statements.

1. Under this plan, a healthcare provider is paid a set amount based on the category of care provided to the patient.

  a. AMA
  b. DRG
  c. ANA
  d. HHS
  e. UNOS

2. Medicare patients who are members of HMOs may now, by law,

  a. not make any deductible payment.
  b. select any physician they wish.
  c. appeal a denial of treatment.
  d. have all their nursing home expenses paid.
  e. none of the above.

3. A type of managed care in which the selection of providers is limited to a defined group who are all paid on a modified fee-for-service basis is a(n)

  a. exclusive provider organization.
  b. group practice.
  c. preferred provider organization.
  d. health maintenance organization.
  e. sole proprietorship.

4. A legal agreement in which physicians agree to share a facility and staff but not the profits and losses is a(n)

  a. solo practice.
  b. sole proprietorship.
  c. partnership.
  d. associate practice.
  e. none of the above.

5. The advantage of a corporation is that it

  a. offers protection from loss of individual assets.
  b. may offer fringe benefits.
  c. will remain in effect after the death of a member.
  d. offers the opportunity for a large increase in income.
  e. a, b, and c only.

6. A physician who is board certified may be addressed as

  a. diplomat.
  b. fellow.
  c. partner.
  d. associate.
  e. a and b only.

7. MCOs are able to manage costs by

  a. shifting some financial risk back to the physicians.
  b. shifting some financial risk back to the hospitals.
  c. using a fee-for-service payment method.
  d. a and b only.
  e. a, b, and c.

8. This federal legislation provides healthcare for indigent persons and is administered by individual states.

  a. Medicare
  b. Medicaid
  c. HMO
  d. PPO
  e. COBRA

9. The managed care system

  a. has a gatekeeper to determine who will receive medical treatments.
  b. provides a mechanism for approval for all nonemergency services.
  c. provides care for a fixed monthly fee.
  d. includes HMOs, PPOs, and EPOs.
  e. all of the above.

10. The American College of Surgeons confers a fellowship degree upon its applicants

  a. whenever a surgeon places a request.
  b. when they complete additional training.
  c. when they have documentation of 50 surgical cases during the previous three years.
  d. a, b, and c.
  e. b and c only.

DISCUSSION CASES

1. *Jerry McCall is Dr. William's office assistant. He has received professional training as both a medical assistant and an LPN. He is handling all the phone calls while the receptionist is at lunch. A patient calls and says he must have a prescription refill for Valium, an antidepressant medication, called in right away to his pharmacy, since he is leaving for the airport in thirty minutes. He says that Dr. Williams is a personal friend and always gives him a small supply of Valium when he has to fly. No one except Jerry is in the office at this time. What should he do?*

   a. Does Jerry's medical training qualify him to issue this refill order? Why or why not?

   _____

   _____

   b. Would it make a difference if the medication requested were for control of high blood pressure that the patient critically needs on a daily basis? Why or why not?

   _____

   _____

   c. If Jerry does call in the refill and the patient has an adverse reaction to it while flying, is Jerry protected from a lawsuit under the doctrine of respondeat superior?

   _____

   _____

   d. What is your advice to Jerry?

   _____

   _____

2. *Allison G. has asked her doctor to prescribe a "morning-after" pill to prevent a pregnancy from taking place. Her doctor, Dr. Williams, tells her that he cannot prescribe this pill, which has the ability to abort a pregnancy, based on his own moral beliefs and conscience. Allison tells his medical assistant, Amy, that she thinks it is very wrong of Dr. Williams to impose his religious beliefs upon his patients. She says that he should not have become a physician if he could not separate his personal values from patient care.*

   a. In your opinion, what should Amy say to the patient?

   _____

   _____

   b. Should Dr. Williams let his patients know what his religious beliefs are when they become his patient? Why or why not?

   _____

   _____

   c. Is there an ethical or legal problem with Dr. Williams' action?

   _____

   _____

3. *Dennis tells his father that he wishes to study to be a Physician Assistant (PA). He says, "It's a great field. I can work independently and do almost everything the doctor does without having the high cost of malpractice insurance."*

  a. Is Dennis' statement to his father correct?

  _____

  _____

  b. What does a PA do?

  _____

  _____

  c. Will Dennis work independently of a physician if he becomes a PA?

  _____

  _____

PUT IT INTO PRACTICE

Interview a senior citizen and ask about his or her health insurance needs. Does he or she have difficulty with the paperwork required by the insurance company? Ask what could be done to make this a less difficult task.

WEB HUNT

Discuss the type of information that is available on the website for the American Medical Association (www.ama-assn.org).

CRITICAL THINKING EXERCISE

What would you do if you are processing billing statements for patients and notice that your physician/employer has entered patient charges for relatively minor procedures that were never done?

BIBLIOGRAPHY

Beaman, N., and L. Fleming-McPhillips. 2007. *Comprehensive medical assisting*. Upper Saddle River, NJ: Pearson/Prentice Hall.

Fremgen, B., and S. Frucht. 2010. *Medical terminology: A living language*. Upper Saddle River, NJ: Pearson/Prentice Hall.

Freudenheim, M. 2001. "A changing world is forcing changes on managed care." *New York Times*, (July 2), 1.

Hall, M., and M. Bobinski. 2003. *Health care law and ethics: In a nutshell*. St. Paul, MN: West Publishing.

Managed Care. 2008. *ISBA legal health checkup*. (April, 30), 10.

Stanfield, P. 2002. *Introduction to the health professions*. Boston: Jones & Bartlett.

Stein, R. 2006. "A medical crisis of conscience." *Hartford Courant*, (Aug. 8), D 4.

Tindall, W., W. Williams, J. Boltri, T. Morrow, S. van der Vaart, and B. Weiss. 2000. *A guide to managed care medicine*. Gaithersburg, MD: Aspen.

The Physician–Patient Relationship

5

Learning Objectives

1. Define the glossary terms.
2. Describe the rights a physician has when practicing medicine and when accepting a patient.
3. Discuss the nine principles of medical ethics as designated by the American Medical Association (AMA).
4. Summarize "A Patient's Bill of Rights."
5. Understand standard of care and how it is applied to the practice of medicine.
6. Discuss three patient self-determination acts.
7. Describe the difference between implied consent and informed consent.

Key Terms

Abandonment
Acquired immune deficiency syndrome (AIDS)
Advance directive
Against medical advice (AMA)
Agent
Consent
Do not resuscitate (DNR)

Durable power of attorney
Human immunodeficiency virus (HIV)
Implied consent
Informed (or expressed) consent
In loco parentis
Living will
Minor

Parens patriae authority
Privileged communication
Prognosis
Proxy
Uniform Anatomical Gift Act

CASE OF DAVID Z. AND AMYOTROPHIC LATERAL SCLEROSIS (ALS)

David, who has suffered with ALS for twenty years, is now hospitalized in a private religious hospital on a respirator. He spoke with his physician before he became incapacitated and asked that he be allowed to die if the suffering became too much for him. The physician agreed that, while he would not give David any drugs to assist a suicide, he would discontinue David's respirator if asked to do so. David has now indicated through a prearranged code of blinking eye movements that he wants the respirator discontinued. David had signed his living will before he became ill, indicating that he did not want extraordinary means keeping him alive.

The nursing staff has alerted the hospital administrator about the impending discontinuation of the respirator. The administrator tells the physician that this is against the hospital's policy. She states that once a patient is placed on a respirator, the family must seek a court order to have him or her removed from this type of life support. In addition, it is against hospital policy to have any staff members present during such a procedure. After consulting with the family, the physician orders an ambulance to transport the patient back to his home, where the physician discontinues the life support.

1. What were the primary concerns of the hospital?

2. What was the physician's primary concern?

3. When should the discussion about the patient's future plans have taken place with the hospital administrator?

Few topics are as important as the physician–patient relationship. This relationship impacts the entire healthcare team. All healthcare professionals who interact with the patient must understand their responsibilities to both the patient and the physician. The patient's right to confidentiality must always be paramount.

The first physicians were "medicine men," witch doctors, or sorcerers (Figure 5.1 ■). The physician–patient relationship has come a long way from those early years. In order for the relationship to exist, both physician and patient must agree to form a contract for services. Once a doctor has agreed to treat a patient, the patient can expect that the doctor will provide medical services for as long as necessary (Figure 5.2 ■). In order to receive proper treatment, the patient must confide truthfully in the physician. Failure to do so may result in serious consequences for the patient, and the physician is not liable if the patient has withheld critical information. Medical personnel who work closely with physicians, such as nurses, physician assistants, and medical assistants, must keep in mind that the physician–patient relationship is one to be closely guarded by them also. Any patient information that is either overheard or read is always to be considered confidential.

PHYSICIAN'S RIGHTS

Physicians have the right to select the patients they wish to treat. They also have the right to refuse service to patients. From an ethical standpoint, most physicians treat patients who need their skills. This is particularly true in cases of emergency.

Physicians may also state the type of services they will provide, the hours their offices will be open, and where they will be located. The physician has the right to expect payment for all treatment provided, and a physician can withdraw from a relationship if the patient is noncooperative or refuses to pay bills when able to do so.

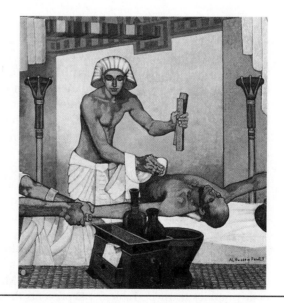

FIGURE 5.1
An Early Physician
(Brian Warling/International Museum of Surgical Science/ Chicago, IL)

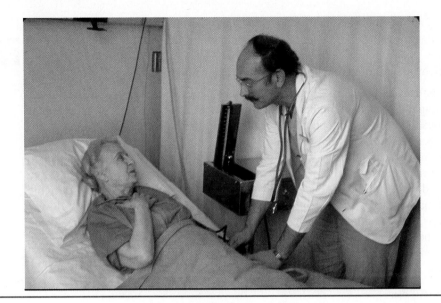

FIGURE 5.2
The Physician–Patient
Relationship

Physicians have the right to take vacations and time off from their practice and to be unavailable to care for their patients during those times. It is legally prudent for physicians to arrange for coverage during an absence. In most cases, other physicians will cover for them and take care of their patients. Physicians should notify their patients when they will be unavailable.

Some physicians now charge for services such as answering after-hours phone calls and filling out insurance forms. Many physicians feel that the large increases in their malpractice insurance premiums and the tighter regulations by HMOs have forced them to charge for services that they previously performed without charge.

PHYSICIAN'S RESPONSIBILITIES

Clearly, a physician's first responsibility is to be professionally competent. In addition, a physician must treat all patients with the same standards regardless of race, gender, sexual orientation, or religion. While a physician has the right to accept or decline to establish a professional relationship with any person, once that relationship is established, the physician has certain responsibilities. For example, federal law and many state laws prohibit hospitals from giving physicians 'kickbacks' of money or other benefits in return for referring patients. In 1994, NME Psychiatric Hospitals pleaded guilty to making unlawful payments to physicians in order to induce them to refer patients to their institutions. NME agreed to pay the federal government $379 million to settle the case (*United States v. NME Psychiatric Hosps., Inc.*, No. 94-0268).

The physician has many other responsibilities, including ethical ones. The American Medical Association (AMA) has taken a leadership role in setting ethical standards for the behavior of physicians. The AMA, organized in 1846, formed its first code of ethics in 1847. Table 5.1 ■ presents the AMA's current statement of principles in its entirety.

	TABLE 5.1
	AMA Principles of Medical Ethics

Preamble

The medical profession has long subscribed to a body of ethical statements developed primarily for the benefit of the patient. As a member of this profession, a physician must recognize responsibility not only to patients, but also to society, to other health professionals, and to self. The following principles adopted by the American Medical Association are not law, but standards of conduct which define the essentials of honorable behavior for the physician.

Human Dignity

I. A physician shall be dedicated to providing competent medical service with compassion and respect for human dignity.

Honesty

II. A physician shall deal honestly with patients and colleagues, and strive to expose those physicians deficient in character or competence, or who engage in fraud or deception.

Responsibility to Society

III. A physician shall respect the law and recognize a responsibility to seek changes in those requirements that are contrary to the best interests of the patient.

Confidentiality

IV. A physician shall respect the rights of patients, of colleagues, and of other health professionals, and shall safeguard patient confidence within the constraints of the law.

Continued Study

V. A physician shall continue to study, apply, and advance scientific knowledge, make relevant information available to patients, colleagues, and the public, obtain consultation, and use the talents of other health professionals as needed.

Freedom of Choice

VI. A physician shall, in the provision of appropriate health care, except in emergencies, be free to choose whom to serve, with whom to associate, and the environment in which to provide service.

Responsibility to Improved Community

VII. A physician shall recognize a responsibility to participate in activities contributing to an improved community and the betterment of public health.

Responsibility to Patient

VIII. A physician shall recognize that responsibility to the patient is paramount.

Patient Access to Medical Care

IX. A physician must support access to medical care for all people.

Source: American Medical Association, Code of Medical Ethics © 2008–2009.

PROFESSIONAL PRACTICE RESPONSIBILITIES

Medical practice responsibilities include such commonplace routines as effective hand-washing techniques before touching any patient. While this may seem to be an issue that hardly needs to be stated, nevertheless, there are serious ethical, legal, and economic implications when healthcare personnel ignore these sensible routines. For example, a survey of over 900 hospitals, cited in the *Chicago Tribune,* reports that medical mistakes kill anywhere from 44,000 to 98,000 Americans every year. According to the report, many often-preventable complications, such as postoperative infections, lead to more than 32,000 hospital deaths and more than $9 billion in extra costs annually. One of the most serious complications is postsurgery sepsis (bloodstream infections). Researchers believe that improved hand washing might reduce these high rates of death.

> ## MED TIP
>
> Failure to practice correct hand washing is considered to be a medical error when it results in patient infection. All healthcare professionals must hold themselves to the same high standards regarding diligent hand washing that we set for physicians. Physicians have many duties upon entering the practice of medicine. Examples of professional duties are described in Table 5.2. ■

TABLE 5.2 Examples of Physicians' Duties		
Conflict of interest	Physicians should not place their own financial interests above the patient's welfare.
Professional courtesy	Historically, there is an unwritten practice among many physicians that they would not charge each other for professional services. However, this practice has lost favor because many physicians are concerned about the lack of documentation when seeing a fellow physician free of charge.
Reporting unethical conduct of other physicians	A physician should report any unethical conduct by other physicians.
Second opinions	Physicians should recommend that patients seek a second opinion whenever necessary.
Sexual conduct	It is unethical for the physician to engage in sexual conduct with a patient during the physician–patient relationship.
Treating family members	Physicians should not treat members of their families except in an emergency.

Duties During a Medical Emergency

A physician cannot ethically or legally turn away a patient who is in an emergency situation. If the physician is unable to adequately treat the patient, then he or she must call for emergency assistance from paramedics (a 911 call). For instance, allergy specialists may be unable to give life-saving medications to a stroke victim, because the drugs won't be available in their offices. However, allergy specialists can handle victims who are in respiratory distress as well as, or better than, some other medical specialists. It is especially important to remember that patients cannot be turned away from a hospital or physician's office if they are indigent or uninsured.

> ## MED TIP
>
> Remember that all physicians receive the same basic medical training regardless of their medical specialty. They and their staff should be able to assist with basic CPR.

Duty to Treat Indigent Patients

In U.S. hospitals, there has been, in the past, a "dumping crisis" of indigent patients who lack medical insurance. There are many stories of deaths occurring after a patient has been shuffled from a private hospital emergency room to a public hospital that accepts indigent patients. While the hospital treatment may not be to blame for the death, the long delay in treatment while the patient is being transferred might. The Comprehensive

Omnibus Budget Reconciliation Act (COBRA) contains an amendment (EMTALA) that prohibits "dumping" patients from one facility to another. It is now a federal offense to do this. (See EMTALA discussed further in Chapter 8.) This amendment does not mandate treatment, but it does require a hospital to stabilize a patient during an emergency situation.

Does a physician have a duty to treat a patient who is unable to pay? According to the Summary of Opinions of the Council on Ethical and Judicial Affairs of the AMA (2008–2009), a physician has the right to select which patients to treat. However, physicians do not have the same freedom to drop patients once they have agreed to treat them. The healthcare professional has the right to earn a living and charge for services, but from an ethical standpoint, a physician cannot abandon any patient, even in a nonemergency situation. Abandonment might expose the patient to dangers due to lack of oversight of medications and treatment.

Duty Not to Abandon a Patient

Once a physician has agreed to take care of a patient this is considered to be a contract that may not be terminated improperly. Physicians may be charged with **abandonment** of the patient if they do not give formal notice of withdrawal from the case. In addition, the physician must allow the patient sufficient time to seek the service of another physician. This does not mean the physician may never withdraw from a case. Physicians may decide they can no longer accept responsibility for the medical treatment of a patient because the patient refuses to come in for periodic checkups or take prescribed medications and treatments. They may even offer referral suggestions. Abandonment could occur if the physician does not give enough notice to the patient so that other arrangements for medical care can be made.

MED TIP

There are occasions, such as during vacations, when a physician will ask another physician to "cover" or take charge of his or her patients. This is not considered to be abandonment.

Abandonment is considered to be a civil wrong or tort. It can be considered to be a breach of contract and even negligence. The courts have found the physician–patient relationship to be that of a contract when they enter into a mutual agreement. The physician agrees to diagnose and treat the patient until the relationship is over. The patient agrees to pay the physician for these services. If the physician, who has already agreed to this mutual contract, does not allow the patient to make an appointment for treatment, then abandonment may exist.

MED TIP

Office receptionists and nurses need to use care when denying patients an appointment. In some cases, office personnel believe they are serving the best interests of the physician by not overloading his or her schedule, but they may be setting up the physician for a charge of abandonment.

Abandonment with negligence occurs when the physician terminates the relationship in an unreasonable way as compared to the way other physicians would act in the same circumstances. For example, if a physician refused to see a patient for follow-up care after a surgical procedure because the patient or the patient's insurance company did not pay the bill, the physician could be liable for damages due to negligence and abandonment.

It is a frustration for physicians when patients do not comply with the treatment plan. Patients can also be frustrated when they do not experience a cure from a physician. The patient may then terminate the physician–patient relationship by not making any more appointments to see the physician. However, physicians and their office staffs must be vigilant about maintaining the relationship until it is terminated in a formal manner such as a letter sent by certified mail.

MED TIP

Sending a letter by certified mail is the best method physicians can use to protect themselves from a charge of abandonment when they have to sever a relationship with a patient.

Abandonment does not just apply to the physician–patient relationship. Licensed providers of healthcare such as dentists, podiatrists, physician assistants, and nurse practitioners are all subject to this principle. There are difficult situations relating to abandonment that arise when medical personnel have started to provide emergency care such as CPR. For example, once emergency medical technicians (EMTs) have started to give treatment, they may not stop until someone else takes over for them or the patient expires. In fact, all persons who administer CPR are taught to continue to provide this procedure until someone else relieves them or they cannot perform CPR any longer.

Hospitals are also liable for abandonment, especially in emergency situations. In some cases, an emergency patient may have to be transferred to another hospital that can better handle his or her care, such as one having a burn unit. However, an emergency patient must be stabilized, usually with intravenous medications, before being transferred to other facilities.

The Noncompliant and Incompetent Patient

A patient who is noncompliant and also incompetent presents a special concern for physicians and hospitals. Hospitalized patients who are noncompliant may discharge themselves **against medical advice** of their physicians, but the incompetent patient poses a unique problem because he or she may not be able to understand the need for treatment and may even pose a threat to another person. In this case, a physician will submit an emergency application to a judge, who can then order an emergency hospital admission for the patient. Most states require that within 72 hours a formal (due process) hearing be held. At this hearing, the patient's medical condition is evaluated along with the loss of any of his or her rights. A decision may be made to either allow the patient to return home or to continue to be hospitalized. Additional hearings are held as long as the incompetent patient is hospitalized.

MED TIP

Note that abbreviations used for the American Medical Association (AMA) and Against Medical Advice (AMA) are the same. Be careful not to confuse the two.

Duty to Treat Patients with AIDS

Acquired immunodeficiency syndrome (AIDS) is a disease resulting in infections that occur as a result of exposure to the **human immunodeficiency virus (HIV)**, which causes the immune system to break down. Testing for HIV is useful, since medications are available that can slow or even stop the advancement of the disease. Because there is a strong stigma attached to this disease, it is important to respect the confidentiality of anyone having an HIV or AIDS test. Patients must give their informed consent for the test.

MED TIP

Note that testing positive for HIV does not necessarily mean that a person has, or will develop, AIDS. Positive test results, if leaked to an employer, can lead to loss of job, on-the-job harassment, or other serious consequences, even though such actions may be illegal.

Ethical Considerations When Treating AIDS Patients

A physician who knows that the patient may endanger the health of others has certain ethical obligations, which include the following:

1. Persuading the patient to inform his or her partner(s).
2. Notifying authorities if there is a suspicion that the patient will not inform others.
3. As a last resort, notifying the patient's partner(s).

MED TIP

As with all legal/ethical issues, when in doubt about a notification obligation, it is wise to check the laws in your state regarding the requirement and/or consult an attorney. Many states only require information about a new case of AIDS and do not require names to be provided.

It is unethical to refuse to treat, work with, or provide housing for a person who is HIV- or AIDS-infected. In addition, the Americans with Disabilities Act (ADA), a federal law, protects HIV and AIDS patients from discrimination.

Physicians have been faced with the dilemma of honoring the confidentiality of their patients and then risking being sued for failure to warn or protect third parties who may have been exposed to HIV/AIDS through the activity of the patient. This is of particular concern when the patient is a child. The child may be shunned by friends or others who are afraid of being exposed to the virus. In *Doe v. Borough of Barrington,* the court cited the plaintiffs' brief for numerous examples of hysteria caused as a result of AIDS. These included a Florida family with hemophiliac children who tested positive for AIDS, driven out of town after their house was firebombed; a teacher with AIDS who was removed from teaching duties; and children with AIDS who were denied schooling in Colorado (*Doe v. Borough of Barrington,* 729 F. Supp. 376, N.J. 1990). The physician, by law, must make a full report to the state about any patient who is HIV- or AIDS-positive, despite the potentially serious consequences to the patient by reporting the case.

> ### MED TIP
> Patients with AIDS, or who are HIV-positive, need to be treated with the same compassion and care that would be given to any patient with a life-threatening illness.

Exposure of Healthcare Workers to a Patient's Blood

Unfortunately, needlestick injuries in healthcare settings are common even when physician and healthcare workers take special precautions, such as using gloves. After exposure to an HIV-positive patient's blood, a physician or healthcare worker has a 0.3 percent risk of contracting HIV, according to the CDC estimates. In one study of medical school residents, it was found that almost 70 percent reported they had received a needlestick during their medical training. Understandably, healthcare workers who have received needlestick injuries wish to know if the patient's blood contained the HIV or AIDS virus.

If the patient refuses to be tested for HIV or AIDS, can the physician order blood work to test for the virus without the patient's consent? This presents both legal and ethical concerns. HIV testing without the patient's consent is illegal. However, some states have allowed HIV testing without the patient's consent when a serious situation warrants the testing. From an ethical standpoint, HIV testing in spite of the patient's objection violates the patient's autonomy and privacy.

Restriction on HIV-Infected Healthcare Workers

Public health concerns about HIV-infected healthcare employees has always been an issue. Several ethical questions have been presented:

▶ Should healthcare workers, especially those who perform invasive procedures such as drawing blood specimens, be tested for HIV?

▶ Should HIV-infected healthcare workers inform their patients that they are positive for the virus?

▶ Should the practice of HIV-infected workers be restricted?

As patients/consumers, it is relatively easy for us to answer yes to these three questions. For example, physicians have an ethical obligation that requires that they do no harm to their patients. Further, physicians are obligated to disclose information to their patients that a reasonable person would require in order to make an informed decision about their own testing for the virus. Most patients would certainly want to know if their physician or healthcare worker is infected with HIV. A *Newsweek* poll found that 94 percent of their readers responding to the poll agreed that all physicians and dentists should be required to tell their patients if they are HIV-infected.

The American Medical Association (AMA) recommends that HIV-positive healthcare workers should not perform invasive procedures that pose a risk to their patients and that physicians should always "err on the side of protecting patients." The American Academy of Orthopedic Surgeons recommends that HIV-positive surgeons not perform procedures that involve the placement of internal devices, such as hip replacements, wires, or even blind probing of tissue. Probably the strongest statements come from the Federation of State Medical Boards, which states that it would be professional misconduct for healthcare workers to perform invasive procedures if they *do not* know their HIV-status. Furthermore, the Federation recommends that all state boards require that the names of HIV-infected healthcare workers be reported to them.

There are strong arguments for ignoring confidentiality issues and reporting HIV-positive workers if their actions put patients' health at risk. For example, surgeons, gynecologists, dentists, phlebotomists, surgical nurses, and emergency medical technicians all take part in invasive procedures in which HIV could be transmitted. In addition, removing the HIV-positive healthcare worker from close patient contact could ultimately provide protection from patients' infections and diseases such as tuberculosis.

There are valid arguments against requiring mandatory testing and restricting the activities of HIV-positive healthcare workers. For example, healthcare workers have a right to freedom from discrimination and to privacy. There are statistics that show that the risk of transmitting the HIV to another person is very low. In addition, the cost of testing all healthcare workers for HIV is prohibitive. The CDC has estimated that it would cost more than $250 million for testing alone. This money would have to be diverted from research and other programs. The CDC guidelines also declare that healthcare workers have no ethical duty to disclose their HIV status if they present no significant risk to their patients.

On-the-Job Protection for the Healthcare Worker

There is a relatively low risk of infection for persons working in the fields of medical transcription, secretarial, or office management in which there is little patient contact. There is a greater risk of infection for healthcare professionals, such as a physician, nurse, or medical assistant, as they have direct patient contact. The bottom line for all healthcare organizations is that there should be a clearly stated policy on how to handle all needlestick situations (Figure 5.3 ■) and patients' bodily fluids.

MED TIP

Medical offices, clinics, and hospitals should have special absorbent cleaning material available in case of a blood spill. Directions on what to do when a blood spill or other accident occurs should be placed where they are visible by the entire staff.

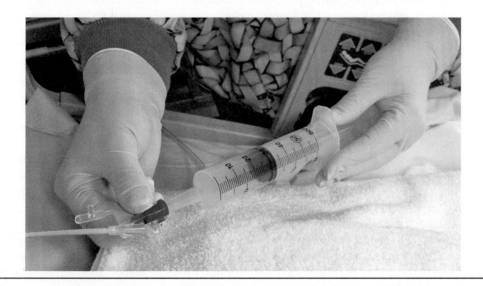

FIGURE 5.3
Needlestick Protection

Duty to Properly Identify Patients

Many medical errors occur because the patient was not properly identified. It is necessary to identify the patient both by stating his or her name and examining any other identification such as a medical wristband. It's always wise to ask patients to identify themselves by name. Patients who are hard of hearing, suffering from Alzheimer's disease, non-English-speaking, or elderly may not understand when you call them by name. There have been cases of incorrect patients in the emergency room (ER) waiting area going in for treatment because they didn't properly hear their name called. It's always wise to ask to examine some identification, such as a driver's license or medical wristband. Some medical offices take the patient's photo for their records.

MED TIP

Remember, if an error is made, such as not properly identifying the correct patient, admit it immediately. Then seek to correct the situation. You may save a life.

Duty to Respect Confidentiality

Medical personnel should use a low voice when speaking to patients over the telephone or speaking about patients to other staff members within hearing distance of any patients in the waiting room. Ideally, a glass enclosure should be present at the front desk in all waiting rooms to separate the receptionist from the patients and provide an additional aid for patient confidentiality. The sign-in sheet or patient register should be designed so those patients who are signing in or registering cannot view other patients' names.

Duty to Tell the Truth

There has always been the dilemma in medicine about whether to tell dying patients the truth about their **prognosis** (prediction for the course of their disease). On the one hand, the truth can be a means for patients to have a sense of control and even empowerment over their remaining time. On the other hand, the truth can act as a traumatic and demoralizing event that may cause the patient to lose the will to live.

There has been a major change in physicians' attitudes concerning truth telling during the past several decades. Originally, many physicians believed in a paternalistic, or protective, approach in which they avoided upsetting their terminally ill patients by telling them the truth about their condition. In a research study conducted in 1961, Donald Oken reported that 88 percent of U.S. physicians surveyed said it was their policy not to tell their patients if they had a terminal malignancy. The physicians believed it would be too upsetting to the patient. In a follow-up study twenty years later, these findings were completely reversed, with 98 percent of the physicians surveyed following a policy of telling the truth to patients. This position of truth telling has continued to the present day. The openness for cancer patients came about, in part, due to the necessity to seek consent for chemotherapy and radiation therapy.

Is this change in honesty for the benefit of the patient? Should physicians inform their Alzheimer's patients if their families want the information withheld? Should elderly patients be lied to when they have to move into a nursing home? Should family members be misled over the phone when called to come into a hospital after a family member has expired? These difficult questions have caused many healthcare professionals to reexamine the truth-telling issue.

For example, a medical ethicist, Joseph Fletcher, states that maintaining the lie of a diagnosis becomes very difficult for everybody on the healthcare team. He believes in focusing on the consequences of an action while protecting the patient. Furthermore, according to Fletcher, medicine has now become too complex to keep secrets from patients. He states that in the long run it is better for the patient if the truth is told.

MED TIP

The physician is the person responsible for discussion of the diagnosis with the patient. There are various interpretations of what constitutes lying. However, most people believe that a lie is a falsehood told in those circumstances in which the other person has a reasonable expectation of the truth.

False results of research studies also have had a negative impact upon patients. For example, a Canadian physician working with researchers at a major U.S. medical school reported fictitious results about a mastectomy study. The researchers falsely claimed, and advised the medical community, that the "less radical" surgical procedure (something other than a mastectomy) was an effective treatment for cancer of the breast. This deception took place over a fifteen-year period until finally they retracted their false claims.

Many believe that when dealing with the issue of truth telling, one should apply principles of justice. In other words, try to determine what a "just" action would be for the patient. Thomas Hackett, in writing about psychological assistance for the dying patient, cites an example of a typical victim in which there was a failure to inform:

> A woman with terminal breast cancer asked her doctor why her headaches persisted. When the doctor said it was probably nerves, she asked why she was nervous. He returned the question. She replied, "I am nervous because all the tests have stopped, nobody wants my blood, and I get all the pills I want. The priest comes to see me twice a week, which he never did before, and my mother-in-law is nicer to me even though I am meaner to her. Wouldn't this make you nervous?" There was a pause. Then the doctor said, "You mean you think you are dying?" She said, "I do." He replied, "You are." Then she smiled and said, "Well, I broke the sound barrier; someone finally told me the truth."

In some circumstances, truth telling is at variance with the medical profession's obligation of confidentiality. For example, in the famous Tarasoff case, the court held that a psychiatrist should have warned Tatiana Tarasoff that one of his patients was threatening to kill her. The patient did fulfill his threat to kill Tatiana Tarasoff. The court stated that the therapist was under an obligation to take reasonable steps, such as breaching confidentiality, to protect all third parties from the ill patient (*Tarasoff v. Regents of the University of California,* 17 Cal. 3d 342, 1976). However, in a later case, the same California court that tried the Tarasoff case stated that the therapist did not have a duty to warn a third party of a threat, because the patient had not made threats against a particular person. While these two cases seem to be at odds with each other, the current thinking is that this later verdict is more reasonable. It is difficult, if not impossible, for a psychiatrist to determine which threats a patient makes will result in murder. In reality, however, many mental health physicians are maintaining a conservative approach by hospitalizing patients who show violent tendencies.

The American Hospital Association's Committee on Biomedical Ethics states:

> Also subject to state law, confidentiality may be overridden when the life or safety of the patient is endangered such as when knowledgeable intervention can prevent threatened suicide or self-injury. In addition, the moral obligation to prevent substantial and foreseeable harm to an innocent third party usually is greater than the moral obligation to confidentiality.

PATIENTS' RIGHTS

The patient has the right to approve or give consent—permission—for all treatment. In giving consent for treatment, patients reasonably expect that their physician will use the appropriate standard of care in providing care and treatment—this means that the physician will use the same skill that other physicians use in treating patients with the same ailments in the same geographic locality. (Standard of care is discussed in more detail in Chapter 3.)

The patient's right to privacy prohibits the presence of unauthorized persons during physical examinations or treatments. This right has long been established. In a precedent-setting 1881 case, the plaintiff, a poor woman named Mrs. Roberts, sued Dr. DeMay for bringing in a third party, by the name of Scattergood, to assist him while she was in labor. Mrs. Roberts claimed that Scattergood "indecently, wrongfully, and unlawfully" laid hands on her and assaulted her. Even though Mrs. Roberts thought Scattergood was a physician, which he was not, he was present without her permission. The court found in the plaintiff's favor and awarded her damages for the "shame and mortification" she suffered (*DeMay v. Roberts*, 9 N.W. 146, Mich. 1881).

Additionally, patients have the right to be informed of the advantage and potential risks of treatment—including the risk of not having the treatment. They also have the right to refuse treatment. Some members of religious groups, such as Jehovah's Witnesses and Christian Scientists, do not wish to receive blood transfusions or other types of medical treatment. Physicians may not treat them against their wishes. However, in the case of a minor child, the court may appoint a guardian who can give consent for the child's procedure.

Confidentiality

Patients expect that the physician and staff will keep all information and records about their treatment confidential. In fact, the Medical Patients Rights Act provides that all patients have the right to have their personal privacy respected and their medical records handled with confidentiality. No information, test results, patient histories, or even the fact that the patient is a patient, can be transmitted to another person without the patient's consent. A breach of confidentiality is both unethical and illegal. See Chapter 9 for a detailed discussion of confidentiality when using electronic transmission of patient's medical information as mandated by the Health Insurance Portability and Accountability Act of 1996 (HIPAA).

MED TIP

Remember that no patient information can be given over the telephone without that person's permission.

Privileged communication refers to confidential information that has been told to a physician (or attorney) by the patient. The physician–patient relationship is considered to be a protected relationship and, as such, keeps the holder of this information from being forced to disclose it on a witness stand.

The American Hospital Association developed a published statement called "A Patient's Bill of Rights," which describes the physician–patient relationship (see Table 5.3 ■). All healthcare professionals must follow these guidelines when working with patients.

Patient Self-Determination Acts (Advance Directives)

Several documents executed by the patient, called self-determination documents or advance directives, state the patient's intentions for healthcare-related decisions and in some cases name another person as **proxy** to make decisions for the patient. A proxy statement is the written authorization given by a person so that a second person can act for him or her.

An **advance directive** is a written statement in which people state the type and amount of care they wish to receive during a terminal illness and as death approaches. These documents include living wills, durable power of attorney, and organ donation. Self-determination documents provide protection for both the patient and the physician.

1. The patient has the right to considerate and respectful care.
2. The patient has the right to and is encouraged to obtain from the physicians and other direct caregivers relevant, current, understandable information concerning diagnosis, treatment, and prognosis.
3. The patient has the right to make decisions about the plan of care prior to and during the course of treatment and to refuse a recommended treatment or plan of care to the extent permitted by law and hospital policy and to be informed of the consequences of this action.
4. The patient has the right to have an advance directive (such as a living will, healthcare proxy, or durable power of attorney for healthcare) concerning treatment or designating a surrogate decision maker with the expectation that the hospital will honor the intent of that directive to the extent permitted by law and hospital policy.
5. The patient has the right to every consideration of privacy.
6. The patient has the right to expect that all communications and records pertaining to his/her care will be treated as confidential by the hospital, except in cases such as suspected abuse and public health hazards when reporting is permitted or required by law.
7. The patient has the right to review the records pertaining to his/her medical care and to have the information explained or interpreted as necessary, except when restricted by law.
8. The patient has the right to expect that, within its capacity and policies, a hospital will make reasonable response to the request of a patient for appropriate and medically indicated care and service.
9. The patient has the right to ask and be informed of the existence of business relationships among the hospital, educational institutions, other healthcare providers, or payers that may influence the patient's treatment or care.
10. The patient has the right to consent to or decline to participate in proposed research studies or human experimentation affecting care and treatment or requiring direct patient involvement, and to have those studies fully explained prior to consent.
11. The patient has the right to expect reasonable continuity of care when appropriate and to be informed by physicians and other caregivers of available and realistic patient care options when hospital care is no longer appropriate.
12. The patient has the right to be informed of hospital policies and practices that relate to patient care, treatment, and responsibilities.

TABLE 5.3

A Patient's Bill of Rights

Source: Reprinted with permission of the American Hospital Association, © 2008.

TABLE 5.4 Advance Directives	Type	Description
	Living will	Document that a person drafts before becoming incompetent or unable to make healthcare decisions.
	Durable power of attorney for healthcare	A legal document that empowers another person (proxy) to make healthcare decisions for an incompetent patient. It goes into effect after the person becomes incompetent and only pertains to healthcare decisions.
	Uniform Anatomical Gift Act	All states have some form of this law. It allows persons 18 years or older and of sound mind to make a gift of any part of their body for purposes of medical research or transplantation.
	Do not resuscitate (DNR) order	This is an order placed into a person's medical chart or medical record. It indicates that the person does not wish to be resuscitated if breathing stops.

The patients obtain assurance that their healthcare wishes will be followed at the point in time when they are unable to express their intent, and physicians have an assurance that they are acting within the guidelines for care set by their patients. Table 5.4 ■ contains a brief summary of advance directives.

Living Will

A **living will** allows patients to set forth their intentions in advance as to their treatment and care. This document contains the patient's desires in the case of a catastrophic situation in which he or she may be incompetent to voice wishes concerning medical treatment. A patient may request that life-sustaining treatments and artificial nutritional support, such as tube feedings, either be used or not be used to prolong life. The patient may also request that no extraordinary medical treatment, such as being placed on a respirator (ventilator), be given. In this case, the physician puts a **Do not resuscitate (DNR)** order in the patient's medical chart in either the hospital or nursing home. This means that cardiopulmonary resuscitation (CPR) cannot be used if the person's heart and breathing stop. This living will document gives patients the legal right to direct the type of care they wish to receive when death is imminent.

Some state statutes will specifically state what conditions need to be present in order for a living will to go into effect. For example, Ohio follows the Modified Rights of the Terminally Ill Act, which states that the person must be terminally ill and/or in a state of permanent unconsciousness. The patient must be in a state that is irreversible, untreatable, and incurable with the prospect of imminent death. This type of regulation protects patients from having their living will implemented when they are briefly unconscious following surgery or a mild stroke.

Ideally, this process is discussed in the physician's office with patients when they are capable of making the decision. Other family members or significant others can also be part of the discussion and decision process. The living will document must be signed by the patient and witnessed by another person. One copy should be kept in the patient's record. Many patients ask their attorneys to also retain a copy. See Figure 5.4 ■ for a sample of a living will document.

Durable Power of Attorney

The **durable power of attorney,** when signed by the patient, allows an **agent** (also called a proxy) or representative designated by the patient to act on behalf of the patient. If the durable power of attorney is for healthcare only, then the agent may only make healthcare-related decisions on behalf of the patient.

Declaration:

This declaration is made this _____ day of _____ (month, year)

I, _____being of sound mind, willfully and voluntarily make known my desires that my moment of death [shall not be artificially] postponed.

If at any time I should have an incurable and irreversible injury, disease, or illness judged to be a terminal condition by my attending physician who has personally examined me and has determined that my death is imminent except for death-delaying procedures, I direct that such procedures that would only prolong the dying process be withheld or withdrawn, and that I be permitted to die naturally with only the administration of medication, sustenance, or the performance of any medical procedure deemed necessary by my attending physician to provide me with comfort care.

In the absence of my ability to give directions regarding the use of such death-delaying procedures, it is my intention that this declaration shall be honored by my family and physician as the final expression of my legal rights to refuse medical or surgical treatment and accept the consequences from such refusal.

Signed _____

Date:_____

City, County and State of Residence _____

The declarant is known to me personally and I believe him or her to be of sound mind. I saw the declarant sign the declaration in my presence, or the declarant acknowledged in my presence that he or she had signed the declaration, and I signed the declaration as a witness in the presence of the declarant. I did not sign the declarant's signature above for or at the direction of the declarant. At the date of this instrument, I am not entitled to any portion of the estate of the declarant according to the laws of intestate succession or to the best of my knowledge and belief, under any will of declarant or other instrument taking effect at declarant's death or directly financially responsible for declarant's medical care.

Witness _____ Date: _____

Witness _____ Date: _____

FIGURE 5.4
Sample Living Will

Power of Attorney made this _____ day of _____, _____

                                                           (month)   (year)

1. I, _____

   (insert name and address of principal)

   hereby appoint _____

   (insert name and address of agent)

   as my attorney-in-fact (my "agent") to act for me and in my name (in any way I could act in person) to make any and all decisions for me concerning my personal care, medical treatment, hospitalization, and healthcare and to require, withhold, or withdraw any type of medical treatment or procedure, even though my death may ensue. My agent shall have the same access to my medical records that I have, including the right to disclose the contents to others. My agent shall also have full power to make a disposition of any part or all of my body for medical purposes, authorize an autopsy, and direct the disposition of my remains.

2. The powers granted above shall not include the following powers or shall be subject to the following rules or limitations (here you may include any specific limitations you deem appropriate, such as your own definition of when life-sustaining measures should be withheld; a direction to continue food and fluids or life-sustaining treatment in all events; or instructions to refuse any specific types of treatments that are inconsistent with your religious beliefs or unacceptable to you for any other reasons, such as blood transfusion, electroconvulsive therapy, amputation, psychosurgery, voluntary admission to a mental institution, etc.).

   _____

   _____

   _____

   (The subject of life-sustaining treatment is of particular importance. For your convenience in dealing with that subject, some general statements concerning the withholding of life-sustaining treatment are set forth below. If you agree with one of these statements, you may initial that statement, but do not initial more than one):

   _____
   (initialed)   I do not want my life to be prolonged nor do I want life-sustaining treatment to be provided or continued if my agent believes the burdens of the treatment outweigh the expected benefits. I want my agent to consider the relief of suffering, the expense involved, and the quality as well as the possible extension of my life in making decisions concerning life-sustaining treatment.

FIGURE 5.5
Sample Durable Power of Attorney

_____ I want my life to be prolonged, and I want life-sustaining treatment to be
(initialed) provided or continued unless I am in a coma that my attending physician
believes to be irreversible, in accordance with reasonable medical
standards at the time of reference. If and when I have suffered irreversible
coma, I want life-sustaining treatment to be withheld or discontinued.

_____ I want my life to be prolonged to the greatest extent possible without regard
(initialed) to my condition, the chances I have for recovery, or the cost of the
procedures.

3. This power of attorney shall become effective on _____

(insert a future date or event in your lifetime, such as a court determination of your disability, when you want this power to first take effect)

4. This power of attorney shall terminate on _____

(insert a future date or event, such as a court determination of your disability, when you
want this power to terminate prior to your death)

5. If any agent named by me shall die, become incompetent, resign, refuse to accept the
office of agent, or be unavailable, I name the following (each to act alone and succes-
sively, in the order named) as successors to such agent:

_____

_____

_____

6. I am fully informed as to all the contents of this form and understand the full import of this
grant of powers to my agent,

Signed _____

(principal)

The principal has had an opportunity to read the above form and has signed the form or
acknowledged his or her signature or mark on the form in my presence.

_____ Residing at: _____

(witness)

FIGURE 5.5
Sample Durable Power of Attorney *(continued)*

Because the power of attorney is "durable," the agent's authority continues even if the patient is physically or mentally incapacitated. This document is in effect until canceled by the patient. A copy of the durable power of attorney should also be kept with the patient record. Both a living will and durable power of attorney for healthcare are recommended for all people. See Figure 5.5 ■ for a sample of a durable power of attorney for healthcare document.

Uniform Anatomical Gift Act

The **Uniform Anatomical Gift Act** allows persons 18 years or older and of sound mind to make a gift of any or all body parts for purposes of organ transplantation or medical research. The statute includes two specific safeguards. First, a physician who is not involved in the transplant must determine the time of death. Second, no money is allowed to change hands for organ transplantation.

The donor carries a card that has been signed in the presence of two witnesses. In some states, the back of the driver's license has space to indicate the desire to be an organ donor, with space for a signature.

If a person has not indicated a desire to be a donor, the family may consent on the patient's behalf. Generally, if a member of the family opposes the donation of organs, then the physician and hospital do not insist on it, even if the patient signed for the donation to take place. See Figure 11.3 for a sample donor card.

Questions that are frequently asked about advance directives include the following:

1. To whom should the advance directives be given? Copies of the advance directives should be given to the personal physician, close relatives, and a close friend. In addition, a copy should be placed in the medical chart if the patient is hospitalized or in a nursing home.

2. Where should advance directives be stored? They should be kept with the patient's personal papers in the home or nursing home setting. It is not recommended that they be stored in a safety deposit box, as they will not be accessible in an emergency.

3. How can the advance directive be changed or amended? Any revisions can be made by drawing through the outdated statement in the original document. After a revision is made, it should be dated and signed. An amended copy should be given to the personal physician, family member, and friend.

4. Can the advance directive be revoked? People can revoke their documents by destroying them and asking anyone holding a copy to do the same. Ideally, the request to destroy the advance directive should be sent in writing to all those who hold a copy.

5. What does the law say about advance directives? A federal law, the Patient Self-Determination Act (PSDA) was passed in 1991. Congress has strongly supported a person's right to self-determination before becoming incompetent. However, a patient's request for assisted suicide will not be honored in any states except Oregon and Washington.

MED TIP

It is recommended that all persons place in writing their wishes about what type of treatment they should receive if they become incompetent. The advance directive should be specific about treatments such as CPR, tube feedings, and the use of ventilators.

Classification	Definition	
Minor	A person under the age of 18 (termed *infant* under the law). The signature of a parent or legal guardian is needed for consent to perform a medical treatment in nonemergency situations.	
Mature minor	A person judged to be mature enough to understand the physician's instructions. Such a minor may seek medical care for treatment of drug or alcohol abuse, contraception, venereal disease, and pregnancy.	
Emancipated minor	A person between the ages of 15 and 18 who is either married, in the military, or self-supporting and no longer lives under the care of a parent. Parental consent for medical care is not required. Proof of emancipation (for example, marriage certificate) should be included in the medical record.	

TABLE 5.5

Classification of Minors' Competencies

RIGHTS OF MINORS

A **minor** is a person who has not reached the age of maturity, which in most states is 18. In most states, minors are unable to give consent for treatment, except in special cases involving pregnancy, request for birth control information, abortion, testing and treatment for sexually transmitted diseases, problems with substance abuse, and a need for psychiatric care. The courts have held that the consent of a minor to medical or surgical treatment is not sufficient. The physician must secure the consent of the parents or someone standing in for the parents (*in loco parentis*) or run the risk of liability.

In some cases the state must take over the care for minors who cannot care for themselves. The principle of *parens patriae* **authority** occurs when the state takes responsibility from the parents for the care and custody of minors under the age of 18. This principle may also occur when persons are mentally incompetent to take care of themselves. If the child is removed from his or her parents, then two rights must be protected through due process: the rights of the child and the rights of the parents. It is not a simple matter for the state to remove a child from the custody of the parents. The state must prove that the parents are neglecting the child or are not capable of caring for the child. Then a hearing must take place in juvenile court.

Mature minors and emancipated minors are considered competent and can provide consent for other types of treatment as well. The varying degrees of minors' competency are described in Table 5.5 ■.

PATIENTS' RESPONSIBILITIES

In addition to the patients' rights, they also have certain obligations. Patients are expected to follow their physician's instructions. They must make follow-up appointments to monitor their treatment and medication use if requested by their physician. Patients must be absolutely honest with the physician about such issues as past medical history; family medical history; and tobacco, drug, and alcohol use. Finally, patients and parents of minor children are expected to pay the physician for medical services (Figure 5.6 ■).

Consent

Consent is the voluntary agreement that a patient gives to allow a medically trained person the permission to touch, examine, and perform a treatment. The two types of consent, informed consent and implied consent, are discussed in the following section.

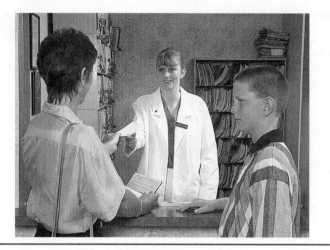

FIGURE 5.6
**A Parent or Guardian is
Responsible for a Minor's
Medical Bills**

The Doctrine of Informed Consent

Informed (or expressed) consent means that the patient agrees to the proposed course of treatment after having been told about the possible consequences of having or not having certain procedures and treatments (Figure 5.7 ■). The patient's signature on the consent form indicates that the patient understands the limits or risks involved in the pending treatment or surgery as explained by the physician. The goal of informed consent is to protect patients' rights to decide for themselves about their own healthcare treatment. In addition, informed consent is meant to disclose information to the patient so that he or she can make a reasoned decision.

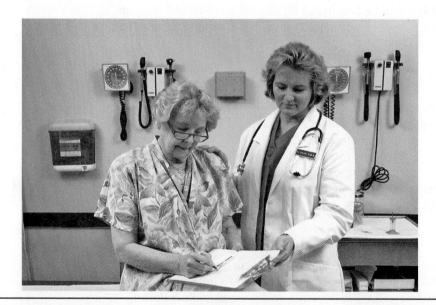

FIGURE 5.7
**Patient Signs
a Consent Form**

The physician, who is solely responsible for providing information to the patient, must carefully explain that in some cases the treatment may even make the patient's condition worse. The Doctrine of Informed Consent requires the physician to explain the following in understandable language:

▶ The patient's diagnosis, if known

▶ The nature and purpose of the proposed treatment or procedure

▶ The advantages and risks of treatment

▶ The alternative treatments available to the patient, regardless of their cost and whether they will likely be covered by the patient's insurance

▶ Potential outcomes of the treatment

▶ What might occur, both risks and benefits, if treatment is refused

In addition, the physician must be honest with the patient and explain the diagnosis, the purpose of the proposed treatment, and the probability that the treatment will be successful. The purpose of this explanation is that the patient can then make a knowledgeable decision about whether to go ahead with the treatment or procedure. In an emergency situation in which the patient cannot understand the explanation or sign a consent form, the physician providing the care is protected by law.

According to recent studies, a few physicians have withheld options for treatment from their patients. A University of Chicago research study found that 29 percent of the 1,144 surveyed physicians would have problems referring a patient to another doctor for some legal procedures. In some cases, such as for contraceptives or end-of-life issues such as withholding chemotherapy, they had ethical problems making the referral. The advice to patients is to be aware that they may not get all the information about treatments they are legally due.

In a case in Alaska, the court determined that the physician did not fulfill his duty to disclose the risks of breast reduction surgery when he failed to warn the patient about the risk of scarring. In answer to the patient's questions, the physician said that she shouldn't worry and she would be happy with the results. The patient wasn't happy, and she sued the physician and won (*Korman v. Mallin,* 858 P.2d 1145, Alaska 1993).

Is it difficult to know if or when the patient is fully informed? There are two standards to use to determine if the patient understands what he or she is being told. The first standard is based upon what the physician tells the patient. Many courts will use a "reasonable physician standard," meaning that the physician must tell the patient what a "reasonable physician in the same specialty" would tell him or her under the same circumstances. This allows for a type of mass-produced consent form for many treatments and surgical procedures. However, in addition to having a patient sign this mass-produced consent form, the physician must also explain the procedure, risks, and alternatives. The second standard is "the reasonable patient standard," which means that the patient must receive the information that other patients receive but, in addition, must be provided the opportunity to communicate questions to the physician. Healthcare professionals such as nurses and medical assistants should not replace the physician in obtaining a signed informed consent form. However, they are in an ideal situation in either the office or hospital to alert the physician when they believe that the patient is confused about the procedure.

MED TIP

In many cases, patients will be more comfortable discussing their fears with a trusted caregiver rather than with their physician. These patient fears must then be conveyed to the physician, and documented on the patient chart, even if a consent form has been signed.

It is very difficult to fully inform a patient about all the things that can go wrong with a treatment. However, the physician must make a reasonable attempt to do so in order for the patient to make an informed decision about treatment.

The Canterbury decision is a classic example of two crucial components of informed consent: patients *granting consent* because they have the right to control what is done to their bodies and insisting on *information* so they can make an intelligent decision. For patients to be able to consent in an intelligent manner, they must be given information by the physician that a "reasonable person" in the patient's situation would wish to receive. As such, the amount of information is not based on what the physician believes is relevant, but on what the patient believes he or she needs to hear. The "reasonable person standard" was used in a 1959 case, *Canterbury v. Spence.* Nineteen-year-old Jerry Canterbury, who suffered from back pain, underwent a surgical procedure to treat a suspected ruptured vertebral disk. On the day following surgery, he fell off the hospital bed while he was trying to urinate and subsequently became paralyzed from the waist down. Emergency surgery reversed some of his paralysis, but he continued to have urological problems. Canterbury sued both the physician (Spence) and the hospital, claiming that he was not fully warned about the risk of falling out of bed and of paralysis. The physician based his defense on a therapeutic privilege claim that he did not think the disclosure of the risk of falling out of bed was necessary. The judge in the district court ordered a directed verdict and told the jury that they must find in favor of the hospital and physician. Upon appeal, a higher court sent the case back to the lower court so that a jury could hear the evidence and make a decision. The court was not clear on whether the fall or the surgery had caused the patient's paralysis. The court also declared that a physician cannot use the therapeutic privilege to justify withholding information the patient requires to make an informed decision. In an unusual decision, the jury also found in favor of the hospital and physician (*Canterbury v. Spence,* 464 F.2d 772, D.C. 1972).

MED TIP

Except in emergency situations, the process of obtaining consent cannot be delegated by the physician to someone else. If the emergency involves risk to the patient's life or the patient is unable to communicate, consent may be implied under the rationale that the patient would have consented to emergency treatment.

Except in cases of emergency, all patients must sign a consent form before undergoing a surgical procedure. This signed form indicates that the patient has been instructed concerning the risks associated with the procedure. If, after the physician has carefully explained the treatment, the patient acknowledges understanding the explanation and risks and signs the consent form, then, generally, there is some protection from lawsuits. However, patients have sued and won cases in which they were presented the risks of a procedure and signed the form, and then the treatment failed.

A patient's informed consent is limited to those procedures to which the patient has consented. For example, in the case of *Mohr v. Williams,* a woman consented to have an operation on her diseased right ear. After she was unconscious under the anesthetic, the ear surgeon determined that the right ear was not diseased enough to warrant an operation, but the left ear was seriously diseased. He proceeded to operate on the left ear without reviving her to seek permission. The operation was skillfully performed and successful. However, the plaintiff sued for battery and won. The physician appealed that verdict, but the appellate court determined that because the surgery was unauthorized, even though successful, it constituted an assault (*Mohr v. Williams,* 104 N.W.12, Minn. 1905). In another early case, a physician was sued when he received consent to repair a woman's hernia but also removed both ovaries (Zoterell v. *Repp* 153 N.W. 692, Mich. 1915).

Procedures in which an informed consent form should be signed include the following:

- Minor invasive surgery
- Organ donation
- Radiological therapy, such as radiation treatment for cancer
- Electroconvulsive therapy
- Experimental procedures
- Chemotherapy
- Any procedure with more than a slight risk of harm to the patient

In some circumstances—such as HIV testing, procedures involving reproduction, and major surgical procedures—state laws require that the patient sign an informed consent form. This signed document represents a legal statement in which the patient certifies that the risks, benefits, and alternatives to treatment have been thoroughly explained. The document is an indication that the informed patient enters the treatment of their own free will and not by means of coercion.

MED TIP

Remember that the patient grants informed consent to the physician. Simply explaining a procedure to the patient does not constitute informed consent. The patient must understand the explanation and agree to the procedure.

Certain categories of patients are judged to be incapable of giving an informed consent. These include minors (other than emancipated minors), the mentally incompetent, persons who do not understand English or the language of the physician transmitting the information and had no interpreter present, and emergency patients who are unconscious.

Implied Consent

A physician should obtain written consent before treatment whenever possible. However, the law may assume or "imply" a patient's consent. Implied consent can be difficult to interpret because it is based on another person's interpretation. **Implied consent** occurs when patients indicate by their behavior that they are accepting of the procedure. The patient's nonverbal communication may indicate an implied consent for treatment or examination. Because consent means to give permission or approval for something, when a patient is seen for a routine examination, there is implied consent that the physician will touch the person during the examination. Therefore, the touching required for the physical examination would not be considered the crime of battery.

In a famous precedent-setting case involving implied consent, the court declared that a woman had given consent for a vaccination when she extended her arm (*O'Brien v. Cunard S.S. Co.,* 28 N.E. 266, Mass. 1891). Implied consent is also assumed in medical emergencies when the patient cannot respond to give consent. In this case, the law assumes that if the patient were able, consent would be given for the emergency procedure. In an Iowa case, the court determined that implied consent existed when a surgeon removed the mangled limb of a patient run over by a train because the procedure was necessary to save the patient's life (*Jackovach v. A. L. Yocum, Jr.*, 237 N.W. 444, Iowa, 1931).

MED TIP

Both expressed and implied consent should be an informed consent. This means that patients must know, or be informed, about what they are providing consent for.

Exceptions to Consent

There are exceptions to the informed consent doctrine that are unique to each state. Some of the more general exceptions follow:

1. A physician need not inform a patient about risks that are commonly known. For example, physicians need not tell patients that they could choke swallowing a pill.

2. A physician who believes the disclosure of risks may be detrimental to the patient is not required to disclose them. For instance, if a patient has a severe heart condition that may be worsened by an announcement of risks, the physician should not disclose the risks.

3. If the patient asks the physician not to disclose the risks, then the physician is not required to do so.

4. A physician is not required to restore patients to their original state of health, and in some cases, may be unable to do so.

5. A physician may not be able to elicit a cure for every patient.

6. A physician cannot guarantee the successful results of every treatment.

Refusal to Grant Consent

Adult patients who are conscious and considered to be mentally capable have a right to refuse any medical or surgical treatment. The refusal must be honored no matter what the patient's reasoning: concern about the success of the procedure, lack of confidence in the physician, religious beliefs, or even mere whim. Failure to respect the right of refusal could result in liability for assault and battery. In *Erickson v. Dilgard,* the hospital requested the court to authorize a blood transfusion over the patient's objection. The court held in favor of the patient who refused a blood transfusion, even though the refusal could have resulted in the patient's death (*Erickson v. Dilgard,* 252 2d 705, N.Y.S. 1962). The hospital and medical personnel have a responsibility to use reasonable care to protect the patient from touching (assault and battery) when consent has not been granted.

ROLE OF THE HEALTHCARE CONSUMER

Today's healthcare consumer is better informed about medicine and treatments than ever before due to an abundance of literature, television programming, and information available on the World Wide Web. However, wise consumers will not self-medicate or offer their medications to family members and friends for their use. Healthcare personnel must carefully question all patients/consumers about over-the-counter (OTC) medications they may be taking. Many OTC medications, such as aspirin, can have a negative interaction with prescribed medications. Dietary supplements such as herbs and vitamins should also be declared by the patient. The consumer must alert the medical staff to any allergies and adverse reactions to medications.

Healthcare consumers must be honest with their physicians about prescriptions they may be taking that were prescribed by other doctors. Every patient/consumer should carry a small card listing all medication names and dosages in the event the names are needed for a patient history or in an emergency situation. They should ask questions about their medications and the treatments they are receiving. If they do not understand what they are told, then they should be persistent with the physician or healthcare professional until they do understand the instructions.

The patient/consumer can assist the physician in prevention of medical errors. Before undergoing any surgical treatment, it is important that the patients, their personal physicians, and their surgeons all are clear on what will be done. Many fail-safe approaches have been instituted by medical professionals to prevent errors. For instance, performing surgery at the wrong site, such as the right knee instead of the left knee, is rare. But to prevent this type of injury to the patient, the American Academy of Orthopedic Surgery urges all its members to sign their initials directly on the site to be operated upon before the surgery.

MED TIP

It is important to remember that many patients do not understand medical terminology. They are often ashamed to admit that they either do not understand or cannot hear the instructions. It is the healthcare professional's duty to make sure that the patient is fully informed.

POINTS TO PONDER

1. Does it surprise you to find out that physicians have the right to select the patients they wish to treat?

2. Can a physician receive a payment from a hospital for referring patients to that particular institution? Why or why not?

3. If a deceased relative signed a statement (Uniform Anatomical Gift Act) requesting that any or all body parts be used for organ transplantation or medical research, can a family member overturn that statement?

4. Do you believe that it is appropriate for a physician to report the unethical conduct of a fellow physician?

5. Do you think that physicians should treat their own family members? Why or why not?

6. Can a nurse obtain consent from a patient for a surgical procedure if the physician is extremely busy handling an emergency case?

7. What can you say to your patient's employer who calls to find out if the employee's medical condition has improved?

DISCUSSION QUESTIONS

1. Explain what it means when one physician "covers" for another.

2. Describe the three advance directives that a patient can use. When are they appropriate?

3. Denny O'Malley is being treated by Dr. Williams after having fallen off a ladder at work. His employer calls to find out how Denny is doing. Can Dr. Williams discuss Denny's progress with his employer? Why or why not?

REVIEW CHALLENGE

Short Answer Questions

1. What might happen if a physician ignores a patient's refusal to grant consent?

   _____

   _____

2. A woman opens her mouth for the physician to examine her throat. Is this a form of consent? If so, what form of consent is this?

   _____

   _____

3. A 4-year-old child opens his mouth for the physician to examine his throat. In your opinion, has the child granted consent?

   _____

   _____

4. A physician makes the following statement to Sarah: "Your blood pressure is only slightly elevated. This blood pressure medication is guaranteed to reduce your blood pressure a few points." In your opinion, is this a safe comment to make? Explain your answer.

   _____

   _____

5. Why does a patient need to know the consequences of NOT having a procedure or treatment?

   _____

   _____

6. Why is a Durable Power of Attorney called "durable."

   _____

   _____

7. You are working in a nursing home as a nurse's aide. But your long-term goal is to become a nurse. You have become very skilled in performing CPR due to an excellent educational program. As you are about to move a patient to her bed, she stops breathing and has no pulse. You immediately begin CPR as you have been trained. A nurse in the room with you says that you must stop since the woman has a DNR order. You have been taught that once you begin CPR you must continue until you no longer can continue. What do you do?

   _____

   _____

8. You are in an internship in a physician's office in the final two weeks of a medical assisting program. Just as a patient is brought into the office he collapses in front of you, stops breathing, and has no pulse. You call for help because you are afraid that, even though you have been trained in CPR, you have never performed it on a patient. It would take several minutes for someone else to begin CPR. Please comment.

   _____

   _____

Matching

Match the responses in column B with the correct term in column A.

Column A

_____ 1. agent
_____ 2. minor
_____ 3. standard of care
_____ 4. implied consent
_____ 5. privileged communication
_____ 6. informed consent
_____ 7. exception to consent
_____ 8. right to be informed
_____ 9. durable power of attorney
_____ 10. abandonment

Column B

a. commonly known risks
b. consent granted by inference
c. document that allows an agent to represent a patient
d. same skill that is used by other physicians
e. representative acts on patient's behalf
f. withdrawing medical care without notice
g. person under 18 years of age
h. "A Patient's Bill of Rights"
i. knowledgeable consent
j. confidential information

Multiple Choice

Select the one best answer to the following statements.

1. A patient rolling up a sleeve to have a blood sample taken is an example of
   a. standard of care.
   b. informed consent.
   c. implied consent.
   d. advance directive.
   e. agent.

2. A condition in which a patient understands the risks involved by not having a surgical procedure or treatment performed is known as
   a. standard of care.
   b. informed consent.
   c. implied consent.
   d. advance directive.
   e. agent.

3. The Uniform Anatomical Gift Act is applicable for
   a. persons up to the age of 18.
   b. persons 18 years of age and older.
   c. persons who are mentally handicapped.
   d. very few people.
   e. the purpose of selling organs.

4. Which of these refers to a physician using the same skill that is used by other physicians in treating patients with the same ailment?
   a. privileged communication
   b. informed consent
   c. implied consent
   d. standard of care
   e. none of the above

5. The physician's rights include
   a. the right to decline to treat a new patient.
   b. the ability to receive payment from hospitals for referring patients.
   c. the right to protect fellow physicians who are guilty of a deception.
   d. the right to publish confidential information about a patient if it is in the physician's best interest.
   e. all of the above.

6. In what document are patients able to request the type and amount of artificial nutritional and life-sustaining treatments that should or should not be used to prolong their life?
   a. Uniform Anatomical Gift Act
   b. Medical Patients Rights Act
   c. living will
   d. standard of care
   e. euthanasia

7. The patient's obligations include
   a. honesty about past medical history.
   b. payment for medical services.
   c. following treatment recommendations.
   d. a and c only.
   e. a, b, and c.

8. Exceptions to informed consent include
   a. telling the patient about the risk involved in not having the procedure.
   b. the discussion of sensitive sexual matters.
   c. not having to explain risks that are commonly known.
   d. all of the above.
   e. none of the above.

9. The doctrine of informed consent
   a. can be delegated by the physician to a trusted assistant.
   b. may have to be waived in the event of an emergency situation.
   c. does not have to be signed by every patient.
   d. could result in a lawsuit for assault and battery if not performed.
   e. b and d only.

10. A newspaper reporter seeks information from a receptionist about a prominent personality who has been hospitalized. What information can be given to the reporter?
    a. none
    b. the basic fact that the person is a patient
    c. the name and phone number of the attending physician
    d. a very brief statement about the person's medical condition
    e. there are no restrictions

DISCUSSION CASES

1. *Dr. Williams has just telephoned Carl, her office nurse, explaining that she is behind schedule doing rounds at one of the hospitals. She has asked Carl to do her a favor and interpret Mrs. Harris's EKG, sign her name, and fax the report to Mrs. Harris's internist, who is expecting the results. Carl learned to take and read EKGs while he was in nursing school. Dr. Williams' EKG machine includes new technology that interprets EKGs. Carl will not have any difficulty carrying out Dr. Williams' request.*

   a. Given the scope of Carl's education and training, would this "favor" fall within his scope of practice?

   _____

   _____

   b. Would any portion of Dr. Williams' request fall within the scope of practice for Carl?

   _____

   _____

   c. Does Dr. Williams' request violate the physician–patient relationship? Why or why not?

   _____

   _____

   d. What, if anything, should Carl say to Dr. Williams?

   _____

   _____

2. *Terry O'Rourke, a 25-year-old patient of Dr. Williams, refuses to take her medication to control diabetes and is not following her dietary plan to control her disease. After repeated attempts to help this patient, Dr. Williams has decided that she can no longer provide care for Terry. The office staff has been advised not to schedule Terry for any more appointments.*

   a. Is there an ethical and/or legal concern regarding this situation?

   _____

   _____

   b. Is there anything else that either Dr. Williams or her staff should do to sever the patient relationship with Terry?

   _____

   _____

   c. Is this a breach of contract on the part of Dr. Williams? Explain your answer.

   _____

   _____

3. *Dr. Williams has been treating a popular performer who has just committed suicide.*

   a. What statement can Dr. Williams or her staff give to reporters when they call Dr. Williams' office?

   _____

   _____

   b. What can Dr. Williams or her staff say to the mother of the deceased patient when she calls for information?

   _____

   _____

PUT IT INTO PRACTICE

Interview someone you know who has recently been a patient. Ask that person to tell you what he or she believes are the patient's responsibilities. Do these statements agree with those in the textbook? How do they differ?

WEB HUNT

Search the website of the U.S. Department of Health and Human Services (www.hhs.gov) and examine "The Patient's Bill of Rights in Medicare and Medicaid." What does the document have to say about the confidentiality of health information?

CRITICAL THINKING EXERCISE

What should you do if you know that your employer owns an MRI facility along with two other persons and your patients are being referred to this facility?

BIBLIOGRAPHY

American Hospital Association. 2008. *A patient's bill of rights.* Chicago: American Hospital Association.

American Hospital Association. 2008. *Patient care partnership.* Chicago: American Hospital Association.

American Medical Association. 2008–2009. *Code of medical ethics: Current opinions on ethical and judicial affairs.* Chicago: American Medical Association.

Beaman, N., and L. Fleming-McPhillips. 2007. *Comprehensive medical assisting.* Upper Saddle River, NJ: Pearson/Prentice Hall.

Black, H. 2009. *Black's law dictionary* 8th ed. St. Paul, MN: West Publishing.

CDC National AIDS Clearinghouse. 2002. Rockville, MD: CDC National AIDS Clearinghouse.

Fletcher, J. 1954. *Morals and medicine.* Boston: Beacon Press.

Flynn, E. 2000. *Issues in health care ethics.* Upper Saddle River, NJ: Prentice Hall.

Hackett, T. 1976. "Psychological assistance for the dying patient and his family." *Annual Review of Medicine.* 27; 372–3.

Hall, M., and M. Bobinski. 2003. *Health care law and ethics in a nutshell.* St. Paul, MN: West Publishing.

Levine, C. 2004. *Taking sides.* New York: McGraw Hill.

Lo, B., and R. Steinbrook. 1992. Health care workers infected with the human immunodeficiency virus: The next steps. *JAMA*, 267: 1000–1005.

Manier, J. 2007. "Many doctors withhold options from patients, study says." *Chicago Tribune*, (Feb. 8), 7.

Mappes, T., and D. DeGrazia. 2001. *Biomedical ethics.* New York: McGraw Hill.

Munson, R. 2007. *Interventon and reflection: Basic issues in medical ethics.* New York: Wadsworth.

Oken, D. 1961. "What to tell cancer patients: A study of medical attitudes." *JAMA* 175 (April 1): 1120–1128.

Study: Hospital lapses killing 32,000 yearly. 2003. *Chicago Tribune,* sec. 1 (October 8) 16.

Veatch, R. 2002. *The basics of bioethics.* Upper Saddle River, NJ: Prentice Hall.

Professional Liability and Medical Malpractice

6

Learning Objectives

1. Define the glossary terms.
2. Define the four Ds of negligence for the physician.
3. Discuss the meaning of *respondeat superior* for the physician and the employee.
4. Discuss the meaning of *res ipsa loquitur.*
5. Explain the term *liability* and what it means for the physician and other health-care professionals.
6. List ten ways to prevent malpractice.
7. State two advantages of arbitration.
8. Discuss three types of damage awards.
9. Describe two types of malpractice insurance.
10. Explain the law of agency.

Key Terms

Affirmative defense
Alternative dispute resolution (ADR)
Arbitration
Arbitrator
Assumption of risk
Borrowed servant doctrine
Cap
Claims-made insurance
Comparative negligence
Compensatory damages
Contributory negligence

Damages
Defensive medicine
Dereliction
Direct cause
Duty
Feasance
Federal Rules of Evidence
Fraud
Law of agency
Liable
Malfeasance
Malpractice

Mediation
Misfeasance
Negligence
Nominal damages
Nonfeasance
Occurrence insurance
Proximate
Punitive damages
Res ipsa loquitur
Res judicata
Rider
Settlement

THE CASE OF JOHN F. AND THE HMO

John, a 34-year-old father of two children, is a member of an HMO in Texas. John has made several trips to an area clinic recommended by his HMO to seek medical attention since finding blood in his bowel movements. He has been taking large amounts of aspirin for persistent headaches but did not realize that this could cause internal bleeding. John was always seen at the clinic by a physician assistant, Robert M., but never by a physician. Robert didn't ask John about taking any nonprescription medications. John didn't realize that he should mention his over-the-counter medication (aspirin) consumption. Robert tells John to take an antacid preparation to control the bleeding, but does not order any tests. He tells John to return if he is not any better. Two days later, John is rushed to the area emergency room with a bowel hemorrhage.

1. What responsibility, if any, does Robert have for John's emergency condition?

2. Does the clinic have a responsibility to provide its HMO members with the services of a physician?

3. What responsibility, as a healthcare consumer, does John have for his own medical condition?

ven when procedures or treatments are conducted with the best intentions and skill, they don't always turn out as expected. Unfortunately, we are living in a litigious society, and when medical accidents happen, the patients and their family may look for someone to blame. Healthcare professionals need to be on constant alert for practices that could result in injury to the patient. Not only is the injury a painful process, it can also be a life-threatening one. All healthcare professionals must realize that they are responsible for their actions. The physician/employer also assumes responsibility for the employees through the doctrine of *respondeat superior.* While people have always been liable for their own conduct, the courts are now finding that everyone associated with negligent actions is liable for damages (monetary award to the plaintiff).

The topics of negligence and malpractice are briefly discussed in Chapter 2. This chapter concentrates on professional liability and how to prevent malpractice from happening. Included in this chapter are numerous examples of court cases to illustrate the wide variety of lawsuits and negligence cases that name physicians and hospitals as defendants. While most of the cases reflect legal actions against physicians, all people working in the medical profession can be sued. Examples are also provided of other healthcare professionals who have been named in lawsuits such as nurses, medical assistants, dental assistants, laboratory technicians, nursing assistants, paramedics, pharmacists, physical therapists, physician assistants, and respiratory therapists (Figure 6.1 ■).

MED TIP

All healthcare workers are responsible for their actions even though the doctrine of *respondeat superior* states that an employer is also liable for injury to a patient.

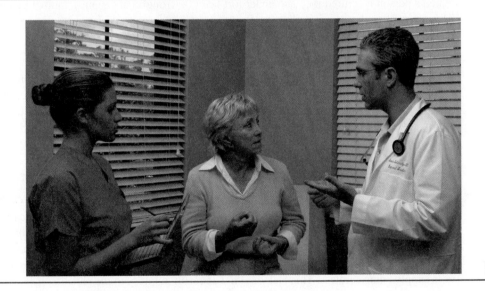

FIGURE 6.1
Members of Healthcare Team Explain Medical Information to a Patient

PROFESSIONAL NEGLIGENCE AND MEDICAL MALPRACTICE

Professional misconduct or demonstration of an unreasonable lack of skill with the result of injury, loss, or damage to the patient is considered **malpractice.** Malpractice acts consist of professional misconduct, improper discharge of professional duties, and failure to meet professional standards of care that result in harm to another person. A physician is held to a different but not higher standard of care than a nurse, medical assistant, physician assistant, or phlebotomist. In the United States, physicians and most licensed professionals such as nurses and physician assistants are held to a national standard of care. This standard is set by observing what a competent peer in another location would do in a similar circumstance. It's important to note that this high level of practice and "standard of care" is actually the minimum that is considered acceptable. Some malpractice is relatively clear and easy to determine, such as when a surgical instrument left in a patient during an operation shows up on x-ray. However, many cases are not as clear. There are cases in which the physician or other healthcare professional has performed a procedure that would normally be beneficial but does not have the expected outcome. Because each patient is unique, each may react differently to a medical treatment. If there is a negative result, the patient and family are naturally upset. But is this negligence? A court of law is often asked to determine the answer.

Negligence, which is often an unintentional action, occurs when a person either performs or fails to perform an action that a reasonable professional person would or would not have performed in a similar situation.

MED TIP

When a person is injured they sue under tort law ("a wrongful act against another person"). The unintentional tort of negligence is the most often cause of lawsuits for healthcare professionals.

Charges of negligence against a physician or other healthcare professional arise because the patient or family is not happy with the outcome of the treatment or procedure. A jury in a negligence trial would have to determine if a reasonable professional person would have done the same action. Malpractice is the wrongdoing or negligence committed by a professional person, such as a medical professional.

MED TIP

Healthcare professionals are expected to use "reasonable skill" when providing care and treatment to patients. This means that not everyone will perform an action in exactly the same way, as each person's skill level will vary by small amounts. However, an "unreasonable lack of skill" is unacceptable, since it demonstrates that a person does not have the required skills or is simply being careless. This lack of skill can result in injury to the patient.

For most people, the tort (civil wrong) of negligence and malpractice is often considered to be the same thing. Every mistake or error, however, is not malpractice. Therefore, when a treatment or diagnosis does not turn out well, the physician is not necessarily negligent. Rather, physicians must act within the standard of care appropriate for their profession, with attention to their special field or their particular level of medicine.

All healthcare providers are held to this same standard in their field of practice. Physicians and healthcare workers who fail to act reasonably in the same circumstances are negligent.

Medical malpractice often involves more than just a poor outcome for the patient. It may reflect an inexcusable lapse in judgment by a medical professional that results in serious injury and even death for the patient. In fact, there is consistent evidence that nearly 90,000 Americans die each year, not from their medical condition, but from preventable medical errors. Medication errors are one of the leading types of medical errors. Medical malpractice claims may arise when a physician acts in an unacceptable manner when compared to how other physicians with similar training would act. However, an unsuccessful or unanticipated result from a surgical procedure or medical treatment does not, in itself, mean that malpractice has been committed.

MED TIP

The medical model that said, "If we train people enough, they won't make a mistake. But if they do make a mistake, we will punish them." doesn't seem to work anymore. The best solution to avoid errors is to always double-check all orders and healthcare decisions that physicians and other healthcare professionals make. Technology is also helping to ease the problem by using electronic prescriptions in place of handwritten ones; this has eliminated many medication errors. And, most important, never perform a procedure for which you are not trained.

THE TORT OF NEGLIGENCE

Both actions and inactions (omissions) can be considered negligence. Failure to provide clear instructions regarding treatment or a medication's use is an omission that could result in a disastrous outcome for the patient. Providing incorrect information is also considered negligence.

MED TIP

Remember that you can be sued even if you are right. Patients can be injured through no fault of the medical personnel.

Professional liability malpractice claims are classified in three ways: malfeasance, misfeasance, and nonfeasance. These terms all stem from the word **feasance,** which means doing an act or performing a duty.

Malfeasance refers to performing a wrong and illegal act. For example, it is malfeasance for a nurse or medical assistant to prescribe a medical treatment or medication. Only the physician can prescribe medications and treatments. Medical personnel must be especially aware of malfeasance when they offer advice such as, "Try giving your child aspirin to bring down the fever." The term malfeasance is often used when a public official has done something illegal.

Misfeasance is the improper performance of an otherwise proper or lawful act. An example of misfeasance occurs when a poor technique is used by a nurse, medical assistant, or phlebotomist to perform a venipuncture and the patient suffers nerve damage.

Nonfeasance is the failure to perform a necessary action. For instance, it would be nonfeasance if a medical assistant or nurse is trained in cardiopulmonary resuscitation (CPR) but does not administer this life-saving technique when a patient collapses in the physician's waiting room and requires CPR.

TABLE 6.1 **The Four D's of Negligence**	▶ Duty–takes place when there is an obligation established between the physician and the patient.
	▶ Dereliction of duty–the physician or healthcare provider failed to provide a correct standard of care to the patient and, therefore, has not met the duty.
	▶ Direct or proximate cause–the dereliction or breach of duty was the direct cause of the patient's injury.
	▶ Damages–injuries caused by the defendant for which compensation (financial or otherwise) is due.

The Four Ds of Negligence

In order to obtain a judgment for negligence against a physician (defendant), the patient (plaintiff) must be able to show all four of what are called the "four Ds"—duty, dereliction of duty, direct or proximate cause, and damages. See Table 6.1 ■ for the four D's of negligence.

Duty

Duty is the responsibility established by the physician–patient relationship. It is the obligation that one person has to another person—for instance, not to perform a medical procedure that is known to be harmful to a patient. The patient must prove that a relationship had been established. When the patient has made an appointment and has been seen by the physician, a relationship has been established. Further office visits and treatment also establish that the physician has a duty or obligation to the patient. There is also a duty to warn the patient of problems that could be associated with treatments or medications. A special type of duty arises, for example, when a patient tells a psychiatric counselor he or she intends to harm another person. In this situation, the psychiatric counselor has a duty to warn the other person.

MED TIP

The determination of duty in a court room is the responsibility of the judge, not the jury. For example, if the parents of a child who drowned sued an off-duty nurse who stood by and did nothing, the case would be dismissed by the judge because an off-duty nurse does not have a legal obligation (duty) to do anything, except in the state of Vermont.

The duty of "due care" uses the reasonable person standard, which means that everyone has a duty to act as a reasonable, prudent person of average intelligence would under the same or similar circumstances. Those in special professions, such as physicians, physician assistants, nurses, and medical assistants, are held to a standard of care exercised by similar professionals in the same or a similar community or geographic area. This standard never varies for a particular professional, so a physician is held to the same standard as another reasonable and prudent physician, a nurse is held to the same standards as other nurses, and so on.

There is a duty to care for a hospitalized patient once the patient enters the nursing floor. A phone call from admitting or the emergency room, stating "You are getting a new patient," usually precedes the patient's arrival. If all the beds are filled on the nursing unit, the nurse may state, "We don't have room for a new patient." But once the patient arrives on the nursing unit, there is an obligation, or legal duty, to care for that patient.

Dereliction or Neglect of Duty

Dereliction, or neglect, of duty is a physician's failure to act as any ordinary and prudent physician (a peer) would act in a similar circumstance. To prove dereliction or neglect of duty, a patient would have to prove that the physician's performance or treatment did not comply with the acceptable standard of care. For example, if a physician does not properly inform patients about all the risks associated with surgical procedures, then the physician has neglected, or breached, his or her duty to the patients. If the outcome of a procedure is one that the patient did not anticipate or was not informed about, then this may constitute grounds for a lawsuit claiming dereliction of duty.

Direct or Proximate Cause

Direct cause is the continuous sequence of events, unbroken by any intervening cause, that produces an injury and without which the injury would not have occurred. Direct or **proximate** cause means that the injury was proximately or closely related to the physician's (defendant's) negligence. It does not necessarily mean the closest event in time or space to the injury, and it may not be the event that set the injury in motion. Proximate cause means that there were no intervening forces between the defendant's action(s) and the plaintiff's (patient's) injury—hence a cause-and-effect relationship. Proximate cause of injury requires the patient to prove that the physician's or agent's (such as a nurse's) dereliction of duty was the direct cause for the injury that resulted.

An example of proximate cause would be if a medical assistant or laboratory technician, who works under the direct supervision of a doctor, performs a venipuncture on a patient to obtain a blood sample, and subsequently the patient complains of a loss of feeling in the arm that was used for the venipuncture. To prove proximate cause, the plaintiff (patient) would have to prove that there was no intervening cause, such as a tennis injury or damage from an accident, that occurred between the time the blood was drawn and the time the nerve damage happened.

MED TIP

Proximate cause refers to the *last* negligent act that contributed to a patient's injury, without which the injury would not have resulted.

Preponderance of Evidence   One side of a case must demonstrate a greater weight of evidence than the other side. The plaintiff must prove that it is more likely than not that the defendant, in this case the physician, has caused the injury. If the defendant demonstrates more convincing evidence than does the plaintiff, then the case will be found for the defendant. If both sides demonstrate equally convincing evidence, then the case will usually be found in favor of the defendant. Remember that the burden of proof remains on the plaintiff.

MED TIP

To have a preponderance of evidence to find in favor of the plaintiff, the jury believes that it is at least 51 percent likely the defendant caused the injury.

Res Ipsa Loquitur   The doctrine of ***res ipsa loquitur,*** meaning "the thing speaks for itself," applies to the law of negligence. This doctrine tells us that the breach (neglect) of duty is so obvious that it doesn't need further explanation, or it "speaks for itself." For instance, leaving a sponge in the patient during abdominal surgery, dropping a surgical instrument onto the patient, and operating on the wrong body part are all examples of *res ipsa loquitur.* None of these would have occurred without the negligence of someone. *Res ipsa loquitur,* often called *res ipsa* or RIL, is so obvious that expert witnesses are usually not necessary.

Under the doctrine of *res ipsa loquitur,* an exception to the burden of proof rules occurs since the burden of proof now falls to the defendant, who must prove that, based on evidence, the patient's injury was not caused by negligence. The judge decides in pretrial hearings if a case can be tried on the basis of *res ipsa.* Three conditions must be present:

1. The injury could not have occurred without negligence.
2. The defendant had total and direct control over the cause of injury, and the duty was within the scope of the duty owed to the patient or injured party.
3. The patient did not, and could not, contribute to the cause of the injury.

For example, a patient under anesthesia when the alleged injury occurred could not have contributed to the cause of the injury. However, if, before receiving the anesthetic, the patient neglected to inform the physician about a condition that could be adversely affected by the procedure or anesthesia, such as a diabetic condition or eating a full meal, then this may rule out *res ipsa loquitur,* because the patient may have contributed to the cause.

In order to have a civil malpractice lawsuit, the plaintiff (patient) must show that:

1. A relationship had been established between the patient and the physician.
2. This relationship established a duty of the physician to the patient.
3. This duty required the physician to perform at a particular standard of care.
4. The duty was breached by the physician.
5. The patient received an injury as a result of the physician's breach of duty.
6. The physician's breach of duty was the proximate cause of injury to the patient.

Damages

Damages refer to any injuries caused by the defendant. Patients seek recovery, or compensation, for a variety of damages:

- Permanent physical disability
- Permanent mental disability
- Loss of enjoyment of life
- Personal injuries
- Past and future loss of earnings
- Medical and hospital expenses
- Pain and suffering

If the patient does not receive any injury, then there is no negligence case. For example, if the risks involved in having a particular surgical procedure, such as the risk of infection, were not explained to a patient and the patient did not suffer an injury (infection, in this case) then there is no negligence case.

The court may award compensatory damages to pay for the patient's injuries. Other monetary awards fall into the categories of special compensatory, punitive, and nominal damages. Some states have placed a limit, or **cap,** on the amount of money that can be awarded in a medical malpractice case.

Compensatory damages are payment for the actual loss of income, emotional pain and suffering, or injury suffered by the patient. These losses are past, current, and future and include lost wages and profits. The court will consider the amount of physical disability, loss of earnings to date, and any future loss of earnings to determine the amount of the monetary award. Special compensatory damages, also called exemplary damages, refer to a monetary award to compensate the patient for losses that were not directly caused by the negligence. For example, the patient might incur additional medical expenses for physical therapy to regain strength after being bedridden due to the original injury. Non-economic reasons include disfigurement, disability, and loss of consortium.

In some states the plaintiff's attorney may receive as much as 33 1/3 percent of the payment, plus expenses. In some states, where there is no cap, or limit, on the amount of money that can be awarded, the plaintiff may receive millions. In some cases, these large payments have meant that physicians' medical malpractice insurance premiums have increased to a point where physicians cannot afford them and, thus, have had to leave their practices.

Punitive damages, also called exemplary damages, are monetary awards by a court to a person who has been harmed in an especially malicious or willful way. This monetary award is not always related to the actual cost of the injury or harm suffered. Its purpose is to serve as punishment to the offender and a warning to others not to engage in malicious behavior. Punitive damages can result in a large cash amount. The punitive awards have been growing substantially over the past decade and may reach into the millions. For example, a person who practices medicine without a license may receive punitive damages in order to serve as a warning to that person and others that this is an especially harmful practice.

Nominal damages refer to a slight or token payment to a patient to demonstrate that, while there may not have been any physical harm done, the patient's legal rights were violated. The award may be as little as one dollar. However, most states currently require actual damages in the form of compensatory payments rather than just nominal damages or payments.

Wrongful-Death Statutes   If a patient's death has been caused by the physician's negligence, the deceased person's dependents and heirs may sue for wrongful death. Some states have wrongful-death statutes that allow the deceased person's beneficiaries (estate) and dependents to collect money from the offender to compensate for the loss of future earnings to the estate. A plaintiff in a wrongful-death suit does not have to prove that he or she was completely dependent on the deceased person for support, but only that the death resulted in a financial loss. To win such a case, the plaintiff must prove that the defendant's actions were the "proximate," or immediate, cause of death.

Medical malpractice cases are state specific. Some states, such as Iowa, Missouri, and Pennsylvania, allow the surviving spouse and children of a wrongful-death victim to sue for compensatory damages for the pain and suffering they experienced upon the death of their loved one. However, many states have placed a cap on the amount of money that can be awarded in wrongful-death cases.

There are no federal malpractice laws. In common law practice, the government is immune from wrongful-death suits, although some state governments now allow suits brought against state employees.

FRAUD

Unlike negligence, which is an unintentional action that could lead to patient injury, **fraud** is the deliberate concealment of the facts from another person for unlawful or unfair gain. Fraud in healthcare includes a wide range of illegal actions: illegal billing for services that may or may not have been rendered; receiving kickbacks for making referrals for Medicare and Medicaid patients; dishonesty when conducting medical research; embezzlement, particularly in the medical office; and the illegal sale of drugs.

Fraud in the healthcare setting is one of the fastest growing criminal areas. This is especially true in the medical office. Therefore, it is paramount that medical assistants remain vigilant when performing their duties. There have been many medical office cases in which medical assistants were requested by their physician/employers to perform fraudulent acts. In every case, the medical assistant could have refused to perform the actions that were either beyond his or her scope of practice or obviously fraudulent.

In the case of *People v. Gandotra,* Dr. Gandotra hired three medical assistants to provide care for patients in his clinic. One of the medical assistants prescribed controlled substances (Diazepan and Fiorinal with Codeine no. 3) to patients and to undercover federal agents. Dr. Gandotra billed the state of California under his provider number for the medical assistant's unauthorized services. The court stated that the medical assistants were not licensed to practice medicine or write prescriptions. Evidence was also presented that Dr. Gandotra had presented claims for payment for services that were never rendered. His wife, Rita, processed some of the fraudulent claims. As a result of the fraudulent billing practices, Dr. Gandotra and his wife were both charged and convicted of felonies. They paid a fine of $30,000. The medical assistants were not charged with criminal action (*People v. Gandotra,* 14 Cal. Rptr. 2d 896, 11th Cal. App. 1992).

In *People v. Scofield,* the Aetna Casualty and Surety Company charged that Scofield, the patient, along with a physician, presented the company with a fraudulent insurance claim. A medical assistant, who handled the overload of medical insurance work for the office, was employed by the physician. The physician instructed her that his patients were to be billed for treatments three times a week, regardless of whether actual treatment was given. A second medical assistant stated during the grand jury hearing that the same physician told her that his personal injury patients were not put in the regular bookkeeping system; these patients had separate cards. She was told to prepare bills for these patients showing treatments that were not reflected on the actual patient records. The physician told her that it was office policy to submit fraudulent bills to insurance companies for at least $100 to $300 worth of treatment, and then the defendant (Scofield, the patient,) and "we" (the physician and the medical assistant) would each get $100. The court determined that the medical assistant did prepare the bills with guilty knowledge of their fraudulent nature and purpose. However, she was not convicted of aiding in the actual fraud. In this case, Scofield was sentenced to serve 90 days in the county jail. The physician was not charged in this trial. The significance of this case for medical personnel is that the two medical assistants are clearly named even though they were not charged in the fraud (*People v. Scofield,* 95 Cal. Rptr, 405, Cal. App. 1971).

In *United States v. Busse, Dey, Lupulescu, and Failla,* the defendants were charged with participating in a scheme to generate fraudulent billings to Blue Cross and Blue Shield of Michigan from their five medical/chiropractic health clinics. The chiropractors (Busse and Dey) would see the patients and then refer them to the medical side of the clinic, knowing that no physician would be present to examine them. Instead, several medical assistants became involved in the case when they used Dr. Lupulescu's "standing medical orders" (SMOs) to take the patient's medical history, record the patient complaints, and order medical tests, including EKGs, ultrasound, and blood and urinalysis tests. Blue Cross and Blue Shield were then billed for all of these tests. Dr. Lupulescu visited the clinic one afternoon a week to see only the returning patients. His new patients were routinely seen only by the medical assistants, who would then order the tests in conjunction with his SMOs. He was indicted on 68 counts and was convicted on 48 counts. Dr. Lupulescu was sentenced to fifteen concurrent four-year prison terms and fined $6,000. Dr. Dey was sentenced to five concurrent 18-month terms and fined $5,000. Dr. Busse was convicted of aiding in the fraud but was not sentenced to prison or fined. Mr. Failla, the business manager of the clinics, was also convicted of criminal action. The medical assistants were not charged with fraud (*U.S. v. Busse, Dey, Lupulescu, and Failla,* 833 F.2d 1014, U.S. App. 1987).

It appears that the medical assistants involved in the above cases were aware of the fraudulent activities taking place in their office or clinic, but they were not charged in these cases.

Some of the most frequently cited areas of medical-related fraud include:

▶ Billing fraud which includes billing for services not needed, billing for nonexistent patients, or billing for products not needed or supplied.

▶ Overutilization of services such as treatments, including office visits, laboratory tests, therapy, and prescriptions that are not necessary.

▶ Pharmacy fraud of billing for prescriptions and supplies that were not delivered or providing lower-priced generic drugs and billing for higher-priced medications.

▶ Durable equipment and supplies which includes billing the patients for equipment, such as wheelchairs and other devices, and unnecessary supplies.

▶ Legal scams such as workers' compensation fraud and false injury claims.

▶ Kickbacks which are improper payments in order to induce physicians and other healthcare professionals to refer patients to a facility such as a hospital or insurance company.

MED TIP

An allied healthcare professional must use caution when submitting patient claims for medical reimbursement. Filing a false claim for programs such as Medicare or Medicaid is a federal crime. The employee's physician/employer could be severely fined and even lose his or her license for this type of fraudulent act.

OFFICE OF INSPECTOR GENERAL

One of the major players in the war against healthcare fraud, such as false insurance claims, is the Office of the Inspector General (OIG). This office was created to protect the programs under the Department of Health and Human Services (HHS), such as Medicare and Medicaid, from fraudulent activities. For example, healthcare payers will use the diagnosis and procedure codes submitted by billing and coding personnel when making a decision to pay or deny a claim. It is important to determine if an incorrect coding is the result of an error or a deliberate fraud. In a case such as this the OIG, if consulted, would provide an advisory opinion. If the coding was found to be in error, then it would have to be corrected, The party requesting the OIG's opinion could be prosecuted if the error is not corrected. The OIG reports problems with healthcare programs to the Secretary of State and Congress and makes recommendations on how to correct them. The Office of Counsel to the Inspector General

▶ Provides legal services to the OIG.

▶ Represents the OIG in civil cases tried under the False Claims Act.

▶ Imposes money penalties on healthcare providers found guilty of fraud.

▶ Issues fraud alerts.

There are numerous federal statutes to avoid waste, fraud, and abuse in the healthcare industry. The major areas of concern are:

1. Additional costs to federal healthcare programs such as Medicare and Medicaid

2. Quality of patient care

3. Access to care

4. Freedom of choice

5. Competition

6. Healthcare providers' abuse of professional judgment

In general, most of the federal cases revolve around money—wrongful receipt of state or federal funds, presenting false claims for reimbursement, or improper referral relationships (kickbacks and discounts). In many cases there have been stiff fines and/or criminal penalties. False claims, which result in the loss of billions of dollars each year, carry a stiff fine with a minimum of $5,500 up to a maximum of $11,000 for *each* false claim submitted. In addition to this penalty, the provider can be found liable for up to three times the amount lawfully claimed. Since office staff, including nurses, are often the persons designated to submit the insurance claims for payment, they need to be fully aware of the consequences of providing false information.

See Table 6.2 ■ for the federal government's definition of what constitutes a "false claim."

An example of a false claim is a podiatrist who knowingly submitted claims to Medicare and Medicaid for "nonroutine" surgical procedures when what he had actually done was to trim the toenails and remove corns and calluses from patients.

The OIG accepts public comments relating to alerts. The address is Department of Health and Human Services, Office of Inspector General, 330 Independence Avenue, SW, Room 5246, Washington, DC 20201.

MED TIP

Remember that every person has the right to say "no" when asked to perform an activity that is unethical, illegal, or against his or her own value system.

Violation of Statutes

Every medical provider, including physicians, hospitals, nursing homes, and pharmacists, should be familiar with statutes that affect their particular discipline. For example, in the case of *Osborne v. McMasters*, a drugstore clerk employed by McMasters sold a bottle without a "poison" label to Osborne who then unknowingly took the poison and died. The poison label was required by law (statute). A verdict was returned against the defendant who then appealed the decision. The original judgment was held (affirmed) because the statute required McMasters to use reasonable care to protect customers from taking the wrong drug. This was found to be a breach of statutory duty that resulted in injury to the plaintiff and was the proximate cause of death to Osborne (*Osborne v. McMasters*, 41 N.W. 543 Minn. 1889).

TABLE 6.2	
FALSE CLAIMS (as defined by the federal government)	▶ A claim for payment for services or supplies that were never provided
	▶ A claim using a diagnosis code other than the true diagnosis code to obtain reimbursement for services
	▶ A claim indicating a higher level of service than that which was provided
	▶ A claim for a service that the provider knew was not necessary
	▶ A claim for services provided by an unlicensed individual

Immunity for Charitable Organizations

In the past, under common law, tort immunity was granted to all charitable organizations on the theory that the charity was only working for the public good and not for profit. However, this immunity has now been rejected in almost all states. The more current belief is that charity is now a large-scale operation and should also include the expense of liability insurance as part of doing business.

In the case of *Abernathy v. Sisters of St. Mary's,* a patient suffered injuries as a result of negligence by the hospital. The plaintiff originally lost the case on summary judgment. However, upon appeal Abernathy won based on the court's statement that charitable organizations should not expect immunity from the law. The court stated "Immunity encourages neglect and irresponsibility, while liability promotes care and caution" (*Abernathy v. Sisters of St. Mary's,* 446 S.W.2d 599 MO. 1969).

DEFENSE TO MALPRACTICE SUITS

After the plaintiff's case has been presented, the defendant can put forward a defense, called an **affirmative defense,** which allows the defendant (usually a physician or hospital), to present evidence that the patient's condition was the result of factors other than the defendant's negligence. The attorney for the physician will suggest defenses grounded on law and truth that can be used to support the physician's side in a lawsuit relating to negligence. The most frequently used defense to negligence is denial. Other defenses include assumption of risk, contributory negligence, comparative negligence, borrowed servant, statute of limitations, and Good Samaritan laws.

MED TIP

It is easier to prevent negligence than it is to defend it.

Denial Defense

The burden of proof, with the exception of *res ipsa loquitur,* is on the plaintiff (patient), who must prove that the defendant (physician) did the wrongful or negligent action. Therefore, the most common defense in a malpractice lawsuit is denial on the part of the physician. A physician may deny that he or she performed a procedure. In some cases patients are upset about the side effects of a treatment and will sue for negligence. Even though unexpected side effects are undesirable, they are not generally the result of negligence. Signed informed consent documents can assist a physician in proving that he or she did explain potential side effects. It is up to a jury to determine if the plaintiff proved the defendant most likely caused the injury. The physician may bring in expert witnesses to substantiate that the standard of care was met.

Assumption of Risk

Assumption of risk is the legal defense that prevents a plaintiff from recovering damages if the plaintiff voluntarily accepts a risk associated with the activity. For example, when people continue to smoke after reading health warnings found on cigarette packaging or they are advised not to smoke by a physician, then they accept the risk when they smoke. A medical professional who agrees to treat a person with a communicable disease knows and assumes the risk of contracting the disease. A patient who understands the risks associated with open-heart surgery and signs a consent form has assumed those risks from complications of the surgery (but not due to negligence).

In order for this defense to be valid, the plaintiff must know and understand the risk that is involved, and the choice to accept that risk must be voluntary. Patients should be asked to sign an authorization for all procedures indicating that they understand the risks involved, accept those risks, and give their consent for treatment.

MED TIP

The physician is solely responsible for explaining the risks of a treatment or procedure. If a physician does delegate this function to a nurse, medical assistant, or physician assistant, the physician still retains overall responsibility.

Contributory Negligence

Contributory negligence refers to conduct on the part of the plaintiff that is a contributing cause of an injury. If it is determined that the patient was fully, or in part, at fault for the injury, the patient may be barred from recovering monetary damages, depending on how the state allocates damages.

For example, in *Jenkins v. Bogalusa Community Medical Center*, a patient being treated for arthritis was told not to get out of bed without ringing for assistance. He nonetheless attempted to get out of bed and fell, fracturing his hip; he subsequently died from an embolism following hip surgery. The court ruled that he contributed to his own death by failing to follow instructions (*Jenkins v. Bogalusa Comm. Medical Ctr.*, 340 So.2d 1065, La. Ct. App. 1976).

MED TIP

The *Jenkins v. Bogalusa Community Medical Center* case illustrates the importance of specific and timely charting. Instructions given to the patient should always be noted in the patient's record.

Comparative Negligence

Comparative negligence is a defense very similar to contributory negligence in that the plaintiff's own negligence helped cause the injury. However, contrary to contributory negligence, which is a complete bar to recovery (meaning the plaintiff will recover nothing), comparative negligence allows the plaintiff to recover damages based on the amount of the defendant's fault. For instance, if a physician is 60 percent at fault and the patient is 40 percent at fault and the patient suffers $100,000 in damages, the physician will be required to pay $60,000.

A defense of comparative negligence has been used in cases in which the physician may be proven negligent, but the patient, in failing to continue with follow-up care by the physician, was also negligent, which added to the patient's injury.

Borrowed Servant

The **borrowed servant doctrine** is a special application of *respondeat superior.* This occurs when an employer lends an employee to someone else. The employee remains the "servant" of the employer, but under the borrowed servant doctrine, the employer is not liable for any negligence caused by the employee while in the service of a temporary employer.

For instance, if a hospital (the employer) allows an operating room nurse to assist a surgeon while in the operating room, the surgeon is "the captain of the ship" and directs the work of the operating room nurse. Thus, under the borrowed servant doctrine, the surgeon, not the hospital, is legally responsible for the nurse's actions. However, the employee still maintains responsibility for his or her actions.

Another example of a "borrowed servant" occurs when a hospital or nursing home hires a nurse or assistant from an agency. Some courts have stated that the borrowed servant doctrine is in effect and the employer of the nurse, the agency, cannot be held liable. Other courts have used a "dual agency doctrine" stating that the nurse is an agent of both the agency and the hospital and, thus, both are liable for his or her actions. In the case of an agency nurse or aide who goes into a patient's home to provide care, the agency and the employee are both liable.

MED TIP

A healthcare professional should have an understanding of what is right and wrong under the law. Arguing that a negligent act was unintentional is not a defense. Remember that ignorance of the law is not a defense.

Statute of Limitations

The statute of limitations protects a healthcare provider by limiting the time frame for a lawsuit to be filed. As discussed in Chapter 3, all states have statutes of limitations. If too many years have passed since the events causing the injury, it is difficult to gather witnesses, and the witnesses may have difficulty in correctly recalling what happened. In general, the statute of limitations for negligence is from one to three years, depending on the state.

An exception to the statute of limitations is the rule of discovery. The statute of limitations does not begin to "run" until the injury is discovered. In addition, it will not begin to "run" if fraud is involved. In a Michigan case, a patient who had a thyroidectomy suffered paralyzed vocal cords after the surgery. He was told it was due to a calcium deficiency when, in fact, the vocal cords had been accidentally cut during surgery. The statute of limitations would have run out in this case; but because fraud (hiding the presence of the cut vocal cords) occurred, the statute did not begin to "run" until the patient discovered the fraud (*Buchanan v. Kull,* 35 N.W.2d 351, Mich. 1949).

Res Judicata

The term *res,* by itself, means "a thing, an object, or subject matter" such as the contents of a will. *Res judicata* means "the thing has been decided" or "a matter decided by judgment." Thus, if a court decides a case, then the case is firmly decided between the two parties, and the plaintiff cannot bring a new lawsuit on the same subject against the same defendant. For example, according to *res judicata,* when a patient has sued a hospital and won the case for an injury caused by a medication error, then that patient cannot sue that hospital again for the same error.

PROFESSIONAL LIABILITY

In the largest sense of the term, everyone is legally responsible or **liable** for his or her own actions. Even children have caused injury to others. All homeowners, business owners, and healthcare employers are responsible for accidents and other harmful acts that take place on their property or premises.

Civil Liability Cases

As discussed, physicians and other medical professionals may be sued under a variety of legal theories, including negligence and *respondeat superior.* Unfortunately, a fear of such lawsuits has influenced the practice of medicine. Some physicians and hospitals have been reluctant to withdraw or withhold treatment at the specific directive of the patient or family. A clearly stated refusal for continued treatment by an informed patient should relieve the physician and hospital of the duty to continue treatment. In fact, if treatment is continued after it has been refused by the patient, the healthcare provider could be liable for battery. In a 1990 case, a federal appellate court ruled that a physician who implanted a Hickman catheter into a minor child, based on a court order, could be sued for the death of the child two weeks later from a massive pulmonary embolus. The court ruled the physician committed battery because the court order was not properly obtained and therefore was invalid. The father of the child, who had opposed the Hickman implant, was eventually awarded $2 million (*Bendiburg v. Dempsey,* 19 F.3d. 557, 11th Cir. 1994).

MED TIP

Medical personnel must listen to and respect the patient's wishes.

Physical Conditions of the Premises

Medical offices, clinics, and hospitals are required to exercise the same standard of care as any other business that has a public facility and grounds. An institution may be liable when regulatory standards have been violated, such as when an accident occurs in a clinic that has not followed regulations for maintaining a safe environment for patients. The institution may not be liable, however, if the plaintiff was aware of a situation that could cause an injury and then chose to ignore it. For example, if someone walks on a wet floor in spite of the caution sign, it is at his or her own risk.

MED TIP

Lawsuits involving the physical condition of hospitals and other medical facilities have involved such cases as broken steps, malfunctioning elevators and doors, and defective carpets. Every staff member must take responsibility for reporting and correcting defects that could cause injury.

In the case of *Rowland v. Christian,* the plaintiff was injured by a cracked water faucet handle on Christian's property. The issue in this case was to determine if an owner, who is aware of a concealed condition that presents an unreasonable risk of harm to others, must warn of the danger or repair the condition. The court found in favor of the plaintiff by ruling that a landowner owed a duty of ordinary care to any persons who are invited onto property as well as trespassers. The result of this case encourages landowners of buildings, such as hospitals, medical offices, and clinics, to warn of conditions, such as wet floors or construction (*Rowland v. Christian,* 443 P.2d 561, 1968).

Illegal Sale of Drugs

In most healthcare settings, access to controlled substances such as morphine and Demerol may be available. One of the reasons to carefully screen all healthcare employees before employment is to determine if there is any history of drug possession or abuse. There are documented instances of physicians and employees, ranging from nurses to housekeeping personnel, who have been found guilty of stealing narcotic drugs from the workplace and either using them personally or selling them. Easy access to narcotics, coupled with a lack of proper security measures, can result in the loss of a license, severe penalty, and even prison for the offender.

In some cases, narcotics that were meant for an ill patient have been stolen and then documented as having been administered to the patient. The patient suffers as a result of this deception.

> ### MED TIP
>
> It's important to always be alert for any indications of drug abuse among coworkers. Even though it may be difficult to report a co-worker's abuse, it is necessary in order to get help for the drug abuser and to protect patients and the reputation of the facility.

Promise to Cure

A promise to cure a patient with a certain procedure or form of treatment is considered under contract law rather than civil law. In a Michigan case, a physician promised to cure a bleeding ulcer, and even though the physician was not negligent in the care of the patient, he was found liable for breach of contract when the treatment was unsuccessful. After this case, many states passed laws requiring that all promises to cure must be in writing (*Guilmet v. Campbell,* 385 Mich. 57, 188 N.W.2d 601, 1971).

> ### MED TIP
>
> Always use caution when speaking to patients. A comment such as "I'm sure you'll be fine." could be taken as a verbal contract.

Law of Agency

The **law of agency** governs the legal relationship formed between two people when one person agrees to perform work for another person. For instance, in a medical office, the list of agents for the physician includes physician assistants, nurses, medical assistants, technicians, and even the cleaning staff if they are hired and paid directly by the physician. In order to protect the physician/employer from liability for negligence under the doctrine of *respondeat superior,* the healthcare professional should

- Have a written job description that clearly defines the responsibilities, duties, and skills necessary for the job.
- Use extreme care when performing his or her job.
- Carry out only those procedures for which he or she is trained.
- Be honest about any errors or inability to perform a procedure.

One exception to the law of agency is the relationship between the pharmacist and the physician. A pharmacist is *not* an agent of the physician because the pharmacist is not hired, fired, or paid directly by the physician. Therefore, the law of agency, or *respondeat superior,* has not been established.

Altered Medical Records

The **Federal Rules of Evidence** allow medical records into courts as evidence under the Uniform Business Records Act. Any time that a medical record has the appearance of being altered or changed, it causes suspicion about the defendant's motives. The defendant, at the advice of his or her attorney, may end by settling a lawsuit in which there was no malicious intent to lie, but simply a poor charting technique. A **settlement,** or agreement between both parties outside of the courtroom, may result in a payment or other form of satisfaction. A settlement does not indicate guilt or innocence of the defendant. It usually indicates that the defendant believes that he or she may not win the lawsuit.

MED TIP

Never completely obliterate any notation on a chart. If a chart note is placed on an incorrect chart, then cross through the notation with one line and state "Incorrect Chart." Always add your name after the correction.

It is poor technique to leave spaces on the chart so that another person can add statements later. While this may be done simply because another staff member was not ready to chart, it gives the appearance that information was added back into the chart at a later date in order to attempt to deceive.

Deliberate attempts to alter the medical record, to fabricate a medical record with someone else's name, or to lose a medical record can result in a defendant, such as a physician or hospital, losing a negligence case. In some of these cases the physician or hospital had no knowledge that the record was being altered. However, under the principle of *respondeat superior,* the employer is held responsible for the employee's action.

Some lawyers, especially after losing a case, have been known to go back several weeks later to request another copy of the medical records. They will check to see if the record has been altered in any way since the trial ended. In one case, an LPN was found not to be negligent in the first case, but was found guilty upon appeal when the attorneys noted that the medical record had been changed after the trial ended. Even though the LPN had not made any of the changes, and was apparently not guilty of the original charges, nevertheless, upon appeal the original decision was overturned. The judge wonders "why alter the record if you are innocent?"

MED TIP

The moral is to NEVER alter a medical record.

Who Is Liable?

Under the doctrine of *respondeat superior,* or "let the master answer," discussed in Chapter 3, the employer is liable for the consequences of the employee's actions committed in the scope of employment. The employer may not have done anything wrong, yet still is liable. For example, if a medical assistant in a physician's office injures a patient while taking a blood sample, the physician/employer can be liable for the action even if the medical assistant was properly selected, well trained, and suitably assigned to the task. *Respondeat superior* does not assign responsibility to anyone other than the employer. Therefore, the immediate supervisor, if he or she is not the employer of the medical assistant, is not the responsible party.

The doctrine of *respondeat superior* was implemented for the benefit of the patient, not the employee. It is not meant to protect the employee. Thus, the patient can sue both the physician and employee. If both are found liable by the court, the plaintiff may seek to collect money from either party; however, the plaintiff cannot collect twice. The employer, if not at fault but forced to pay the plaintiff, can turn around and sue the employee for those damages (*St. John's Reg. Health Ctr. v. American Cas. Co.,* 980 F.2d 1222, 8th Cir. 1992).

Liability Insurance

In order to protect against the risk of being sued and ultimately held liable for the plaintiff's injuries, most physicians carry liability and malpractice insurance. Liability insurance is a contract by which one person promises to compensate or reimburse another if he or she suffers a loss from a specific cause or a negligent act. Many insurance plans are contingent on the insured person's practicing good safety habits. For example, liability coverage for buildings may be contingent on having a good fire alarm system.

In most cases, employers have a general liability policy to cover acts of their employees during the course of carrying out their duties. Some physicians carry a **rider,** or addition, to the policy that covers any negligence on the part of their assistants. For example, if a patient falls and breaks a bone while getting off the exam table, even though a medical assistant had warned the patient to sit up slowly and use the footstool, the insurance company might settle, or come to an agreement about the case, even though negligence was not found.

The two major types of liability insurance are claims-made insurance and occurrence insurance.

▶ **Claims-made insurance** covers the insured party for only the claims made during the time period the policy is in effect (or policy year). For example, if an injury occurred in one year but the claim for liability insurance coverage was made a year later, then the claim would be denied. It is therefore important with claims-made insurance to file claims reports in a timely manner, especially by the time of the policy's year end.

▶ **Occurrence insurance** (also called claims-incurred insurance) covers the insured party for all injuries and incidents that occurred while the policy was in effect (policy year), regardless of when they are reported to the insurer or the claim was made. Under this type of policy, if an injury occurred in one year when the policy was in effect, but the claim against the physician was made two years later, the occurrence liability insurance would cover the claim. With occurrence insurance, it is important to clearly document when an event took place.

Malpractice Insurance

Because physicians treat the human body, not all medical outcomes are predictable or desirable—sometimes, through no fault of the physician. Therefore, physicians carry malpractice insurance to cover any damages they must pay if they are sued for malpractice and lose. All licensed medical professionals, such as nurses and pharmacists, should carry malpractice insurance. Unlicensed healthcare personnel, such as medical assistants, are usually covered under their physician/employer's policy. However, due to the litigious nature of today's medical practice, many medical assistants also carry their own malpractice insurance coverage.

Physicians' malpractice insurance is expensive. Depending on the type of medical practice, it can cost more than $100,000 a year. Coverage for obstetricians and orthopedic surgeons is among the most expensive. Most physicians carry a rider to these policies that covers malpractice suits based on injuries caused by employees and assistants during the course of carrying out their duties. Such coverage is important, again, because of the doctrine of *respondeat superior.*

Practicing Defensive Medicine

Unfortunately, many physicians find themselves in the position of practicing a type of medicine that will help to protect them from lawsuits. This is referred to as **defensive medicine.** It means that more and more tests and procedures will be ordered for each patient in order to avoid a lawsuit. The result of this practice is twofold: The patient will have to undergo additional, and often painful, tests and procedures, and the cost of healthcare will increase. In addition, the use of specialists by primary care physicians has greatly increased. Some medical specialties such as orthopedics and obstetrics are especially prone to litigation. The result is that in some parts of the country there is now a lack of specialists, such as obstetricians, because the cost of their malpractice insurance has become too expensive. The use of specialists has also meant that, in some cases, there is a reduced relationship between the primary care physician and the patient, resulting in a greater propensity for patients to sue if displeased with their medical outcomes.

Defensive medicine becomes problematic if a physician becomes reluctant to attempt some of the more risky, yet potentially effective, procedures for fear of a lawsuit. A more conservative approach might result in a poor outcome, and even death, of the patient.

A research study was conducted to determine if a physician's behavior affected whether he or she would have a lawsuit filed against him or her. The result of this limited study showed that physicians in a hospital setting who took time to talk with the patients in an unhurried manner, sit on the side of their bed, and even hold their hand while talking with them were almost never sued, even when there might have been some unexpected problems. On the other hand, physicians who merely stood in the doorway and asked how the patient was feeling and then quickly walked away were much more prone to a lawsuit if the patient was dissatisfied with the outcome of his or her illness.

Physicians are aware of the need to hire employees who are skilled in their professional duties as well as able to project a warm and caring attitude toward their patients. In some cases, an unhappy employee will reflect negatively on a patient's attitude toward the physician even if he or she is quite competent.

While it is usually a physician who practices defensive medicine, it can often be another healthcare professional who documents what has been done. Narrative documentation that is performed once a shift in either a hospital or nursing home does not always convey exactly what was done for the patient. For example, stating in the medical record "Patient required one-on-one monitoring" is clearly inaccurate because it is not possible unless there is a person assigned to only that patient. If there is once-a-month documentation, such as is commonly done in some nursing homes, the court may find that there is a "lack of monitoring" the patient because it appears that he or she was only monitored on that one date.

MED TIP

While there is not a law that states, "If you didn't document it, you didn't do it," it's difficult to defend a practice that isn't documented.

ALTERNATIVE DISPUTE RESOLUTION

Using methods other than going to court to solve civil disputes is called **alternative dispute resolution (ADR).** The process of **arbitration,** which involves submitting a dispute to a person other than a judge, is becoming a popular means for resolving a civil dispute. This third person, called an **arbitrator,** issues a binding decision after hearing both sides present witnesses and facts or evidence relating to their cases. However, for the arbitrator's decision to be binding, both parties (the patient and physician) must agree ahead of time to accept the decision of the arbitrator. The selection of an arbitrator must be agreed upon by both sides. This can be a time-consuming process.

In addition to arbitration, other methods include mediation and a combination of the two methods referred to as med-arb. **Mediation** involves using the opinion of a neutral third person for a nonbinding decision. The mediator listens to both sides of the dispute and then assists the parties in finding a solution. Using the arbitration, mediation, or a combination of the two methods for deciding a civil case can save money and time.

LIABILITY OF OTHER HEALTH PROFESSIONALS

Not all cases of employee negligence are covered under the doctrine of *respondeat superior*. Also, physicians are not the only medical professionals liable for negligence. The following discussion summarizes some cases illustrating negligence lawsuits against other medical professionals.

Dental Assistant

In a South Carolina case, a patient sued a dental clinic and a dental assistant after the assistant, who was not supervised by the dentist, cut the patient's tongue with a sharp instrument. The court held that the dental assistant performed a breach of duty to the patient. The clinic was also held liable (*Hickman v. Sexton Dental Clinic*, P.A. 367 S.E.2d. 453, S.C. CT. App. 1988).

Laboratory Technician

Medical employees who make repeated errors are not only liable for their errors but also subject to discharge. For instance, in *Barnes Hospital v. Missouri Commission on Human Rights*, a hospital fired a laboratory technician for inferior work performance when he mismatched blood on three occasions. The employee alleged that racial discrimination was the reason for his dismissal. The Supreme Court of Missouri determined that the evidence did not support racial discrimination and upheld the lower court's finding that he was justly discharged (*Barnes Hospital v. Missouri Commission on Human Rights*, 661 S.W.2d 534, Mo. 1983).

Using improper technique or reagents to conduct laboratory tests can be a breach of duty. In *Insurance Co. of N. Am. v. Prieto*, a federal appellate court found a hospital liable when a laboratory technician used sodium hydroxide instead of sodium chloride to perform a gastric (stomach) cytology (cell) test. (*Insurance Co. of N. Am. V. Prieto*, 442 F.2d 1033 6th Cir. 1971).

Medical Assistant

In the case of *Landau v. Medical Board of California*, Dr. Landau appealed a lower court's decision to remove her medical license. The lower court found her guilty of allowing her medical assistant to evaluate and remove lesions for biopsy from patients. Dr. Landau was found guilty of gross negligence by allowing an untrained and unlicensed medical assistant to remove tissue, such as moles, from patients for biopsy purposes. The court stated that Dr. Landau's failure to follow up with two of the patients constituted an extreme departure from standard of care and had serious consequences—one of the patients died. Dr. Landau's license to practice medicine was revoked. The medical assistant was not charged (*Landau v. Medical Board of California*, 71 Cal. Rptr. 2d 54, Cal. App. 1998).

In the above case, the medical assistant did not refuse to perform the task given to her by Dr. Landau. However, she was, in fact, named in the litigation although the principle of *respondeat superior* was ultimately followed.

> ## MED TIP
>
> Medical assistants cannot count on never being named or prosecuted in a lawsuit.

Nurse

When nurses exceed their scope of practice, they violate their nursing license and may be performing tasks that are reserved by statute for another healthcare professional, such as a physician. Due to the shortage of nurses, their responsibilities are ever-increasing, which may lead to actions that result in malpractice. However, nurses have not generally been involved in lawsuits for exceeding their scope of practice, or license, unless they also acted negligently.

There have been many lawsuits against hospitals in which nurses were cited for errors, failing to perform CPR, and failing to alert the physician regarding their patient's condition. A research study of 43,329 nurses conducted by the University of Pennsylvania found that, in many cases, nurses felt overwhelmed and worried about the quality of care they provided to their patients. Some of this "burnout" is blamed on the shortage of nurses.

Nursing supervisors have been found negligent for not establishing procedures for the nursing staff that are designed to protect patients. In an Illinois case, the director of nursing was found negligent for failing to develop standards to prevent accidents involving excessive temperatures while bathing patients (*Moon Lake Convalescent Center v. Margolis*, 435 N.E.2d 956, Ill. App. Ct. 1989).

> ## MED TIP
>
> Remember that "nurse" means a person is a registered nurse (R.N.). The general public often gives all persons wearing a white uniform the title "nurse." A person who is not an R.N. must correct anyone who addresses him or her as "nurse."

In *Quinby v. Morrow,* a patient recovered damages against a surgeon, the instrument nurse, and the hospital for a burn suffered when a hot metal gag was placed in the patient's mouth, causing third-degree burns (*Quinby v. Morrow,* 340 F.2d 584, 2d Cir. 1965).

A nurse was found negligent in a Florida case when she continued to inject a saline solution into an unconscious patient after she noticed the solution's ill effects on the patient (*Parrish v. Clark,* 145 So. 848 Fla. 1933).

A nurse was held liable in a Massachusetts case where a patient who had received a strong sleeping medication fell out of the hospital bed, fracturing her hip. The nurse had left the bedside rails down and, thus, had failed to exercise due care (*Polonsky v. Union Hospital,* 418 N.E.2d 620, Mass. App. Ct. 1981).

Nursing Assistant

A nursing assistant in a Mississippi nursing home was attempting to lift a patient into a whirlpool bath using a hydraulic lifting device. The seat on the device became disconnected, causing the patient to fall and fracture a hip. The nursing assistant was found negligent for improperly connecting the seat to the lift device (*Kern v. Gulf Coast Nursing Home, Inc.,* 502 So.2d 1198, Miss. 1987).

Paramedic

Most states have statutes that provide civil immunity for paramedics who provide emergency life-saving care. In *Morena v. South Hills Health Systems,* the Pennsylvania Supreme Court held that paramedics were not negligent when they transported a shooting victim to the nearest hospital rather than a hospital five miles away that had a thoracic surgeon. The court stated that paramedics were not capable of determining the extent of the patient's injury (*Morena v. South Hills Health Systems,* 462 A.2d 680, Pa. 1983).

Pharmacist

A pharmacist in New York violated statutes covering the sale of controlled substances. He was found negligent relating to the sale of codeine cough substances, and his license was revoked to protect the public (*Heller v. Ambach,* 433 N.Y.S.2d 281, 1979).

Physical Therapist

A physical therapist who refused to allow an 82-year-old nursing home resident to use the bathroom before beginning a therapy session was found to be negligent. The therapist appealed the disciplinary process in the nursing home. The state supreme court ruled that a nursing home has a policy of allowing patients to use the bathroom when they wish, and therefore the therapist was negligent of the patient's health and welfare (*Zucker v. Axelrod,* 527 N.Y.S.2d 937, 1988).

Physician Assistant (PA)

The role of the physician assistant, as determined in the 1970s, was meant to assist a physician in the primary care of the patient. Today many physicians hire a licensed PA to help them with their patient care. The physician (employer) provides oversight of the PA's practice. The PA is able to legally perform more procedures than a registered nurse, but PAs cannot perform all the duties of a physician. A PA, in most states, is able to assess and evaluate patients' conditions, perform physical examinations, suture wounds, change dressings, and prescribe and administer medications. However, a problem can result when there is no physician oversight such as when an HMO or a prison hires only the PA.

In the case of *Mandel v. Doe,* the county entered into a "Memo of Understanding" with its health department to provide medical care to the inmates of the county prison. This plan called for the PA to be supervised by a doctor, but the practice developed to the point where the PA was subject to no supervision or review. The court found that there was no final review of the PA's actions, therefore, the county was liable for any negligence on the part of the PA as it had given the PA the power to act (*Mandel v. Doe,* 888 F.2d 783, 11th Cir., Cal. 1989).

Respiratory Therapist

All healthcare professionals are required to report unusual situations to their supervisors. If they do not, they are negligent in their duties. In an Indiana case involving an inhalation therapist and a nurse, the court found the two negligent in failing to report to their supervisor that an endotracheal tube had been left in a patient longer than the usual three to four days. The patient suffered injury from the tube and needed several surgical procedures to remove scar tissue and open her voice box. Subsequently, the patient required a tracheotomy to breathe and was only able to speak in a whisper at the trial (*Poor Sisters of St. Francis v. Catron,* 435 N.E.2d 305, Ind. Ct. App. 1982).

> ### MED TIP
>
> The message in the above cases warns the healthcare professional to only practice within the scope of your training. There are times when a healthcare professional must refuse to perform a task.

It's wise to talk to risk management about the need to complete an incident report whenever an unusual situation occurs. This report, which accurately reflects the time, date, and facts of the situation, can be subpoenaed by the court in the event of a negligence lawsuit.

> ### MED TIP
>
> Be aware that any written records that you personally keep at home, such as a journal, can also be subpoenaed.

TORT REFORM

Malpractice reform, also referred to as tort reform, is a controversial issue. According to the National Conference of State Legislatures, 32 states have passed reforms in which some of them limit an injured person's ability to sue. In some states there is a cap on damage awards. Physicians, insurance companies and other business interests want reform that will help to shield them from the high costs of lawsuits. On the other hand, patient advocate groups believe that entering into a lawsuit is the only choice left for many people who have been harmed by the health care they received. Some of the tort reforms have resulted in jury awards that are too small to make the lawsuit worthwhile by the time the attorneys have been paid.

Malpractice cases have caused some physicians to leave their practice of medicine even though they were not found to be negligent. Malpractice cases may take years before the case makes it into a courtroom or settlement. One physician writes about a lawsuit in which she was sued by the patient's family after the mother's death from an aggressive colon cancer that was unexpected and very fast. The physician states that she treated the patient as she would wish to be treated. She believes that the patient's children were coping with many emotions over their mother's death and that filing a malpractice suit helped them cope with their anger and frustration. This physician said, "I loved my patients and my practice, but this made me wary and mistrustful of them—and myself." Even though her insurance company would likely cover any settlement, the experience was devastating for this physician. A trial date was scheduled four years after the patient's death occurred. During the intervening four years, this physician closed her primary care practice of almost 30 years. Eleven days before the trial, the plaintiff's lawyers asked to withdraw from the case. The family asked for a continuance of the case which the judge denied. Finally the family agreed to drop the case since it appeared unlikely that they would win. This physician cited all the wasted time in the more than four years since the death occurred, the emotional anguish, and the $150,000 spent by her insurance company in the run-up to the trial. Not to mention giving up her 30-year practice.

MALPRACTICE PREVENTION

You have a legal duty not to inflict harm to the patient. Take everything that you do seriously even when you think it is not an issue. And always be careful what you say in front of the patient. General guidelines for malpractice prevention also include concerns for safety, communications, and documentation.

General Guidelines

- Always act within your scope of practice.
- Make certain that all staff have a clear understanding of what conduct is unlawful.
- Provide in-service training on what is meant by standard of care and professional conduct.
- Do not make promises of a cure or recovery.
- Treat all patients with courtesy and respect. Unfortunately, some patients tend to sue people they do not like. (Figure 6.2 ■)
- Avoid having patients spend more than 20 minutes in the waiting room. Explain the reason for any delays in treatment.
- Always carefully identify the patient before beginning treatment. When a patient identification bracelet is available, use that to identify the patient as well as addressing the patient by name.
- Never attempt to provide care beyond the scope of your training or experience.
- Physicians should avoid diagnosing and prescribing medications over the telephone whenever possible.
- Provide ongoing continuing education and training for all staff.
- Do not criticize other staff members or your employer in public areas where patients could overhear your comments.

Safety

- Always make sure that patients use their assistive devices, such as canes and walkers, when they are in your facility. Don't let them leave these devices in the waiting room.
- Have periodic inspections of all equipment.
- Check electrical cords to make sure they are grounded.
- Keep all equipment in safe condition and ready to use.

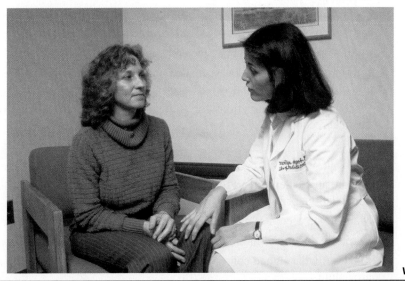

FIGURE 6.2
Malpractice Prevention Includes Treating Patients with Courtesy and Respect

▶ Keep floors clear and clean.

▶ Open doors carefully to avoid injuring someone on the other side of the door.

▶ Provide a mechanism to ensure that all doors and windows, and drawers if necessary, are locked.

▶ Lock up all controlled substances (narcotics).

▶ Place warning signs regarding wet floors, fresh paint, construction, and other slippery or unsafe conditions.

▶ Handle biohazardous waste and sharps such as needles by placing them in the correctly labeled containers.

▶ Know and follow Occupational Safety and Health Administration (OSHA) safety guidelines.

▶ Have a disaster plan and provide periodic drills, including fire, for the staff.

Communication

▶ Make yourself very clear about what you are saying. For example, "This does not seem to be the correct dose." rather than "This does not seem right."

▶ Maintain confidentiality concerning all patient information and conversations and never discuss within hearing distance of other patients.

▶ Return telephone calls to patients as soon as possible.

▶ Refrain from criticizing other medical professionals.

▶ Discuss all fees before beginning treatment.

▶ Provide emergency telephone numbers for patients to use when the office is closed.

▶ Take all patient complaints seriously.

▶ Use a coding system, such as the last four digits of the patient's Social Security number, on the patient registration log rather than the patient's name.

▶ Listen carefully to all the patient's remarks. Communicate the patient's concerns to the entire healthcare team.

▶ If the physician must withdraw from a case, fully inform the patient of the withdrawal in writing and provide enough notice (30 to 60 days) for the patient to acquire another physician.

▶ Call patients at home, either the afternoon of outpatient (day) surgery or the following day, to check on their progress. Document this phone call.

▶ Follow up on all missed and canceled appointments.

▶ Inform patients of all risks associated with any treatment and assure they understand and, in writing, agree to accept the risks.

▶ Place all special instructions for patients in writing and maintain one copy for the medical record.

Documentation

▶ Prepare an incident report to document any unusual occurrence in the medical office, clinic, laboratory, or hospital.

▶ Maintain an accurate log in the patient's chart of all telephone conversations.

▶ Carefully document in the patient's medical record all prescription and refill orders.

▶ Make sure that signed consent forms are obtained before beginning any treatment or procedure.

▶ Document all missed appointments and cancellations in the patient's medical record.

▶ Document whenever it is necessary to withdraw from caring for a patient.

▶ Keep all paperwork current.

▶ Make sure that the physician has read and initialed all diagnostic test reports before filing them.

▶ Do not do "blame charting" by criticizing a physician or other staff member.

NEVER alter the medical record! Make any corrections by using the acceptable method of drawing a single line through the error, write correction above the error, date the change, and initial it. If using an electronic medical record, make corrections according to the standards set by your physician/employer.

▶ Do not delete or alter what another person has charted in the medical record, even if it is clearly incorrect. Contact the supervisor or risk manager with this information.

▶ Enter all telephone orders from physicians on the patient's chart. If there is a concern that the physician may not countersign the order, then have another staff nurse on the phone line who will then sign the chart as a witness.

▶ Carefully document patient discharge notes on the medical chart. Give the patient a written copy of all discharge instructions.

▶ Never leave any spaces for a "late entry" in the medical record. It is a better practice to actually write a late entry when time allows and mark it as such. Remember to accurately note the time and date when the late entry was made. Never add personal notes such as "Too busy to chart yesterday."

▶ Don't just document, "Dr. called . . . " Be sure to include the physician's name such as "Dr. Williams called . . . "

POINTS TO PONDER

1. Is it true that if a patient is injured through no fault of yours, you could still be sued for negligence?

2. If you are trained in CPR and fail to use it on a patient in your facility, could you be sued for malpractice (nonfeasance)?

3. Do all four Ds of negligence need to be present in order to obtain a judgment of negligence against a physician?

4. Does the doctrine of *res ipsa loquitur* apply to all health-care professionals or only to physicians?

5. Can an employee be sued even if the employer (physician) is liable under the doctrine of *respondeat superior*?

DISCUSSION QUESTIONS

1. List five ways to prevent malpractice based on good communication.

2. Give examples of malpractice cases involving healthcare workers, other than physicians, as discussed in this chapter. Discuss the main issues in the case. It is not necessary to memorize the case citations.

3. Name and discuss the four Ds of negligence.

4. Discuss the *law of agency* and why it is an important concept for the healthcare worker to understand.

5. Explain the difference between malfeasance, misfeasance, and nonfeasance.

6. What is an exception to the statute of limitations?

7. Why do you need a thorough understanding of the law as it impacts your employer's practice?

8. State ten steps that may protect a physician and staff from liability.

REVIEW CHALLENGE

Short Answer Questions

1. What are six guidelines for malpractice prevention relating to safety?

_____   _____

_____   _____

_____   _____

2. What is the difference between claims-made and occurrence insurance?

_____

_____

3. Give two examples of assumption of risk.

_____

_____

4. Is the rule of discovery an exception to the statute of limitations?

_____

_____

5. Discuss the difference between comparative negligence and contributory negligence.

_____

_____

6. What is the role of the Office of Inspector General?

_____

_____

7. What are six examples of fraud in medical practice?

_____   _____

_____   _____

_____   _____

8. You drop a sterile packet of gauze on the floor. The inside of the packet is still considered sterile; however, the policy in your office is to resterilize anything that drops on the floor. This is the last sterile packet on the shelf and the physician is waiting for it. The chances are very slight that any infection would result from using the gauze within the packet. What do you do?

_____

_____

Matching

Match the responses in column B with the correct term in column A.

Column A

_____ 1. liable
_____ 2. rider
_____ 3. tort
_____ 4. proximate
_____ 5. misfeasance
_____ 6. nonfeasance
_____ 7. *res ipsa loquitur*
_____ 8. *res judicata*
_____ 9. cap
_____ 10. dereliction

Column B

a. "the thing has been decided"
b. improper doing of a lawful act
c. legally responsible for one's actions
d. "the thing speaks for itself"
e. neglect
f. add-on to an insurance policy
g. failure to perform a necessary action
h. limit
i. a civil wrong
j. direct cause of injury

Multiple Choice

Select the one best answer to the following statements.

1. Carl Simon, a pharmacy technician, fills a prescription for Coumadin, a blood-thinning agent, for Beth White. He hands Beth the prescription without giving her any instructions. Beth has been taking large doses of aspirin for arthritis. The combination of aspirin and Coumadin could cause excessive bleeding when Beth takes them together. What is the legal term to describe a potential liability that Carl may have committed?

   a. malfeasance
   b. misfeasance
   c. nonfeasance
   d. arbitration
   e. standard of proof

2. Emily King mistakenly administers syrup of ipecac, which causes vomiting, instead of syrup of cola, which soothes the stomach lining, to Jacob Freeman. Jacob immediately begins to vomit. Which term could be used to describe Emily's action?

   a. *res judicata*
   b. *res ipsa loquitur*
   c. nonfeasance
   d. misfeasance
   e. rider

3. Which of the four Ds is violated when a physician fails to inform the patient about the risks of not receiving treatment?

   a. duty
   b. dereliction
   c. direct cause
   d. damages
   e. none of the above is correct

4. A phlebotomist draws blood from Sam Ford's right arm. Sam experiences pain and numbness in that arm immediately after the blood is drawn. This is an example of what legal doctrine?

   a. duty
   b. feasance
   c. *res judicata*
   d. proximate cause
   e. rider

5. Allan Walker continues to smoke after his physician warns him that smoking carries the risk of lung cancer. His physician documents this admonition in Allan's medical record. When Allan develops lung cancer, he sues his doctor for malpractice. Allan states that he did not know about the risk of continued smoking. What malpractice defense might apply in this case?

   a. denial
   b. assumption of risk
   c. contributory negligence
   d. borrowed servant
   e. b and c both apply

6. Once the court has decided a case and the appeals process is over, there can be no new lawsuit on the same subject between the same two parties. This is referred to as

   a. statute of limitations.
   b. *res ipsa loquitur*.
   c. *res judicata*.
   d. contributory negligence.
   e. comparative negligence.

7. To cover their employees, some physicians carry additional insurance that is added onto the physician's liability insurance. This is called a

   a. liability.
   b. rider.
   c. tort.
   d. cap.
   e. standard of proof.

8. In a medical office, the list of agents for the physician includes the

   a. nurse, medical assistant, and LPN.
   b. technicians.
   c. cleaning staff.
   d. a and b only.
   e. a, b, and c.

9. The doctrine of *respondeat superior* does not apply between the physician and the

   a. nurse.
   b. medical assistant.
   c. phlebotomist.
   d. pharmacist.
   e. physical therapist.

10. Using a third person to help settle a dispute in a nonbinding decision is called

   a. mediation.
   b. arbitration.
   c. malpractice lawsuit.
   d. civil lawsuit.
   e. none of the above.

DISCUSSION CASES

1. Jessica Mass, a phlebotomist, drew a blood sample from Glenn Ross, a 30-year-old patient of Dr. Williams, to test for AIDS. As Glenn was leaving the office, his friend Harry came in and they greeted each other. Jessica took Harry into an exam room, and in the course of making conversation, he told her that he was a good friend of Glenn's. He asked Jessica why Glenn was seeing the doctor. Jessica responded that it was just for a routine test for AIDS.

     When Harry arrived back home, he called Glenn and told him what the phlebotomist had said. Glenn called Dr. Williams and complained about Jessica's action and said that he planned to sue Dr. Williams. Dr. Williams dismissed Jessica. Dr. Williams told Jessica that if Glenn did bring a lawsuit against her and she lost, then she would sue Jessica.

     a. What should Jessica have done or said when Harry asked about Glenn's reason for being in the office?

     _____

     _____

     b. Did Dr. Williams have a legal right to sue Jessica if she was sued and lost?

     _____

     _____

     c. What important right did Jessica violate?

     _____

     _____

2. Denise, an LPN, works in a nursing home on the 3:00 P.M.–11:00 P.M. shift. She is instructed to prepare medications to give to her own patients to be given as they eat their evening meal. She is also told that it is the policy of the nursing home that she will also prepare all the medications to be distributed in the morning by the LPN who will pass medications at both breakfast and lunch the next day. Denise is told that the reason for doing this is because she will have more time as the evening shift is not as busy as the morning shift. Denise does not want to object because she really needs the job.

     a. What are the potential problems with this policy?

     _____

     _____

     b. What should Denise do?

     _____

     _____

     _____

     c. If a patient is harmed by receiving the incorrect medicine, who would be charged with the negligence?

     _____

     _____

3. *David, an 89-year-old war hero with no living relatives, drove himself at night to a local hospital when he experienced shortness of breath and a headache. When he entered the emergency room (ER) he was placed in a wheelchair and briefly seen by an ER doctor. He was told that he could not be admitted because he was a veteran and had to go to a VA hospital, which was 90 minutes away, for treatment. David was wheeled into the hallway to wait for transportation to a VA hospital. The night shift was very busy. After sitting in the hall for 5 hours, David complained that he needed to lie down. The ER staff, who had been trying to move him to a VA hospital with no luck, finally transferred him by ambulance to a local nursing home. David had a massive stroke shortly after being admitted to the nursing home and died six weeks later.*

a. Does there appear to be negligence in this case?

_____

_____

b. In your opinion, who might have acted on behalf of David?

_____

_____

c. In your opinion, would contributory negligence be a defense if there is a malpractice lawsuit relating to David's death?

_____

_____

PUT IT INTO PRACTICE

Call an insurance company that handles malpractice insurance. Inquire about the cost and coverage for someone in your profession. Request an informational brochure. Write a summary of the information and report back to your class or your instructor.

WEB HUNT

Using the website for the National Association of Healthcare Quality (NAHQ), (www.nahq.org), discuss the six values (transformational leadership, customer-driven continuous improvement, team work, diversity, integrity, and professional development) they list as they relate to your chosen profession.

CRITICAL THINKING EXERCISE

What would you do if you observe the physician you work for exhibiting signs of carelessness when treating patients and documenting the treatment.

BIBLIOGRAPHY

Aiken, T. 2002. *Legal and ethical issues in health occupations.* Philadelphia: Saunders.

Baker, K., and A. Peterson. 2004. *Corporate ethics and governance in the health care marketplace conference: An interdisciplinary discussion.* Seattle: Williams, Kastner, & Gibbs, PLLC, (Feb. 27).

Beaman, N., and L. Fleming-McPhillips. 2007. *Comprehensive medical assisting.* Upper Saddle River, NJ: Pearson/Prentice Hall.

Becker, A. 2009. "State Disciplines Hospital," *Hartford Courant,* (May 28), 1, 3.

Black, H. 2009. *Black's law dictionary.* 8th ed. St. Paul, MN: West Publishing.

Bonner, L. 2008. "Report Rips N.C. Hospital staff." *Chicago Tribune,* (Aug. 20), 9.

Glannon, J. 2005. *The law of torts: Examples & explanations.* Gaithersburg, MD: Aspen Publishers.

Guido, G. 2001. *Legal and ethical issues in nursing.* Upper Saddle River, NJ: Prentice Hall.

Hall, M., and M. Bobinski. 2003. *Health care law and ethics in a nutshell.* St. Paul, MN: West Publishing.

McWay, D. 2003. *Legal aspects of health care.* New York: Delmar.

Savitsky, J. 2009. "A Patient Dies, and Then the Anguish of Litigation. *New York Times,* (Dec. 29), D5.

Schmalleger, F. 2007. *Criminal justice today.* Upper Saddle River, NJ: Pearson/Prentice Hall.

Taber's cyclopedic medical dictionary. 2009. 21st ed. Philadelphia: F.A. Davis Company.

Public Duties of the Physician and the Healthcare Professional

7

Learning Objectives

1. Define the glossary terms.
2. Describe the public duties of a physician.
3. Discuss the guidelines that should be used when completing a legal record or certificate.
4. List the information that must be included in a death certificate.
5. Describe the cases in which a coroner or health official would have to sign a death certificate.
6. List ten reportable communicable diseases.
7. Discuss the Child Abuse Prevention and Treatment Act of 1974.
8. Describe eight signs that indicate a child, spouse, or elderly person may be abused.
9. Discuss the federal legislation of controlled substances.
10. List and explain the five schedules of drugs.
11. Explain how an Employee Assistance Program (EAP) can help troubled employees.

Key Terms

Addiction

Autopsy

Bureau of Narcotics and
Dangerous Drugs (BNDD)

Compounding

Controlled Substances Act
of 1970

Coroner

Data

Dispensing

Drug Enforcement
Administration (DEA)

Employee Assistance
Program (EAP)

Food and Drug
Administration (FDA)

Forensic medicine

Habituation

Inquest

Material Safety Data Sheet
(MSDS)

Morbidity rate

Mortality rate

Postmortem

Probable cause

Public duties

Restraining or protective
order

Retailing

Vital statistics

THE CASE OF BRIAN B. AND THE MEDICAL FILE

Brian B. is taken into an exam room in the office of Dr. K. by the medical assistant, Amy. Amy gets into an animated discussion with Brian about their mutually favorite baseball team. As Amy leaves the exam room she accidentally places Brian's medical file on the counter. While Brian waits for Dr. K., he reads through his file folder. He is shocked to discover that his recent test for AIDS came back positive. Brian panics and runs out of the office before seeing Dr. K. The doctor tries to reach Brian by phone but there is no answer. Dr. K. then sends a letter marked "Confidential" to Brian and explains that he must be treated for his disease and also needs to inform his sexual partners about his diagnosis. Brian does not respond to the letter.

1. What else can Doctor K. do to meet his obligation to report a communicable disease?

2. What responsibility does the medical assistant, Amy, have relating to this problem?

3. How might Brian be encouraged to report his condition to his sexual partners?

I n order to protect the health of all citizens, each state has passed public health statutes that require certain information be reported to state and federal authorities. These statutes help protect the public from unsanitary conditions in public facilities such as restaurants and restrooms, and they require the examination of water supplies. Physicians and other healthcare workers must inform the government when a situation may affect public health, such as in the case of communicable diseases.

PUBLIC HEALTH RECORDS AND VITAL STATISTICS

Important events, or **vital statistics,** in a person's life, such as birth and death dates, are used by the government, public health agencies, and other institutions to determine population trends and needs. The reporting agencies and services include the Department of Health and Human Services, Centers for Disease Control and Prevention, the National Center for Health Statistics, and the Public Health Service. The **mortality rate,** also called the death rate, is the ratio of the number of deaths to total population in a given location. The **morbidity rate** is the number of sick people or cases of disease in relationship to a specific population. The Mortality and Morbidity Weekly Report, a list of illness and death rates for a variety of illnesses, is published every week by the Centers for Disease Control (CDC) in Atlanta, Georgia. The CDC is always on the lookout for outbreaks of disease in major cities and all the states. Therefore, the CDC needs to have accurate input from physicians and healthcare officials of statistics relating to deaths and illness.

The physician's duty to report these events is a duty owed the public—**public duties.** These duties include reports of births, stillbirths, and deaths; communicable illnesses or diseases; drug abuse; certain injuries, such as rape, gunshot, and knife wounds; animal bites; and abuse of children, spouses, and older adults. Additional information includes data such as marriages, divorces, and induced termination of pregnancies.

Office personnel such as nurses, medical assistants, and school nurses may carry out many of these reporting duties. The collection of this information should be taken seriously. The **data**—or facts, figures, and statistics—represent information about the individual patient's life. In addition, some of the data is of a highly sensitive nature, such as the facts concerning rape, abuse, and death.

MED TIP

Even though office staff may actually perform the paperwork requirements of the law, the ultimate responsibility for reporting health statistics and abuse remains with the physician.

Recommendations for completing legal records such as birth and death certificates are summarized in Table 7.1 ■.

Births

Physicians, primarily those assisting at births, issue the certificate of live birth that will be maintained during a person's life as proof of age. A valid birth certificate is required to receive many government documents such as a Social Security card, passport, driver's license, and voter registration.

A physician must sign the certificate of live birth. For a hospital birth, the certificate is filed by the hospital at the county clerk's office in the state in which the birth took place. If the delivery occurs at home, the midwife or person in attendance at the birth can

TABLE 7.1	1. Request information from the state registrar for specific requirements on completing certificates.
Recommendations for Completing Legal Records and Certificates	2. Type all documents when possible. If the record is completed manually, then print using black ink.
	3. Make sure that *all* blank spaces are completed.
	4. Verify all names for correct spelling.
	5. Use full original signature, not rubber stamps.
	6. File original certificates or reports with the appropriate registrar. Copies or reproductions are not acceptable.
	7. Avoid abbreviations.
	8. Do not alter the certificate or make erasures.
	9. Keep a copy in the patient's file.

file the birth certificate at the county public health department. While the time frame to submit a birth certificate varies somewhat from state to state, in most cases it must be done within the first week of the baby's life. Some states impose a criminal penalty if the birth and death certificates are not properly completed and handled. If the birth has not been registered within a year, then the physician, midwife, or other person in attendance at the birth may have to go to court to provide proof of the birth.

Physicians and others who attend a birth, such as midwives, are required to report certain diseases in newborns. Ophthalmia neonatorium is a serious eye condition present at birth that causes inflammation, swelling, redness, and an unnatural discharge in an infant's eyes. If untreated, it may result in blindness. Evidence of this disease must be reported within twelve hours after birth. A test for the condition of phenylketonuria (PKU) is another test required by state health departments on newborns. PKU can be treated with dietary restrictions. In addition, some states also require testing for sickle cell anemia.

MED TIP

Some states impose a criminal penalty if a birth and death certificate are not handled correctly.

Deaths

Physicians sign a certificate indicating the cause of a natural death. The Department of Public Health in each state provides the specific requirement for that state. For example, in the case of a stillbirth before the twentieth week of gestation, the physician must file both a birth and death certificate in some states. In other states, neither is required if the fetus has not reached the twentieth week of gestation. And in some states only a death certificate is required for a stillbirth after the twentieth week. In the case of a live birth with a subsequent death of the infant, both a birth certificate and a death certificate are necessary in all states.

The physician who had been attending the deceased person usually signs the death certificate, stating the time and cause of death. The physician must include the following information on the certificate:

▶ The date and time of death

▶ The cause of death: diseases, injuries, or complications

▸ How long the deceased person was treated for the disease or injury before dying

▸ The presence or absence of pregnancy (for female decedent)

▸ If an autopsy took place

In most states, a death certificate must be signed within 24 to 72 hours after the patient's death. After the physician has signed the certificate, it is given to the mortician, who files it with the state or county clerk's office.

MED TIP

Because funeral arrangements and burial cannot take place until the death certificate is signed, it is important that the physician sign as soon as possible.

The death certificate provides proof that a death has occurred. It is often required to confirm information concerning veteran's benefits, Internal Revenue Service (IRS) information, insurance benefits, and other financial information when settling an estate. If a funeral home provides the burial, they will often obtain copies of the death certificate for the family to submit to agencies, such as the IRS. The death certificate must be signed as soon as possible after a person's death. The time and date of the death are important facts and must be accurate.

In some deaths, a coroner or health official must sign a certificate. See Table 7.2 ■ for a listing of cases that need a coroner's signature.

A coroner or medical examiner completes the death certificate if the deceased has not been under the care of a physician. A **coroner** is the public health officer who holds an investigation, or **inquest,** if the death is from an unknown or violent cause. In some states, the coroner will also investigate an accidental death, such as one resulting from a fall. A medical examiner is a physician, usually a pathologist, who can investigate an

---

Cases	TABLE 7.2
▸ No physician present at the time of death	**Cases Needing a Coroner's Signature**
▸ A violent death, including homicide, suicide, or accident	
▸ Death as a result of a criminal action	
▸ An unlawful death such as assisted suicide	
▸ Death from an undetermined cause (unexpected or unexplained)	
▸ Death resulting from chemical, electrical, or radiation injury	
▸ Death caused by criminal abortion, including self-induced	
▸ Death occurring less than 24 hours after hospital admission	
▸ No physician attending the patient within 36 hours preceding death	
▸ Death occurring outside of a hospital or licensed healthcare facility	
▸ Suspicious death, such as from a fall	
▸ Death of a person whose body is not claimed by friends or relatives	
▸ Death of a person whose identity is unknown	
▸ Death of a child under the age of 2 years if the death is from an unknown cause or if it appears the death is from Sudden Infant Death Syndrome (SIDS)	
▸ Death of a person in jail or prison	

unexplained death and perform autopsies. An **autopsy,** which is a **postmortem** or after-death examination of the organs and tissues of the body, may have to be performed to determine the cause of death.

Unless the death results from suspicious causes, such as a homicide, an autopsy cannot be performed on a body without the consent of the surviving person who has the "first right" to the body. This person is usually a family member who is responsible for burying the deceased person.

Communicable Diseases

Physicians must report all diseases that can be transmitted from one person to another and are considered a general threat to the public. The report can be made to the public health authorities by phone or mail. The communicable disease report should include the following:

- Name, address, age, and occupation of the patient
- Name of the disease or suspected disease
- Date of onset of the disease
- Name of the person issuing the report

The list of reportable diseases differs from state to state, but all states require reports of tuberculosis, rubeola, rubella, tetanus, diphtheria, cholera, poliomyelitis, AIDS, meningococcal meningitis, and rheumatic fever. In addition, some diseases, such as influenza, need to be reported if there is a high incidence within a certain population. Sexually transmitted diseases (STDs) or venereal diseases, such as syphilis, gonorrhea, and genital warts, must also be reported to protect the public. Employees in food service, day care, and healthcare occupations are more carefully monitored for contagious diseases by public health departments.

A listing of childhood vaccines and toxoids that are required by law (the National Childhood Vaccine Injury Act of 1986) are found in Table 7.3 ■.

TABLE 7.3 **Required Children's Vaccines**	• Diphtheria, pertussis (whooping cough), tetanus toxoid (DPT) • Measles, mumps, rubella (MMR) • Poliovirus vaccine, live • Poliovirus vaccine, inactivated • Hepatitis B vaccine (HBV) • Tuberculosis test

Many pediatricians also recommend that every child receive *H. influenzae* type b vaccine (HiB), hepatitis A vaccine, varicella (chicken pox) vaccine, and pneumococcal (pneumonia) vaccine (PCV7). In most states, newborn infants also receive erythromycin applied to both eyes and a Vitamin K injection to prevent hemorrhagic diseases of the newborn.

The National Childhood Vaccine Injury Act, passed by Congress in 1986, requires a physician or healthcare administrator to report all vaccine administrations and adverse reactions to vaccines and toxoids. The physician must report information directly relating to the vaccine and toxoid, such as the manufacturer and lot number. In addition, the name and address of the person administering the vaccine and the date of administration should be documented in the patient's record.

Duty to Report AIDS, HIV, and ARC Cases

All states have statutes or regulations that require healthcare providers to report cases of acquired immunodeficiency syndrome (AIDS) to the local or state department of health. Most states also require that human immunodeficiency virus (HIV) and AIDS-related complex (ARC) cases be reported as well. Who should report the cases varies. In some states, it is the duty of the attending physician or laboratory that performs the test. Other states may require hospitals, clinics, blood banks, and other facilities to report positive cases.

To date, Minnesota is the only state that has a self-reporting provision requiring healthcare workers who are diagnosed with HIV to report the fact to the health department or commissioner of health within thirty days of learning the diagnosis. In addition, the Minnesota law requires healthcare workers to report, within ten days, other healthcare workers who are infected (Minn. Stat., §214.18(2),(4).).

Many states have confidentiality statutes that allow notification of an HIV patient's spouse, needle-sharing partner, or other contact person who is at risk of the infection (California Health and Safety Code 121015). A physician who wishes to notify a contact person under one of these laws should always discuss such plans with the patient first. The physician may wish to remind the patient of the moral obligation to others. Patients should always be informed that there are some statutes that impose criminal liability on someone who is an HIV carrier and knowingly engages in activities that could spread the virus to others (Fla. Stat. §Ann. 384.24.).

Disclosure to Patients of Health Workers' HIV Status

Many people believe that healthcare workers have a moral obligation to disclose their own HIV-positive status to their patients. However, healthcare providers have argued that it is an unnecessary invasion of their privacy as there is little evidence that HIV is transmitted from healthcare providers to patients. The most notorious case occurred when a Florida dentist, who later died of AIDS, allegedly infected at least one of his patients. This patient later died of AIDS. The accused dentist practiced invasive procedures such as tooth extractions and fillings without practicing universal safety precautions such as wearing gloves and a mask. The allegations in this case have never been proven.

In 1985 a law went into effect that mandated the testing of all blood and tissue donors to protect any potential surgery and hemophiliac patients from the transmission of HIV. In addition, the requirement to use standard precautions was implemented. There are many people who believe that healthcare workers who practice any type of invasive procedures or techniques, such as injections and surgery, should be required to take an HIV test. The alternative is that healthcare workers should be tested if they have a needlestick incident. This HIV testing is currently done in hospitals whenever a needlestick incident occurs.

In spite of the lack of statistics to demonstrate that healthcare workers can infect their patients, patients still have a desire to know if they are at risk of being infected with HIV/AIDS. Because AIDS is a fatal disease, many patients believe they should be told if their physician is HIV-positive.

MED TIP

It is the duty of the physician to report communicable diseases, such as HIV, AIDS, and ARC. However, patients often feel more comfortable sharing personal information with nurses, physician assistants, medical assistants, or laboratory technicians. These healthcare professionals have a duty to report this information to the physician.

Child Abuse

The first child protective agency in the world was established in 1874 when a little 10-year-old girl, Mary Ellen McCormack, explained to the court how her mother beat and abused her. The New York Society for the Prevention of Cruelty to Children began as a result of her story. She became known as "the child who put a face on abuse."

The Child Abuse Prevention and Treatment Act of 1974 requires reporting of all child abuse cases. All states have statutes that define child abuse and require that all abuse must be reported. To begin to investigate questions of neglect and child abuse, the state must have **probable cause,** which is a reasonable belief that something improper has happened. Many states list personnel who are required by law to make an immediate report of any suspected child abuse. These personnel include teachers; health professionals such as physicians, emergency room staff, physician assistants, nurses, and medical assistants; law-enforcement personnel; daycare personnel; and social service workers. Questionable injuries of children, including bruises, fractured bones, and burns, must be reported to local law-enforcement agencies.

The term *battered child syndrome* is sometimes used by healthcare professionals to describe a series of injuries, including fractures, bruises, and burns, done to children by parents or caregivers. This is not a legal term but, rather, a description of injuries (Figure 7.1 ■). Signs of neglect such as malnutrition, poor growth, and lack of hygiene are reportable in some states. In a Minnesota case, the court ruled that the Minnesota Board of Psychology acted correctly when it revoked the license of a psychologist who failed to report the sexual abuse of a child (*In re Schroeder,* 415 N.W.2d 436, Minn. Ct. App. 1987).

Physicians have been held liable if they do not report cases of child abuse. For example, in *Landeros v. Flood,* the state supreme court ruled that the physician should not have returned a battered child to the parents after he treated the child for intentionally inflicted injuries. The court held that the "battered child syndrome" was a legitimate medical diagnosis and the physician should have suspected that the parents would inflict further injury on the child (*Landeros v. Flood,* 551 P.2d 389, Cal. 1976).

Any person who suspects that child abuse is taking place can report the abuse to local authorities without fear of liability. It can sometimes be difficult to determine if a child's injury is accidental or intentional. The persons reporting these cases, acting in

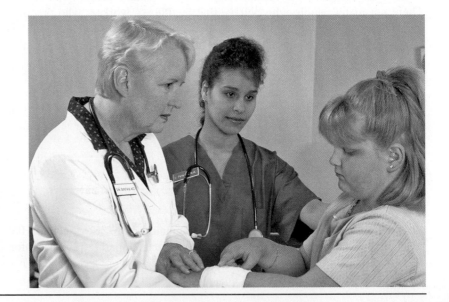

FIGURE 7.1
A Young Child Explains Her Injury to a Physician

the best interests of the child, are protected by law from being sued by parents and others. In the case of *Satler v. Larsen,* a pediatrician reported a case of possible child abuse concerning a 4-month-old comatose infant to the Bureau of Child Welfare. There was not enough evidence to demonstrate that the parents were at fault, and they subsequently sued the physician for defamation. The defamation lawsuit was dismissed, because the physician reported the suspected abuse in good faith (*Satler v. Larsen,* 520 N.Y.S.2d 378, App. Div. 1987).

Most state statutes require that an oral report of suspected abuse be made immediately, followed by a written report. The written report should include:

- Name and address of the child
- Child's age
- Person(s) responsible for the care of the child
- Description of the type and extent of the child's injuries
- Identity of the abuser, if known
- Photographs, soiled clothing, or any other evidence that abuse has taken place

MED TIP

The person reporting a suspected case of child abuse is protected from civil and criminal liability unless that person is the abuser. However, failure to report a suspected case of child abuse may result in a charge of misdemeanor.

Parental neglect occurs when a parent or parents have a religious belief that does not allow medical treatment for their children. States refrain, as much as possible, from interfering with parental rights since the parents are the decision makers for their children. However, the state may have to step in when there is intentional neglect such as when a child is not receiving the medical care that could save his or her life. For example, members of some religious denominations do not allow blood transfusions. If a child suffers from leukemia, a type of cancer of the blood, he or she may need frequent blood transfusions in order to live. A full court hearing may be required to temporarily remove the child from the parent's custody in order to obtain treatment. There have been cases in which parents were charged with murder, manslaughter, or negligent homicide when a child died due to apparent parental neglect.

MED TIP

Parents may have to be asked to leave the exam room while their child is questioned about suspicious bruises and injuries.

Elder Abuse

Elder abuse is defined in the amendment to the Older Americans Act (1987). It includes physical abuse, neglect, exploitation, and abandonment of adults 60 years and older and is reportable in most states. The reporting agency varies by state but generally includes social service agencies, welfare departments, and nursing home personnel. As in the case of child abuse, the person reporting the abuse is, in most states, protected from civil and criminal liability.

Residents of nursing home facilities must be protected from abusive healthcare workers. To do so, some states have made "resident abuse" a crime. In the case of *Brinson v. Axelrod,* a nurse's aide was prosecuted for resident abuse for causing injuries to the hands and face of an elderly resident (*Brinson v. Axelrod,* 499 N.Y.S.2d 24, App. Div. 1986). Another medical employee in a New York case was found guilty of resident abuse when she "held the patient's chin and poured the medication down her throat" after the patient had refused medication (*In re Axelrod,* 560 N.Y.S.2d 573, App. Div. 1990).

The elderly are also protected by the Older Americans Act from financial abuse or exploitation. This is considered a crime in many states.

Spousal Abuse

One of the most difficult situations that healthcare providers confront is when they suspect that a patient suffers from spousal abuse. Laws governing the reporting of spousal abuse vary from state to state. The local police may have to become involved when spousal abuse is suspected, and in some cases a court will issue a **restraining or protective order** prohibiting the abuser from coming into contact with the victim. Questions that are frequently asked of a suspected abused spouse include:

- Are you or your children afraid of your spouse?
- Does your partner threaten, grab, shove, or hit you?
- Does your partner prevent you from spending time with your family or friends?
- Do you stay with your partner because you are afraid of what he or she would do if you broke up?
- Has your partner ever abandoned you in a dangerous place?

Abused spouses are warned that in most relationships the cycle of abuse happens many times. The abuse does not stop.

MED TIP

All medical offices and hospital emergency rooms should have access to a 24-hour abuse hotline, such as a women's support services hotline.

Signs of Abuse

Healthcare workers, social workers, daycare personnel, and nursing home staff should all be on the lookout for victims of abuse. However, physical signs in children, spouses, the elderly, and the mentally incompetent vary. These signs of abuse are found in Table 7.4 ∎.

TABLE 7.4 **Signs of Abuse**	<ul><li>Repeated injuries</li><li>Bruises such as blackened eyes and unexplained swelling</li><li>Unexplained fractures</li><li>Bite marks</li><li>Unusual marks, such as those occurring from a cigarette burn</li><li>Bruising, swelling, or pain in the genital area</li><li>Signs of inadequate nutrition, such as sunken eyes and weight loss</li><li>Venereal disease and genital abrasions and infections</li><li>Makeup used to hide bruises</li><li>Sunglasses worn inside a building or hospital to hide blackened eyes</li></ul>

Healthcare workers must do everything possible to gain the victim's confidence. However, it is not possible to assure the victim that all information will be held in confidence, as abuse cases are reportable by law. This should be clearly explained to the victim at the time of the initial visit.

It is difficult to discuss the abuse with the victim when the suspected abuser is present. Always attempt to speak to the victim in private. If possible, have another healthcare professional present during the interview to act as a witness.

MED TIP

Those persons who are unable to protect themselves, such as children and the elderly, must be protected by healthcare workers and caregivers who become aware of abusive situations.

Substance Abuse

Abuse of prescription drugs is reportable immediately, according to the law. Such abuse can be difficult to determine, as the abuser may seek prescriptions for the same drug from different physicians. A physician will want to see a patient before prescribing medication. A violation of controlled substances laws is a criminal offense. Prescription pads and blanks should always be kept locked up when not in use. Physicians will usually keep a pad in their pocket during working hours. Pads are never left out on exam room counters or desks.

MED TIP

All physicians and healthcare workers should be familiar with the laws relating to controlled substances. Violation of the laws can result in fines, imprisonment, and a loss of license to practice medicine.

Gathering Evidence in Cases of Abuse

Gathering evidence from abuse victims usually takes place in a hospital or emergency room setting. However, a physician may see an abused patient in the office. Precise documentation of all injuries, bruises, and suspicious fluid deposits in the genital areas of children is critical. The court may subpoena these records at a later date. The physician may also be asked to testify in court and offer observations.

Evidence in abuse cases includes the following:

▶ Photo of bruises and other signs of abuse

▶ Female child's urine specimen (containing sperm) or laboratory report indicating the presence of sperm in the urine

▶ Clothing

▶ Body fluids, such as semen, vomitus, or gastric contents

▶ Various samples, such as blood, semen, and vaginal or rectal smears

▶ Foreign objects such as bullets, hair, and nail clippings

Evidence should be handled as little as possible, and by only one employee, to prevent damaging the evidence. All evidence in abuse cases should be clearly labeled and protected with sealed plastic bags or covers.

Chain of Custody for Evidence

It is important to maintain a clear chain of custody for evidence to verify that the specimen has been handled correctly. All evidence must be clearly labeled with the name of the patient, date, and time when the specimen was obtained, and all information regarding evidence should be carefully documented in the patient's medical record. In addition to the time and date, the medical record should include complete documentation of the patient's condition as well as the treatment that was provided. All photographs and x-rays should be carefully labeled with the patient's name, patient registration number, time, and date. Items such as clothing, including underwear, must be retained as evidence and not handled excessively or washed. All evidence should be kept in a locked storage area until it is required.

Care must be taken when turning evidence over to a third party. Always request identification and authorization of the person as well as a receipt which can then be placed into the medical record.

Other Reportable Conditions

Many states require physicians to file a report of certain medical conditions in order to maintain accurate public health statistics. These conditions include cancer, epilepsy, and congenital disorders such as phenylketonuria (PKU) of the newborn that can cause mental impairment if untreated. Because the testing for many of these conditions occurs in the hospital, the reporting responsibility rests on the hospital.

Gunshot Wounds

Gunshot wound laws require reports when injuries are inflicted by lethal weapons or by unlawful acts. In addition, every case of a bullet wound, powder burn, or any other injury arising from the discharge of a gun or firearm must be reported to the police authorities of the city or town where the person reporting is located. The report must be made by the physician treating the patient or an administrative person in charge of a hospital, sanitarium, or other institution.

Forensic Medicine

Forensic medicine is that branch of medicine concerned with the law, especially criminal law, such as in gunshot cases resulting in death. A forensic pathologist is a physician who specializes in the examination of bodies when there are circumstances indicating that the death was unnatural, such as in suicide, accident, or homicide. Their examination usually includes an assessment of the time of death (from data such as the temperature of the corpse and decomposition), and a determination of the cause of death (based on a study of the injuries). They also examine blood, hair, and skin from the victim with those on any weapons, found in automobiles, or on the clothing of suspects.

Forensic pathologists also examine victims of sexual and child abuse. In addition, they consult in cases of attempted poisoning and drug abuse. They are called upon to advise on blood grouping in cases of disputed paternity.

CONTROLLED SUBSTANCES ACT AND REGULATIONS

The **Food and Drug Administration (FDA),** an agency within the Department of Health and Human Services, ultimately enforces drug (prescription and over-the-counter) sales and distribution. The FDA came into existence with the passage of the Food, Drug, and Cosmetic Act of 1938, which sought to ensure the safety of those items sold within the United States.

Drugs that have a potential for **addiction, habituation,** or abuse are also regulated. The **Drug Enforcement Administration (DEA)** of the Department of Justice controls these drugs by enforcing the Comprehensive Drug Abuse Prevention and Control Act of 1970, more commonly known as the **Controlled Substances Act of 1970.** This act regulates the manufacture and distribution of the drugs that can cause dependence and places controlled drugs into five categories that are called schedules: I, II, III, IV, and V. The **Bureau of Narcotics and Dangerous Drugs (BNDD)** is the agency of the federal government authorized to enforce drug control.

Physicians who administer controlled substances, also called narcotics, must register with the DEA in Washington, DC, and the registration must be renewed every three years. A DEA registration number is assigned to each physician. A physician who leaves the practice of medicine must return the registration form and unused narcotic order forms to the nearest DEA office.

An accurate count of all narcotics must be kept in a record such as a narcotics log, and all narcotics records must be kept for two years. The date and the name of the person to whom the drug was administered, along with the signature of the person administering the drug, are recorded. In some states, physicians who prescribe narcotic drugs but do not administer them, such as dentists and psychiatrists, are also required to maintain narcotics logs and inventory records.

Most states limit the administration of narcotics to physicians and nurses. States may be more restrictive, but not less, than the federal government when regulating the administration of controlled substances. For example, a state may require physicians to keep controlled substances records for a longer period of time than the federal regulations require.

All narcotics must be kept under lock and key. According to the U.S. Food and Drug Administration, due to environmental concerns *controlled* (narcotic) drugs should only be "wasted" or destroyed down a toilet or drain, if there are specific instructions on the packaging to do this. Two people should be present when controlled substances are destroyed. Non-narcotic drugs should be removed from their original containers and properly disposed of with other medical waste.

The *controlled drugs* are classified into five schedules based on the potential for abuse, which are summarized in Table 7.5 ■.

A violation of the Controlled Substances Act is a criminal offense that can result in a fine, loss of license to practice medicine, and a jail sentence. Medical office personnel can assist the physician in maintaining compliance with the law by

- Alerting the physician to license renewal dates.
- Maintaining accurate inventory records.
- Keeping all controlled substances in a secure cabinet.
- Keeping prescription blanks and pads locked in a secure cabinet, office, or physician's bag.

Prescriptions of Controlled Drugs

Only those persons with a Drug Enforcement Administration (DEA) registration number may issue a prescription for narcotics. This registration number must appear on all prescriptions for controlled substances. Schedule I drugs require approval by the Food and Drug Administration (FDA) and the DEA for use in research. The sale of these drugs is forbidden. Schedule II drugs require a special DEA order form that is completed in triplicate. One copy is kept in the physician's records, one copy is sent to the narcotics supplier, and one copy is sent to the DEA. Because there is a high potential for abuse and

TABLE 7.5	Level	Description	Comment
Schedule for Controlled Substances	Schedule I	Highest potential for addiction and abuse. Not accepted for medical use. May be used for research purposes. Example: marijuana, heroin, and LSD	Cannot be prescribed.
	Schedule II	High potential for addiction and abuse. Accepted for medical use in the United States. Example: codeine, cocaine, morphine, opium, and secobarbital	A DEA-licensed physician must complete the required triplicate prescription forms entirely in his or her own handwriting. The prescription must be filled within seven days, and it may not be refilled. In an emergency, the physician may order a limited amount of the drug by telephone. These drugs must be stored under lock and key if they are kept on the office premises. The law requires that the dispensing record of these drugs be kept on file for two years.
	Schedule III	Moderate-to-low potential for addiction and abuse. Example: butabarbital, anabolic steroids, and APC with codeine	A DEA number is not required to prescribe these drugs, but the physician must handwrite the order. Five refills are allowed during a six-month period, and this must be indicated on the prescription form. Only a physician may telephone the pharmacist for these drugs.
	Schedule IV	Lower potential for addiction and abuse than Schedule III drugs. Example: chloral hydrate, phenobarbitol, and diazepam	The prescription must be signed by the physician. Five refills are allowed over a six-month period of time.
	Schedule V	Low potential for addiction and abuse. Example: cough medications containing codeine, lomotil.	Inventory records must be maintained on these drugs.

addiction with these drugs, the prescription cannot be refilled. Physicians must take a written inventory of their drug supply every two years. All narcotics-dispensing records must be kept for a two-year period. It requires careful communication between the physician and patient to assure that the patient is not seeking narcotics prescriptions from multiple physicians. In some instances, pharmacies that maintain careful records have been able to pinpoint abuse.

The compounding, dispensing, and retailing of drugs is controlled by the Controlled Substances Act. **Compounding** is the combination and mixing of drugs and chemicals. For example, a pharmacist compounds a drug by filling a physician's prescription that involves preparing and mixing medications. In general, most medications are compounded by the pharmaceutical companies. Hospital-based pharmacists may have to compound certain medications, as for example, for children's dosages. **Dispensing** is defined as distributing, delivering, disposing, or giving away a drug, medicine, prescription, or chemical. Most state statutes authorize professionals, such as nurses, nurse practitioners, or physician assistants to dispense drugs. For example, hospital-based nurses may dispense to their patients medications that have been prepared by a pharmacist, if they have a physician's order. However, nurses may not enter a hospital pharmacy and remove drugs/medications from the hospital's floor stock in order to carry out a physician's orders. **Retailing** is the legal act of selling or trading a drug, medicine, prescription, or chemical.

The term drug, in most state statutes, is similar to the definition found in the Federal Food, Drug, and Cosmetic Act. This states that a drug is intended to affect the structure or function of the body of man or other animals. When applying this definition, the courts have decided that aspirin, laxatives, vitamin and mineral capsules, and whole human blood can be considered drugs under certain circumstances. Therefore, when handling these drugs, even aspirin, nurses and other professionals must be aware that they cannot be compounded or retailed. And a nurse can only dispense these drugs with a physician's order. This means that if a hospitalized or nursing home patient asks a nurse for an aspirin it cannot be dispensed without a prescription from the physician.

MED TIP

A violation of the Controlled Substances Act is a criminal offense. The penalties range from a fine to a long prison sentence.

PROTECTION FOR THE EMPLOYEE AND THE ENVIRONMENT

Employee Assistance Programs (EAPs)

An Employee Assistance Program is a service provided by many institutions, such as hospitals and corporations, for all of their employees and employees' family members. An **Employee Assistance Program (EAP)** may be defined as a management-financed and confidential counseling and referral service. It is designed to help employees and/or their family members assess a problem, such as alcoholism or marital strife, develop a plan to resolve personal problems and determine the appropriate resources to assist in the resolution process. The EAP is geared toward helping employees maintain their job performance while attempting to resolve the difficulty. It is generally administered and staffed by experienced professionals who are trained to understand personal problems and their relation to job performance.

It is estimated that personal problems cost the U.S. economy $70 billion annually. Nearly half of this cost, $30.1 billion, is related to alcohol and/or drug abuse and the resulting loss of productivity. The Department of Health and Human Services estimates that

▶ 4.0 percent of the employed population use some form of illegal drugs daily.

▶ 5 to 10 percent of the workforce suffer from alcoholism. These substance-abusing employees are absent from work sixteen times more often than the average employee, have four times more home accidents, use a third more sickness benefits, and have five times more compensation claims.

A "troubled" employee also means a supervisor will have a problem, and productivity may decline for both employees. The types of problems that an EAP can help with are substance abuse (alcoholism and drug abuse), stress-related (depression and anxiety), family and marital, psychological, and job-related (interpersonal and burnout).

MED TIP

It is important to remember that only trained, objective professionals should counsel employees regarding their personal problems.

Without an effective way to deal with employee problems, a healthcare supervisor may confront the employee, accept continued excuses, provide inadequate counseling, reassign tasks, give verbal warnings, demote or transfer the employee, give a final warning, and eventually resort to termination of the employee. By using an effective EAP, the supervisor

▶ Continues to supervise the employee's job performance.

▶ Receives feedback of the first appointment from the EAP (subsequent appointment counseling sessions are not reported back to the supervisor due to confidentiality issues).

▶ Notes improved performance or states the consequences of poor performance.

▶ Consults the EAP for suggestions of how to work with a difficult employee.

▶ Does not diagnose.

▶ Follows disciplinary documentation procedures.

▶ Is free to focus on job performance.

▶ Continues to talk with the employee, but does not provide counseling.

See Table 7.6 ■. for warning signs that an employee needs an EAP.

Confidentiality is essential for the success of any EAP. Employees who have confidence in the medical staff may discuss personal problems with physicians and nurses. Many of these problems are those that an EAP staff is especially trained to handle, such as alcoholism, drug abuse, and marital problems. If it is necessary for a medical unit, such as in a hospital setting, to receive feedback on the employee condition, then the employee must sign a release allowing the EAP counselor to communicate with the medical unit.

While it is preferable that employees leave their personal problems outside of the workplace, this is often difficult to do. All healthcare workers must have empathy for each other, while still respecting an individual's privacy.

Medical Waste

Hospitals, dental practices, veterinary clinics, laboratories, nursing homes, medical offices, and other healthcare facilities generate 3.2 million tons of hazardous medical waste each year. Much of this waste is dangerous, especially when it is potentially infectious or radioactive. There are four major types of medical waste: solid, chemical, radioactive, and infectious.

TABLE 7.6 **Warning Signs That an Employee Needs an EAP**	▶ Attitude changes ▶ Decrease in output ▶ Inability to carry his/her load ▶ Persistent lateness in completing tasks ▶ Lowered quality of work ▶ Increase in accidents or near accidents ▶ Repeated safety violations ▶ Excessive tardiness ▶ Repeated early departures ▶ Excessive absenteeism	▶ Prolonged lunch hours or breaks ▶ Mysterious absences from workstation ▶ Decline in personal appearance ▶ Mood changes ▶ Conflicts with coworkers ▶ Increase in personal phone calls ▶ Increased use of medical services ▶ Calls from creditors ▶ Garnishments of wages

Solid waste is generated in every area of a facility, including administration, cafeterias, patient rooms, and medical offices. It includes trash such as used paper goods, bottles, cardboard, and cans. Solid waste is not considered hazardous, but it can pollute the environment. Mandatory recycling programs have assisted in reducing some of the solid waste in the United States.

Chemical wastes include germicides, cleaning solvents, and pharmaceuticals. This waste can create a hazardous situation—a fire or explosion—for the institution or community. It can also cause harm if ingested, inhaled, or absorbed through the skin or mucous membranes.

New guidelines from the U.S. Food and Drug Administration advise that non-narcotic drugs should *not* be flushed down the toilet unless information on the drug label specifically instructs one to do this. Ideally, they should be taken out of their original container and then mixed with substances such as coffee grounds to make it undesirable for anyone going through trash. They can then be placed in a sealable bag or empty can and discarded.

Medical personnel have a duty to refrain from pouring toxic, flammable, or irritating chemicals down a drain. These chemicals should be placed in sturdy containers or buckets and then removed by a licensed removal facility. Chemical wastes must be documented on the **Material Safety Data Sheet (MSDS)**, which also provides specific information on handling and disposing of chemicals safely. Clinical laboratories, such as those used by nursing and medical assistant students, must also document their use of chemicals.

MED TIP

Don't flush medications down a toilet unless specifically instructed on the label to do so. Drugs can kill bacteria in septic systems and pass largely untouched through sewage treatment plants. Once in the landfills, drugs can trickle into groundwater.

Radioactive waste is any waste that contains or is contaminated with liquid or solid radioactive material. This waste must be clearly labeled as radioactive and never placed into an incinerator, down the drain, or in public areas. It should be removed by a licensed removal facility.

Infectious waste is any waste material that has the potential to carry disease. Between 10 and 15 percent of all medical waste is considered infectious. This waste includes laboratory cultures as well as blood and blood products from blood banks, operating rooms, emergency rooms, doctor and dentist offices, autopsy suites, clinical training laboratories, and patient rooms. All needles and syringes must be placed in a specially designed medical waste container. The three most dangerous types of infectious pathogens (microorganisms) found in medical waste are hepatitis B virus (HBV), hepatitis A virus (HAV), and the human immunodeficiency virus (HIV), which causes Acquired Immune Deficiency Syndrome (AIDS).

Infectious waste must be separated from other solid and chemical waste at the point of origin, such as the medical office. It must be labeled, decontaminated onsite, or removed by a licensed removal facility for decontamination.

MED TIP

Physicians and healthcare personnel have an ethical responsibility to protect the public from harm caused by medical waste.

POINTS TO PONDER

1. Is it only the responsibility of the physician to report child abuse cases? To whom, in your community, should such a report be made?

2. How soon after death does a death certificate have to be signed?

3. Does a woman have to report a stillbirth if it happens at home?

4. Who signs a death certificate in a death resulting from a fall from a window?

5. Does the physician have to report a case of genital warts, or can this information be kept confidential?

6. Is "battered child syndrome" a legitimate medical diagnosis?

7. Can a physician who, in good faith, reports a suspected case of child abuse be sued by parents?

8. Can a "wasted" controlled substance be poured down a sink?

9. Wouldn't it be better for a person who has personal problems to be counseled by a supervisor or employer who knows him or her than to be counseled by a stranger in EAP? Why or why not?

10. Should healthcare workers be tested to see if they are HIV-positive?

DISCUSSION QUESTIONS

1. What drugs fall under each of the five categories (Schedules) of controlled substances?

2. To what does the term *public duties* refer?

3. What are the physician's public duties?

4. What records must physicians keep if they dispense or administer controlled substances?

5. What is the healthcare worker's responsibility with medical waste?

6. What are some conditions surrounding death that require an autopsy?

REVIEW CHALLENGE

Short Answer Questions

1. What are the four categories of medical waste?

_____   _____

_____   _____

2. What are some of the events that a physician has a duty to report?

_____   _____

_____   _____

_____   _____

3. In a case of child abuse, what does the requirement that the state must have probable cause mean?

_____

_____

4. In your opinion, should patients be told if their physician is HIV-positive?

_____

_____

5. What is a potential legal charge for a person who fails to report child abuse?

_____

_____

6. Violations of laws relating to controlled substances can result in what type(s) of legal action?

_____

_____

7. What can medical office personnel do to assist the physician in maintaining compliance with the Controlled Substances Act?

_____

_____

8. How should non-controlled drugs be wasted?

_____

_____

Matching

Match the responses in column B with the correct term in column A.

Column A

_____ **1.** data
_____ **2.** coroner
_____ **3.** Schedule II drug
_____ **4.** postmortem
_____ **5.** Schedule I drug
_____ **6.** addiction
_____ **7.** inquest
_____ **8.** DPT
_____ **9.** STDs
_____ **10.** public duty

Column B

a. after death
b. statistics
c. physical dependence
d. diphtheria, pertussis, tetanus toxoid vaccine
e. public health official who investigates cause of death
f. report child abuse
g. LSD
h. codeine
i. sexually transmitted diseases
j. investigation to determine cause of death

Multiple Choice

Select the one best answer to the following statements.

1. Vital statistics from a person's life include all of the following except

   a. pregnancies.
   b. marriages and divorces.
   c. animal bites.
   d. sensitive information such as rape and abuse.
   e. all of the above are considered to be vital statistics.

2. A coroner does not have to sign a death certificate in the case of

   a. suicide.
   b. death of elderly persons over the age of 90.
   c. death occurring less than 24 hours after hospital admission.
   d. death from electrocution.
   e. death of a prison inmate.

3. All of the following vaccines and toxoids are required for children by law except

   a. measles.
   b. polio.
   c. hepatitis.
   d. a and b only.
   e. a, b, and c are all required.

4. The Controlled Substances Act is also known as the

   a. Drug Enforcement Administration Act.
   b. Food and Drug Administration Act.
   c. Comprehensive Drug Abuse Prevention and Control Act.
   d. Bureau of Narcotics and Dangerous Drugs Act.
   e. none of the above.

5. Schedule III drugs

   a. can be refilled by an order over the phone from the office assistant.
   b. are allowed only five refills during a six-month period.
   c. require the DEA number of the physician on the prescription.

   d. require the order to be typed on the prescription form.
   e. all of the above.

6. An EAP program may help an employee cope with

   a. marital problems.
   b. alcoholism and drug abuse.
   c. criminal charges.
   d. a and b only.
   e. a, b, and c.

7. Infectious waste

   a. should be separated from chemical waste at the site of origin.
   b. can be safely removed by a licensed removal facility.
   c. consists of blood and blood products.
   d. may contain the HIV and hepatitis A and B viruses.
   e. all of the above.

8. Phenobarbital is an example of a

   a. Schedule I drug.
   b. Schedule II drug.
   c. Schedule III drug.
   d. Schedule IV drug.
   e. Schedule V drug.

9. The best method to "waste," or destroy, a narcotic is to

   a. place it in a medical waste container that is clearly marked.
   b. return it to the pharmaceutical company.
   c. flush it down a toilet only if instructed to do so on the packaging.
   d. do it without any witnesses.
   e. none of the above.

10. Elder abuse is clearly defined in the

   a. Food and Drug Administration Act.
   b. Controlled Substances Act of 1970.
   c. amendment to the Older Americans Act of 1987.
   d. amendment to the Older Americans Act of 1974.
   e. none of the above.

DISCUSSION CASES

1. *A pharmaceutical salesperson has just brought in a supply of nonprescription vitamin samples for the physicians in your practice to dispense to their patients. These vitamins are a new, expensive variety that is being given away to patients who are on a limited income and cannot afford to buy them. The other staff members take the samples home for their families' personal use. They tell you to do the same as the samples will become outdated before the physicians can use all of them. It would save you money.*

    a. What do you do?

    _____

    _____

    b. Is your action legal? Why or why not?

    _____

    _____

    c. Is your action ethical? Why or why not?

    _____

    _____

    d. Does your physician/employer have any responsibility for the dispensing of these free nonprescription vitamins? Explain your answer.

    _____

    _____

    e. What precautions should be taken when storing nonprescription drugs?

    _____

    _____

2. *One of your coworkers recently told you that he is HIV positive. He shared information with you that his partner is very ill with AIDS. You observe, while this man is talking to you, that he has a small draining, open lesion on his left arm. You are concerned about his health and caution him to be careful. The next day you see that he is on a list of CPR instructors who will be testing employees. Your facility still uses an older version of CPR in which there is mouth breathing performed on the "Annie."*

    a. Who should you notify about your concerns?

    _____

    _____

    b. Should you approach your coworker and tell him about your concerns?

    _____

    _____

    c. What legal recourse does your coworker have if he loses his job because of his medical condition?

    _____

    _____

3. *Your friend at work has told you that she is going through a difficult divorce. She says she has developed a drinking problem as a result of the stress. She asks for your advice on what to do.*

  a. What do you tell her?

  _____

  _____

  b. Do you tell anyone else about her drinking problem?

  _____

  _____

  c. What do you do if you see her approach a patient while she is intoxicated?

  _____

  _____

PUT IT INTO PRACTICE

Find a newspaper article that discusses an abusive situation (spousal, child, elder, or drugs). Write your thoughts on what could have been done to prevent this from happening. Discuss the role of the healthcare team in reporting abuse cases.

WEB HUNT

Search the website for the Centers for Disease Control (www .cdc.gov). Provide a definition for the morbidity and mortality tables using the CDC's definition as stated on its website.

CRITICAL THINKING EXERCISE

What would you do if you see a fellow employee "wasting" non-narcotic medications by taking them home?

BIBLIOGRAPHY

American Medical Association. 2008–2009. *Code of medical ethics: Current opinions on ethical and judicial affairs.* Chicago: American Medical Association.

Beaman, N., and L. Fleming-McPhillips. 2007. *Comprehensive medical assisting.* Upper Saddle River, NJ: Pearson/Prentice Hall.

How to dispose of unused medicines. FDA Consumer Health Information at http://fda.gov/consumer/updates/drug_disposal062308.html. June 23, 2008.

Hitner, H., and B. Nagle. 2005. *Basic pharmacology for health occupations.* New York: Glencoe.

Markel, H. 2009. "The child who put a face on abuse." *New York Times*, December 15 (D5).

Physician's desk reference. 2010. New York: Three Rivers Press.

Rybacki, J., and J. Long. 2000. *The essential guide to prescription drugs.* New York: Harper.

Taber's cyclopedic medical dictionary. 2009. 21st ed. Philadelphia: F. A. Davis.

Workplace Law and Ethics

Learning Objectives

1. Define the glossary terms.
2. Discuss the regulations concerning equal employment opportunity and employment discrimination.
3. Describe the regulations affecting employee health and safety.
4. Discuss the regulations affecting employee compensation and benefits.
5. Give examples of regulations affecting consumer protection and collection practices.
6. Describe accommodations that can be made in the workplace for persons with disabilities.
7. List several questions that may be legally asked during an employment interview. List several questions that are illegal to ask during the interview.
8. Discuss guidelines for good hiring practices.

Key Terms

Affirmative action programs

Age Discrimination in Employment Act (ADEA)

Americans with Disabilities Act (ADA)

Autonomy

Bias

Bloodborne pathogens

Civil Rights Act

Clinical Laboratory Improvement Act (CLIA)

Consolidated Omnibus Budget Reconciliation Act (COBRA)

Creditor

Debtors

Discrimination

Drug-Free Workplace Act

Emergency Medical Treatment and Active Labor Act (EMTALA)

Employee Retirement Income Security Act (ERISA)

Employment-at-will

Equal Credit Opportunity Act

Equal Employment Opportunity Act (EEOA)

Equal Employment Opportunity Commission (EEOC)

Equal Pay Act

Ethnocentric

Fair Credit Reporting Act

Fair Debt Collection Practices Act

Fair Labor Standards Act (FLSA)

Family and Medical Leave Act (FMLA)

Federal Insurance Contribution Act (FICA)

Federal Wage Garnishment Law	Patient dumping	Title VII of the Civil Rights Act
Garnishment	Preempt	Truth in Lending Act (Regulation Z)
Just cause	Pregnancy Discrimination Act	Unemployment compensation
National Labor Relations Act	Rehabilitation Act	Vesting
Occupational Safety and Health Act (OSHA)	Right-to-know laws	Workers' Compensation Act
Parenteral	Social Security Act	Wrongful discharge
	Stereotyping	

THE CASE OF JANET K. AND EPILEPSY

Janet K. had suffered from epilepsy since she was an infant. Her condition was well controlled as she entered adulthood, and she was able to complete a nursing program in good health. She particularly enjoyed working as a scrub nurse in the operating room. Upon graduation she applied at the large university teaching hospital where she had performed her clinical work during her nursing program. The hospital knew of her epilepsy history and offered her a job in their medical records department. Janet petitioned to be able to work in surgery but the hospital administrators felt that it was too dangerous for Janet and for the surgical patients if she should have a seizure there.

While working in medical records Janet's seizures began to return. She would have a seizure at least every month even though her medications had been changed. Janet noticed that some of her fellow medical records technicians would stay away from her for fear of not knowing how to help her during a seizure. One afternoon a physician was dictating his case records in a cubicle next to Janet's when she had a seizure. He helped her and then went to the hospital administrator and told her that Janet should not be allowed to work in a hospital since it gave the hospital, with its image of healing, a bad reputation.

Janet was then terminated at the age of 27 due to health issues. She died of a brain tumor five years later.

1. Are there some medical or mental conditions that should prevent a person from working in a hospital or other medical setting? If so, what are they?

2. What should have been done when Janet's coworkers shunned her?

3. Was the physician who helped Janet when she had a seizure correct in asking the hospital administrator to dismiss (fire) her?

4. Should Janet have been given the opportunity to work in surgery? Why or why not?

Applied ethics always involves people. And where better to promote good ethical practices than in the workplace—whether it is a hospital, medical office, clinic, nursing home, hospice, or agency? While it is just common sense to treat people one works with well, it is often the workplace where people suffer discrimination, harassment, and other unethical practices. You will note that many of these laws were established as far back as the 1930s. They are one of the reasons that we have fair standards and protection in the workplace today.

PROFESSIONALISM IN THE WORKPLACE

The profession of medicine, whether practiced by a physician, nurse, medical assistant, or other healthcare professional, is inherently meaningful. A medical or health-related career usually requires several years of education to achieve competence, and, in many cases, it is a career that a person selects for all of their working years. Healthcare professionals can justifiably find pride in their achievements.

Medical professionals do not enter their field of study with the expectation that they will have to compromise their professional behavior. However, it has become increasingly difficult to provide the level of care and concern for patients given the elements of increased documentation and sicker patients staying fewer days in a hospital to recover from illness or surgery. In some cases, very ill patients are being seen in medical offices, emergency room settings, or clinics because they do not have insurance to pay for a hospital stay.

In today's world of specialization, patients may have several physicians managing their care. This can result in the patient's spending less time with any one medical professional. In fact, many patients feel that the care they receive has become depersonalized as they never get to know any one caregiver very well. The reverse is also true, as medical professionals become frustrated that they do not have enough time to really get to know and understand their patients.

The case of Libby Zion illustrates this point. Libby was an 18-year-old college student who was treated in a large, busy New York teaching hospital. She entered the hospital's emergency room with moderate aches and pains suggesting influenza. Libby also exhibited agitated behavior but did not tell the emergency room physician that she used drugs. She was given a sedating medication as well as physical restraints to control her agitated movements. Libby died eight hours after she was admitted. Her parents and several journalists investigated the competence and amount of time spent by the medical personnel who cared for Libby. They also examined information about the long hours that interns and residents work in a teaching hospital. The results of the parents' crusade, media coverage, and a resulting court case meant that there is now a closer look at accountability and supervision in teaching hospitals. Interns and residents now have mandatory rest periods and days off work as a result of the Libby Zion case. More than twenty-five years after Libby's death, her legacy lives on in the important changes made in the care of patients.

Professionalism means that each healthcare professional will monitor the time and care that each patient receives so that the care is effective, as well as efficient. It means that we treat all patients with the same standards regardless of race, color, religion, gender, or national origin. This responsibility should not be left to others.

> **MED TIP**
>
> Efficiency is getting the job done; effectiveness is doing the right job! This is especially true in healthcare.

DISCRIMINATION IN THE WORKPLACE

In spite of knowledge about good healthcare habits, people working in the healthcare field often suffer from many of the same problems that affect their patients. For example, overweight nurses, medical assistants, and other healthcare professionals may experience discriminatory behavior due to their weight. In some cases, overweight or obese health-care professionals are either not hired or else they are placed in an unpopular work setting where they will not be seen or promoted. It is an injustice to discriminate against either a fellow employee or a patient because of their weight.

Some companies and hospital have implemented wellness programs, including weight loss, with the belief that healthy employees are more productive. Ethical concerns about privacy issues arise even from well-meaning wellness programs when electronic data records are kept to track the employee's weight loss.

> **MED TIP**
>
> As simple as this sounds, always treat a coworker as you wish to be treated.

PRIVACY AND THE WORKPLACE

The federal government has taken an active role in attempting to prevent violations of a patient's privacy. The Health Insurance Portability and Accountability Act of 1996 (HIPAA), discussed in Chapter 10, includes stiff fines and other penalties if a patient's privacy is violated. However, in spite of federal regulations, some healthcare workers are still invading a patient's privacy, often just to satisfy curiosity.

For example, 7-year-old Nixzmary Brown was found beaten and starved and left to die in a small room that her brothers and sisters called "the dirty room." Her mother and stepfather were both charged with the crime. According to New York's Health and Hospitals Corporation, dozens of workers, including doctors, nurses, technicians, and clerks, opened the patient's computer file even though they had nothing to do with the case. There were several employees who had a legitimate reason to view the file on a "need to know" basis, but investigators believe that 39 employees opening the file were just too many. It was determined that "sheer curiosity" had driven many of the healthcare workers to open Nixzmary's file. The stepfather was convicted in 2006 of first degree manslaughter and sentenced to 29 years in prison. The mother was convicted in 2008 of first degree manslaughter and sentenced to 43 years in prison.

On October 9, 2009 the governor of the state of New York signed into law "Nixzmary's Law" making the maximum penalty for torturing and murdering a child life in prison without parole. This child's death caused an overhaul of the Child Protective Services system. The 39 hospital employees who violated the child's privacy were suspended for 30 to 60 days without pay and received privacy training before returning to work.

> ## MED TIP
> Opening a patient's medical file should always be on a "need to know" basis. Any other reason may constitute an illegal action.

It is just as inappropriate to look at a coworker's personnel file as it is to illegally examine a patient's file. A co-worker's personnel evaluations and salary levels are privileged information. Viewing personnel records without a "need to know" could result in dismissal from a job.

CULTURAL CONSIDERATIONS

A person's background and experience heavily influence personal beliefs. Ideally, everyone entering the medical profession should examine his or her own cultural background to be sure he or she will be able to provide patient care in sensitive situations.

Because family can be extremely important in some cultures, do not be surprised if your patient brings along the entire family for emotional and physical support. In some cultures, a male must always be present if a female member is being examined or meeting with strangers.

The diversity of the U.S. culture presents many challenges for both the healthcare professional and the patient. **Stereotyping** can occur when negative generalities concerning specific characteristics about a group are applied unfairly to an entire population. For example, a statement such as, "Those people are all welfare cheats" is unfair and incorrect when applied to a large group of people. A **bias,** or unfair dislike or preference against someone, can prevent a healthcare professional from making an impartial judgment. As an example, different cultures have their own practices for personal hygiene. A bias occurs when a healthcare professional doesn't pay any attention to a person who displays poor hygiene or has a body odor.

> ## MED TIP
> It is always wise to keep one's opinions about the use of deodorants, clean clothing, and frequent bathing to oneself, unless the patient's health is suffering as a result of poor hygiene conditions.

People who are **ethnocentric** tend to believe that their cultural background is better than any other. For example, if one is heterosexual, then to decide that gay and lesbian persons are inferior to one's own background is ethnocentric and can result in stereotyping and prejudging people. In order to avoid these negative behaviors:

- Be aware of your coworkers' and patients' beliefs.
- Learn as much as you can about other cultures, races, and nationalities.
- Be sensitive to the feelings of others.
- Evaluate all information before accepting it as a belief.
- Always avoid ethnic jokes. Walk away if a coworker is telling an ethnic or disrespectful joke.
- Be open to differences in other people.

Communication can be a challenge for many people who do not understand English. For example, a nod of the head up and down means "yes" to an American, but it means "no" in some other cultures. Non-English-speaking patients need brochures and handouts in their own language. Many publications are now available in Spanish and other languages. It is imperative that an interpreter be present when explaining important information to a patient. Patients may have to be assisted in finding the best community resource to help them because in some cultures it is unthinkable to ask strangers for help.

MED TIP

Slang terms for dealing with bodily functions should never be used. It's perfectly acceptable to ask a patient if he or she has to use the bathroom.

Since there is often a strong ethnic population in some hospitals and medical practices, it is wise to learn all you can about their beliefs. For example, in some cultures it is considered rude or disrespectful to look directly into a person's eyes or to touch the top of a child's head. Some cultures, including Americans, consider modesty to be extremely important. It is always important to make sure that patients are covered with either a gown or draped sheet when having an examination. In some cultures a woman is not allowed to undress or bare any part of her body in front of a man without her husband's permission. Shaving hair before an examination or surgical procedure is not allowed in some cultures. These cultural restrictions can pose difficult situations that need to be handled carefully and sensitively.

Always attempt to find an interpreter when giving instructions to a non-English-speaking patient. If one is unavailable, the website http://babelfish.yahoo.com/ is helpful in translating English words and phrases into a second language.

MED TIP

It is wise to keep in mind how you would wish to be treated if you were a patient in another country without the use of the language.

Many people, especially the elderly, do not like to be addressed by nicknames such as "dear" or "honey." It is always wise to use a title such as Ms., Mrs., or Mr. unless told otherwise by the patient.

RELIGIOUS CONSIDERATIONS

Respecting religious beliefs of others can be a difficult, but necessary, responsibility for the healthcare professional. Advance directives, consent to treatment, and the use of birth control devices are often influenced by a person's religious beliefs. In some cases, it may mean rejecting medical interventions such as blood transfusions, but in other instances it might mean that a patient rejects all medical care.

From an ethical perspective, the principle of patient **autonomy,** or independence for their beliefs, is always an important consideration. However, all of these, sometimes conflicting, conditions can result in confusion for the medical professional. As long as a person is competent, he or she has the right to make his or her own decisions. Bioethical and legal issues arise when a person is called upon to make this decision, based upon his or her own religious beliefs, for another person such as a child or an elderly or incompetent adult. In these cases a guardianship may have to be established by the courts so that the best interests of the patient are observed. There will always be ethical discussions about where religious boundaries should be drawn and when the state should step in to protect the individual.

MED TIP

It is never appropriate to judge, either with verbal or nonverbal criticism, another person's religious customs and beliefs. An exception occurs when there is evidence of abuse as a result of a religious practice.

There are some beliefs that do not allow a person to receive a blood transfusion. When such a situation occurs a physician may seek a court order for a child to receive blood over the objections of the parent. The case of *Prince v. Commonwealth of Mass-achusetts* reasoned that "Parents may be free to be martyrs themselves. But it does not follow that they are free in identical circumstances to make martyrs of their children" (*Prince v. Commonwealth of Massachusetts*, 321 U.S. 158 1944). An even more difficult situation arises when a pregnant mother refuses a transfusion that could save her life and the life of her unborn child. According to her religious beliefs, the mother may believe that "ingesting blood" may doom her in the eyes of her God. In this case a physician, or hospital administrator, would have to seek a court order to administer the blood transfusion.

MED TIP

Remember that the patient's wishes should be honored if they differ from our own beliefs. The exception to this is when a belief may result in harm to either the patient or the health-care worker. In that case, a supervisor must intervene.

An employer has a legal obligation under the Civil Rights Act (discussed later in this chapter) to make accommodations so that employees can practice their religious observations. For example, members of the Jewish religion must observe Saturday as the Sabbath day on which they may not work. Therefore, it would be improper to set up Friday evening meetings after sundown or Saturday meetings that require all employees to attend. It would also be inappropriate to schedule Sunday morning meetings that Christian employees are required to attend. The law also requires that businesses must provide reasonable accommodations, such as a prayer room or a special cleansing bathroom, for employees to practice their religion, as long as it doesn't interfere with other employees' rights.

EFFECTIVE HIRING PRACTICES

There are many examples of lawsuits relating to hiring practices that would not have happened if the employer had acted within the confines of the law. Fairness is one of the most important elements when supervising employees. In addition, employers can improve the

TABLE 8.1	
Recommendations for Good Hiring Practices	▶ Develop clear policies and procedures on hiring, discipline, and termination of employees.
	▶ Effectively screen potential employees' backgrounds.
	▶ Clearly state in all written materials such as employee handbooks, memos, and manuals, that an employee handbook is not a contract.
	▶ Use a two-tier interview screening process. Have candidates interviewed both by healthcare professionals who will supervise or work with the new employee and by trained human resource or personnel department employees.
	▶ Carefully assess the applicant's skill level by having him or her perform some of the position requirements (i.e., drawing blood samples, teaching, performing surgical setups).
	▶ Develop an application form that asks for appropriate information about the applicant's qualifications.
	▶ Provide a job description to every employee.
	▶ Develop a progressive disciplinary procedure and make the policy known to all employees and supervisors.
	▶ Whenever possible, have human resource personnel present during the firing process. Document what is said during this process.
	▶ Provide in-service training to supervisors on how to conduct job interviews and motivate and discipline employees.
	▶ Become familiar with the legal and illegal questions that can be asked in an employment interview.

quality of their employees by using an effective screening process before the actual hiring takes place. It is imperative to perform thorough background checks on applicants in the healthcare field because they may not confess to a criminal record on an application form. Employers are at risk of lawsuits when they hire employees who are a foreseeable danger to others. Some recommendations for good hiring practices are presented in Table 8.1 ■ .

The employee handbook usually explains behaviors, such as sleeping on the job, that can cause an employee's termination. Management needs to use care when issuing a handbook. Statements in employee handbooks have been interpreted as "implied contracts" in a court of law. In *Watson v. Idaho Falls Consolidated Hospitals, Inc.,* a nurse's aide claimed wrongful discharge and sued her employer, a hospital, for violating provisions in the employee handbook when it terminated her. Employees had been asked to read and sign a revised handbook to show that they understood hospital policies regarding counseling, discipline, and termination. The court stated that management and the employees were under an obligation to follow the policies stated in the handbook. Because it was proved in court that the hospital violated the stated policy in the handbook when it terminated her, Watson won her suit. (*Watson v. Idaho Falls Consol. Hosp. Inc.,* 720 P.2d 632, Idaho 1986).

In another case, a Minnesota court held, in a wrongful discharge suit, that the hospital's employee handbook was clearly an employment contract. The handbook contained detailed statements on conduct and procedures for discipline, which the hospital violated when it fired the plaintiff (*Harvet v. Unity Medical Ctr.,* 428 N.W.2d 574, Minn. Ct. App. 1988). These cases indicate that the employee handbook must be carefully examined for any erroneous or misleading statements.

In addition, employees should be given opportunities to speak and present evidence in their own behalf. Employees should be allowed to see, comment on, or copy anything affecting them in written reviews and personnel file memos.

Questions	Legal/Illegal	
Age?	Legal to ask applicants if they are between the ages of 17 and 70, but *not* to ask their specific age. If their age falls outside these boundaries, then it is legal to ask their birth date.	**TABLE 8.2** **Legal and Illegal Questions**
Birthplace?	Legal, but inadvisable to ask where the applicants, their parents, spouse, or children were born. It is illegal to ask about their national heritage or nationality or that of their spouse.	
Address?	Legal to ask, along with how long the applicant has lived there.	
Married?	Legal to ask, but inadvisable.	
Maiden Name?	Illegal as this could indicate a marriage. May inquire if reference information (educational, employment, license) is under a different name.	
Children?	Illegal to ask. It is also illegal to ask any questions relating to childcare arrangements.	
Height and weight?	Illegal to ask unless it relates to the job requirements.	
Race or color?	Illegal to ask.	
Religion or creed?	Illegal to ask, but it is legal to ask if working on a particular day, such as a Saturday or Sunday, would interfere with applicant's religious practices.	
Ever been arrested?	Illegal to ask because an arrest does not indicate guilt. It *is* legal to ask if the applicant has ever been convicted of a crime or have any pending felony charges. For example, "Have you been convicted within the past year on drug-related charges?"	
Citizenship?	Legal to ask, "Are you a citizen of the United States?"	
Handicaps?	Illegal to ask if an applicant has a handicap or a disease. It is legal to ask if the applicant has any physical impairment that would affect his or her ability to do the job.	
Organizations you belong to?	Legal to ask applicants if they belong to any organizations. Illegal to ask about membership in any specific organization or to require applicants to list the organizations to which they belong.	
Languages?	Legal to ask what languages a person can speak or write. However, it can be perceived as discriminatory and a method to determine a person's national origin.	
Military experience?	Legal to ask if the person has been a member of the armed forces, type of training, and when discharged. Illegal to ask what type of discharge was received (honorable, dishonorable, medical, etc.)	

LEGAL AND ILLEGAL INTERVIEW QUESTIONS

The Equal Employment Opportunity Commission (EEOC) has strict guidelines on the types of questions that can be asked during a job interview. These questions have both ethical and legal considerations. Questions that may be interpreted as discriminatory cannot be asked. In some cases, a question may be legal but still inadvisable for an interviewer to ask. For example, while it is legal under the law to ask if an applicant is married, it is inadvisable because it may be discriminatory. Marriage has nothing to do with job performance. If an unmarried applicant is hired, a married applicant may believe that he or she was not given the job based on marital status. Table 8.2 ■ contains a list of questions you can and cannot ask during an interview.

MED TIP
It is important in a healthcare setting to make careful background checks—especially relating to drug use—before hiring an individual.

FEDERAL REGULATIONS AFFECTING THE MEDICAL PROFESSIONAL

Both state and federal laws regulate the employer (physician) and employee (staff) relationship. In some cases, local laws in a particular city or county may also regulate a medical practice. Therefore, healthcare facilities and medical practices must remain current on regulations affecting employment practices, such as health, safety, compensation, workers' compensation, unions, and discrimination laws. Generally, federal laws apply only to those businesses or organizations that employ a declared number of employees (such as 15, 20, 50 or more), and who work a minimum number of weeks in a period of a year. It is always wise to seek advice from legal counsel or a corporate attorney, if the organization has one on staff, concerning specific cases.

> **MED TIP**
>
> It is a widely accepted policy that all employees, whether working in the healthcare field or elsewhere, should receive time away from their workstation for a lunch break (1/2 hour) and two fifteen minutes breaks during an 8-hour work day. These breaks may be required as part of a union agreement if employees are unionized. These policies may be established in individual states by the Department of Labor.

In most situations, federal laws **preempt,** or overrule, state laws. However, there are some exceptions. One occurs when there is not a federal law relating to a topic, in which case the states can then regulate it. A second exception occurs if the court has already ruled that state law does not conflict with federal law, in which case the state law is enforced. Another exception is called a complete preemption, in which Congress prohibits states from regulating a particular area of law. An example of this is the Employment Retirement Income Security Act (ERISA), which is discussed later in this chapter.

The major categories of federal laws regulating the employer–employee relationships include equal employment opportunity and employment discrimination; employee health and safety; compensation and benefits regulations; consumer protection and collection practices; and federal labor acts. In discussing these regulations, many of the legal terms, such as a law and an act, are interchangeable. The cases discussed in this chapter illustrate the variety of lawsuits relating to these regulations.

> **MED TIP**
>
> Each state has its own individual state and local laws. Always determine the local laws that pertain to your particular area. Local county health departments are a good source of information.

EQUAL EMPLOYMENT OPPORTUNITY AND EMPLOYMENT DISCRIMINATION

The government regulates many aspects of the employment relationship, including laws affecting recruitment, placement, pay plans, benefits, penalties, and terminations. The basis of the law is that people must be judged primarily by their job performance. A discussion of these laws should be prefaced with a look at the historical doctrine of employment-at-will.

Employment-at-Will Concept

The common-law doctrine of employment-at-will has historically governed the employment relationship. **Employment-at-will,** in which there is *no* contract of employment, means that employment takes place at the will of either the employer or the employee. Thus, the employment may be terminated at will, without notice, at any time, and without a reason. Conversely, the employee may quit at any time. The exception to this occurs when there is a specific employment contract between the employer and employee, specifying the duration and terms of employment. Then the relationship *cannot* be terminated during the contract period. The only protection of an at-will employment is that employees cannot be fired for an illegal reason—for example, due to the color of their skin or their age.

This concept of termination for any reason without incurring liability had been widely accepted. However, employment-at-will has begun to lose favor. **Wrongful-discharge** lawsuits, in which the employee believes the employer does not have a **just cause,** or legal reason, for firing the employee, have become more common. An example of this occurs when the employer asks employees to perform procedures for which they are not trained or that are not within the scope of their license. Even if employers win a wrongful-discharge lawsuit, they may ultimately be the losers due to the negative publicity and effect on employee morale. See Table 8.3 ■ for a list of equal employment opportunity and employment discrimination laws.

Title VII of the Civil Rights Act of 1964 (1991)

Title VII of the Civil Rights Act prohibits **discrimination** (unfair or unequal treatment), in employment based on five criteria: race, color, religion, gender, or national origin. This strongly worded act means that employers may not refuse to hire, unlawfully discharge, or in any other way discriminate against employees based on these five criteria. This proposal, which came from the Kennedy administration, is considered one of the most important pieces of all legislation, as it affects employment opportunity and discrimination. This act applies to all organizations that have twenty or more employees working twenty weeks or more during a year.

Title VII affects all aspects of patient care in institutions that receive federal assistance, such as Medicare and Medicaid.

MED TIP

Some of the most frequent violations in the healthcare employment field are related to Title VII issues.

TABLE 8.3
Equal Employment Opportunity and Employment Discrimination Laws

▶ Title VII of the Civil Rights Act of 1964

▶ Civil Rights Act of 1991

▶ Equal Employment Opportunity Act (EEOA) of 1972

▶ Pregnancy Discrimination Act of 1978

▶ Age Discrimination in Employment Act (ADEA) of 1967

▶ Rehabilitation Act of 1973

▶ Americans with Disabilities Act of 1990

▶ National Labor Relations Act (NLRA) of 1935

The **Equal Employment Opportunity Commission (EEOC)** monitors Title VII, and the Justice Department enforces the statute. In some cases, the EEOC defers enforcement to local and state agencies. Employees must exhaust all administrative remedies offered from the EEOC before they can sue their employer under Title VII. The Equal Employment Opportunity Act, the Pregnancy Discrimination Act, and the Civil Rights Act of 1991 have further amended this act.

Title VII also makes sexual harassment a form of unlawful sex discrimination. Sexual harassment is defined as "unwelcome sexual advances, requests for sexual favors, and other verbal or physical conduct of a sexual nature." *Quid pro quo,* a Latin term meaning "something for something," occurs when one valuable thing, such as a sexual favor, is given in exchange for another thing, such as job advancement. An employee who quits a job because sexual harassment created an offensive or hostile work environment may sue the employer for damages.

Affirmative action programs to remedy discriminatory practices in hiring minority group members are also covered under Title VII. These programs, required by federal statute, require that positive steps, such as hiring minority personnel, be taken to remedy past discrimination and to take steps to prevent future discrimination. Courts may mandate that affirmative action programs be implemented if there is evidence that an employer has intentionally discriminated against a particular minority group.

Who Is an Employee Under Title VII?

Title VII only prohibits employers from discriminating against employees. If an employer withholds employment taxes from a person's income, then that person is considered an employee. While some cases are less clear, in general, if the employer can control the details of that person's work then the person is considered to be an employee. In some cases, physicians who have lost medical staff memberships and thus hospital admitting privileges, have been able to sue the hospital under Title VII. An example of this is a federal case in which Dr. Pardazi sued the Cullman Medical Center. The federal case was tried in the 11th Circuit Court, and Title VII was the federal law that won the case for Pardazi (*Pardazi v. Cullman Med. Ct.,* 838 F.2d 1155, 11th Cir. 1988).

Who Is an Employer Under Title VII?

A person who employs the services of another and provides payment for those services is considered an employer. In addition, an employer has the right to control the physical conduct of the employee in performing the service. The statute does not apply to independent contractors. A coworker is not an employer and, thus, is not liable under Title VII. The courts have also found that a parent company of the employer is not liable as the employer under Title VII (*Garcia v. Elf Atochem,* N. Am., 28 F.3d 446, 5th Cir. 1994).

Civil Rights Act of 1991

Congress amended Title VII by passing the Civil Rights Act of 1991. Wrongful discharge suits fall under this law. The **Civil Rights Act** permits the court to award both compensatory damages (for the loss of income or emotional pain and suffering) and punitive damages (to punish the defendant) to mistreated employees. Prior to this amendment, only compensatory damages were awarded.

Title VII provides that a hospital must treat physicians, nurses, other employees, and patients in a nondiscriminatory manner. It also prohibits hospital employees, such as nurses, from discriminating against patients, physicians, or fellow employees. In *Simkins v. Moses H. Cone Hospital,* a federal court held that two hospitals were prohibited from denying physicians appointments to the hospital staff on the basis of race. The court also prohibited these hospitals from refusing to admit patients or segregate patients on the basis of race. (*Simkins v. Moses H. Cone Hospital*, 323 F.2d 959, 4th Cir. 1963).

Equal Employment Opportunity Act (EEOA) of 1972

The Equal Employment Opportunity Act (EEOA) authorizes the Equal Employment Opportunity Commission (EEOC) to sue employers in federal court on behalf of a class of people or an individual whose rights under Title VII have been violated.

Pregnancy Discrimination Act of 1978

Under the **Pregnancy Discrimination Act,** employers must treat pregnant women as they would any other employee, providing they can still do the job. This act has saved jobs for women and allowed them to advance even if they became pregnant or had to take a short leave for childbirth. An employer cannot force a woman to quit her job because she is pregnant. In addition, under this law, a woman cannot be refused a job because she has had an abortion. The pregnant woman is assured of equal treatment in such areas as disability, sick leave, and health insurance. The employer's medical plan must cover pregnancy in the same way it would cover other medical conditions. If the worker is unable to work because of the pregnancy, then she qualifies for sick leave on the same basis as all the other employees.

If the employer offers employee leaves for disabilities, then a similar leave must be offered for pregnancy. Mandatory maternity leaves violate Title VII, because the Pregnancy Discrimination Act of 1978 is an amendment to that statute. In addition, the employer's health plan must provide coverage for the dependent spouses of employees.

A federal district court found that a hospital had violated the Pregnancy Discrimination Act when it fired an x-ray technician upon learning that she was pregnant. The court felt that while it was necessary for the x-ray technician to avoid working in some areas of the x-ray department due to her condition, there were less discriminatory alternatives that the hospital could have used (*Hayes v. Shelby Memorial Hosp.,* 726 F.2d 1543, 11th Cir. 1984).

This statute has many aspects that require special considerations. For instance, one federal court held that an employee who had job absences due to infertility treatments was not protected under this act (*Zatarain v. WDSU-Television, Inc.,* WI 16777 E.D.La. 1995). In a 1994 case, a federal appellate court ruled that a pregnant home-health nurse who refused to treat an AIDS patient could be discharged under this statute (*Armstrong v. Flowers Hosp.,* 33 F.3d 1308, 11th Cir. 1994).

Age Discrimination in Employment Act (ADEA) of 1967

The **Age Discrimination in Employment Act** protects persons 40 years or older against employment discrimination because of age. This law applies to employers who have twenty or more persons working for them. The employer will not be liable for violation of this law if there are extenuating circumstances, such as if the person does not have the ability to perform the job. If two people are up for hiring or a promotion and one of them is over 40, then the employer must be able to show (in writing) why the younger person, if hired or promoted, is more qualified. Education and performance, in addition to other factors, count toward qualification. Mandatory retirement is prohibited under this law except for certain exempt executives.

> ## MED TIP
>
> Note that women and men over forty are protected by both Title VII and this act.

Employers must be cautious about what they say or put into writing in the event that they must terminate a person's employment. For example, in a 1985 age discrimination suit, a 62-year-old supervisor nurse resigned and then sued the hospital because its administration had told her "new blood" was needed and made comments about her "advanced age." She believed these statements made working conditions intolerable. The nurse supervisor won the suit (*Buckley v. Hospital Corp. of America, Inc.*, 758 F.2d 1525, 11th Cir. 1985).

Rehabilitation Act of 1973

The **Rehabilitation Act** prohibits employment discrimination of the handicapped. This act prohibits discrimination based on disability in any institution that receives federal financial assistance. Therefore, a hospital or agency that receives Medicare and Medicaid reimbursement must comply with this law. However, courts have held in favor of plaintiffs, such as hospitals and nursing homes, that are not equipped to care for a special-needs patient such as a violent or aggressive patient who abuses the staff (*Grubbs v. Medical Facilities of America, Inc.*, 879 F. Supp. W.D., Va. 1995).

This act had a major influence on the Americans with Disabilities Act of 1990 because it included a very broad definition of "handicapped." It included people with physical or mental impairment, someone who has had an impairment, and someone who currently has an impairment. This definition protected people with a recognizable handicap, such as a physical handicap, and opened many doors for people with handicaps such as mental disorders who were formerly forgotten. In addition, this law was the beginning of a legal means for people to challenge their denial of employment for physical or mental reasons.

Americans with Disabilities Act (ADA) of 1990

There are 43 million disabled persons in the United States. The **Americans with Disabilities Act (ADA)** prohibits employers who have more than fifteen employees from discriminating against such individuals. Persons with Acquired Immune Deficiency Syndrome (AIDS) are also covered under this act. In order to comply with this act, the employer must make reasonable accommodations, such as lowering telephones, installing ramps, and making elevator floor numbers accessible to wheelchair-bound persons. The exception to this occurs if the accommodations would be an undue hardship for the employer, such as the significant difficulty of installing an elevator in an old building. The term *undue hardship* has caused problems, as there is no clear definition of the term *hardship* or a dollar amount that constitutes hardship. There is a two-year implementation window for employers who must comply with this law. Patients, as well as employees, are also protected under this statute.

Private physicians can be held liable under the ADA for acts that take place in their offices. For example, in 1995 a federal appellate court upheld a lower court decision that an HIV-positive patient could sue his primary care physician for allegedly failing to treat or refer him to another physician (*Woolfolk v. Duncan*, 872 F. Supp. 1381, E.D. Pa. 1995).

In *Tugg v. Towney,* a federal court ruled that the ADA requires a state to provide counselors who use sign language to counsel deaf patients in state mental facilities. According to the court, the facility did not satisfy the ADA statute by merely providing mental health services through the use of interpreters (*Tugg v. Towney,* 864 F. Supp. 1201, S.D. Fla. 1994).

Basic accommodations that can be made for persons with disabilities include:

▶ Parking spaces, clearly marked for the handicapped, near an accessible doorway.

▶ Inclined ramps into buildings or over curbs in parking lots.

▶ Elevator floor numbers that are accessible to wheelchair-bound patients and employees.

▶ Handicap accessible bathrooms with handrails.

▶ Hallways with at least 36 inches of clearance for wheelchairs.

▶ Desks and counters that accommodate a wheelchair.

▶ Telephone adapters for the hearing impaired.

Figure 8.1 ■ shows a sign language teacher with a child who has a hearing impairment.

The National Labor Relations Act of 1935

This act, also called the Wagner Act, established some of the most basic union rights. The **National Labor Relations Act** prohibits employer actions, such as attempting to force employees to stay out of unions, and labels these actions as "unfair labor practices." This act set up the National Labor Relations Board (NLRB) to enforce these labor laws.

See Table 8.4 ■ for a list of employee health and safety laws.

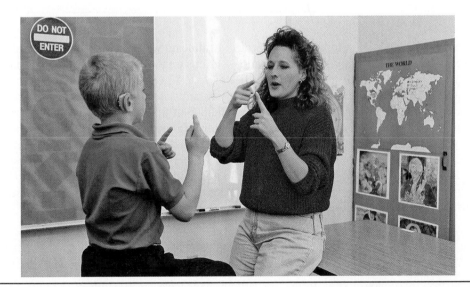

FIGURE 8.1
Sign Language Teacher with a Child who has a Hearing Impairment

(Trevor Baker/Baker Consulting & Design)

TABLE 8.4	
Employee Health and Safety Laws	▶ Occupational Safety and Health Act (OSHA) of 1970
	▶ Clinical Laboratory Improvement Act (CLIA) of 1988
	▶ Health Maintenance Organization (HMO) Act of 1973
	▶ Consolidated Omnibus Budget Reconciliation Act (COBRA) of 1985
	▶ Drug-Free Workplace Act of 1988

EMPLOYEE HEALTH AND SAFETY

Both state and federal laws regulate issues affecting an employee's health and safety. While the state law may be stricter than the federal law, it cannot be more lenient.

Occupational Safety and Health Act (OSHA) of 1970

Under the **Occupational Safety and Health Act (OSHA)**, an employer is required by law to provide a safe and healthy work environment: the employer must protect the worker against hazards. OSHA regulations preempt all other state and local regulations regarding employee safety and health, meaning that states may *not* pass any laws concerning the working environment. In addition, there are **right-to-know laws** in many states which give employees access to workplace safety information such as the use of hazardous or toxic substances.

Employers and office managers should become familiar with OSHA regulations as they apply to their specific fields, not only to protect employees but also to avoid fines for OSHA violations, which can be severe. In addition, the poor publicity and public relations resulting from a serious OSHA violation can damage an office or company's reputation.

MED TIP

It is better to err on the side of being too cautious when implementing OSHA regulations, rather than being too casual.

In 1991, OSHA developed rules to protect healthcare workers from bloodborne diseases. These are known as OSHA Occupational Exposure to Bloodborne Pathogens Standards. OSHA also established severe penalties of up to $7,000 for each violation of these standards by employers. These standards apply to any employee who has occupational exposure, which is defined as a reasonable anticipation that the employee's duties will result in skin, mucous membrane, eye, or **parenteral** (a medication route other than rectal or oral) contact with **bloodborne pathogens** (disease-producing microorganisms) or other potentialy infectious material. Healthcare workers, including physicians, nurses, medical assistants, laboratory workers, and housekeeping personnel, have occupational exposure. The OSHA standards mandate that each employee with occupational exposure must be offered the hepatitis B vaccination at the expense of the employer.

MED TIP

Note that an employee may decline, in writing, to receive the hepatitis B vaccine. See Table 8.5 ■ for a list of potentialy infectious materials.

▶ Body fluid, including semen, amniotic fluid, pleural fluid, and cerebrospinal fluid contaminated with blood ▶ Saliva in dental procedures ▶ Vaginal secretions ▶ Tissues, cells, or fluids known to be HIV-infected ▶ Microbiological waste (kits or inoculated culture media) ▶ Pathologic waste (human tissue) ▶ Any unidentified body fluid	**TABLE 8.5** **List of Potentialy Infectious Materials**

The OSHA standards refer to urine, stool, sputum, nasal secretions, vomitus, and sweat only if there is visible evidence of blood. The OSHA compliance checklist for medical facilities and offices includes: eyewash stations, fire extinguishers, first-aid kits, written training programs, labels for chemical and hazardous waste, sharps containers, exit signs, spill kits, accident report forms, and chemical inventory lists.

MED TIP

In a medical workplace, additional safety issues may arise that are not found elsewhere, including protecting individuals against bloodborne pathogens.

The Hazard Communication Standard (HCS) from OSHA is meant to reduce injuries and illnesses in the workforce by alerting healthcare employees to potential dangers and risks when using hazardous chemicals and materials. Material Safety Data Sheets (MSDS) must be posted wherever hazardous materials are used. Employees are instructed to read the sheets and know how to handle all hazardous products, such as blood and chemicals.

MED TIP

OSHA guidelines are available from the U.S. Department of Labor, Washington, DC.

▶ Evaluate the effectiveness of the laboratory's policies and procedures. ▶ Identify and correct problems. ▶ Ensure the competence and adequacy of staff. ▶ Take corrective action if errors are found. ▶ Integrate corrective procedures into future policies and procedures. ▶ Document employee training and assess competency after the first year. ▶ Maintain the identity and integrity of patient samples during the entire testing process. ▶ Laboratory is subject to inspection every two years if performing moderate or high complexity tests.	**TABLE 8.6** **List of CLIA Laboratory Requirements**

Clinical Laboratory Improvement Act (CLIA) of 1988

The federal government now requires that all clinical laboratories that test human specimens must be controlled. The **Clinical Laboratories Improvement Act (CLIA)**, establishing minimum quality standards for laboratories, has been amended several times. The CLIA 1992 standards mandate that there must be written policies and procedures for a comprehensive quality assurance program that will evaluate the overall ongoing quality of the testing process. See Table 8.6 ■ for a list of CLIA laboratory requirements. (See Figure 8.2 ■ Laboratory technicians at work.)

CLIA testing regulations are mandated for most tests conducted in laboratories. However, there are certain tests that are waived if they are simple to run, almost foolproof, and if an erroneous result would not result in a negative impact on the patient. The Food and Drug Administration (FDA) has the responsibility for categorizing the tests and allowing the waiver (exemption) of testing. In general, tests approved by the FDA for home use are usually waived, although the manufacturer must request the waiver. Tests that require a microscope, calculations, or a judgment call are not waived and must meet CLIA standards. It is always advisable to search the CLIA website at www.hcfa.gov/medicaid/clia and www.cola.org for a complete list of waived tests. If the laboratory test is not on this list then it is not waived and must meet all CLIA requirements.

Health Maintenance Organization (HMO) Act of 1973

The Health Maintenance Organization Act (HMO) requires any company with at least twenty-five employees to provide an HMO alternative to regular group insurance for their employees if an HMO is available in the area.

Many new HMOs were formed in response to this law. HMOs have been able to cut healthcare costs in some areas by focusing on wellness such as well-baby physicals and mammograms. Under an HMO, the patient does not have the same wide choice of doctors as under a traditional healthcare plan. In addition, a patient may have to get a second opinion and permission from the HMO before having a major procedure performed.

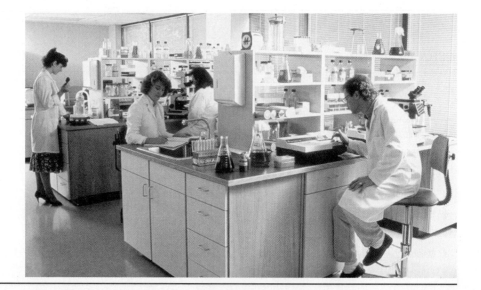

FIGURE 8.2
Laboratory Technologists

Consolidated Omnibus Budget Reconciliation Act (COBRA) of 1985

The **Consolidated Omnibus Budget Reconciliation Act (COBRA)** is an important act that covers a wide range of federal government financing for health insurance coverage continuation *after* an employee has been laid off or left a job.

Millions of Americans are left without any healthcare coverage, many due to job loss. COBRA has helped to decrease this number of uncovered Americans. Under COBRA, a company with twenty or more employees must provide extended healthcare insurance to terminated employees for as long as eighteen months—usually, but not always, at the employee's expense. This insurance may be costly, but some people would be unable to obtain insurance any other way. COBRA has enforcement power as all federal funding may be lost for noncompliance.

COBRA also contains an amendment called EMTALA (Emergency Medical Treatment and Active Labor Act) which prohibits "patient dumping" from one hospital to another if the patient does not have health insurance. EMTALA is more fully discussed later in the chapter.

Drug-Free Workplace Act of 1988

Employers have become increasingly aware of how expensive drug-using employees are in terms of decreased productivity, workplace accidents, and increased healthcare costs. Even under the best security conditions, the nature of some healthcare organizations, such as hospitals, medical offices, and clinics, allows for employee access to various drugs.

MED TIP

To prevent drug abuse, some organizations, such as hospitals, require drug testing as a condition of employment.

Under the **Drug-Free Workplace Act,** employers contracting to provide goods or services to the federal government must certify that they maintain a drug-free workplace. The employer must inform the employee of the intent to maintain a drug-free workplace and of any penalties, such as discharge, that the employee would incur for violation of the policy.

COMPENSATION AND BENEFITS REGULATIONS

These laws influence the compensation (salary) and benefits provided to employees. See Table 8.7 ■ for a listing of compensation and benefits laws.

Social Security Act of 1935

The **Social Security Act** is a federal law that covers all private and most public sector employees. This act laid the groundwork for unemployment compensation in the United States. Social Security is paid by the employer and the employee in equal payroll taxes and Medicare participant premiums. Social Security is composed of several different, but related, programs: retirement, disability, dependent and survivor's benefits, as well as health benefits under Medicare. The amount paid to the retiree or disabled or dependent survivor is calculated based on the worker's average wages earned during his or her working life.

TABLE 8.7	▶ Social Security Act of 1935
Compensation and Benefits Laws	▶ Fair Labor Standards Act (FLSA) of 1938
	▶ Equal Pay Act of 1963
	▶ Unemployment Compensation
	▶ Federal Insurance Contribution Act (FICA) of 1935
	▶ Workers' Compensation Act
	▶ Employee Retirement Income Security Act (ERISA) of 1974
	▶ Family and Medical Leave Act (FMLA) of 1994

Fair Labor Standards Act (FLSA) of 1938

This is the main statute regulating employee benefits. The **Fair Labor Standards Act (FLSA)** establishes the minimum wage, requires payment for overtime work, and sets the maximum hours employees covered by the act may work. The act covers all nonmanagement employees in both for-profit and not-for-profit institutions.

The employer must pay one and one-half times the regular hourly pay rate for any work the employee performs over forty hours in a seven-day (one-week) period. FLSA uses the single workweek to compute the hours of overtime. The law does not permit averaging hours over two or more weeks. Thus, an employee who works thirty-five hours one week and forty-five hours the next—for a weekly average of 40 hours for the two weeks—must still be paid the overtime rate for five hours.

One exception allows hospitals to negotiate an agreement with their employees to establish a work period of fourteen days. In this case, overtime pay would go into effect for employees who work more than eighty hours in the fourteen-day period. It is also acceptable to require fewer than forty hours a week to qualify for overtime payment or a higher rate than one and one-half times the regular hourly pay, but the employer cannot require more hours or pay less than the law requires.

This law affects only full-time hourly employees. Some workers, such as management or salaried employees, are exempt from the minimum wage and overtime requirement of the FLSA. In addition, part-time employees and employees who are part of a time-sharing program generally do not benefit from this law.

Equal Pay Act of 1963

The **Equal Pay Act,** an amendment to the Fair Labor Standards Act (FLSA), makes it illegal for an employer to discriminate on the basis of gender in the payment to men and women who are performing the same job. Equal work means work that requires equal skill, responsibility, and effort under the same or similar working conditions. For example, male orderlies cannot be paid more than female orderlies (*Odomes v. Nucare,* Inc., 653 F.2d 6th Cir. 1981).

MED TIP

Employees generally "earn" a certain number of paid sick days per year based on the number of hours worked. These can be saved up and used when the employee has to take time off for an illness or surgery. Sick days are *not* part of earned vacation days. In general, they cannot be used except for sickness.

Unemployment Compensation

The Social Security Act was the origin of this insurance program. Today, employers pay taxes into a state unemployment compensation plan that covers employees who are unable to work through no fault of their own. The **unemployment compensation** laws provide for temporary weekly payments for the unemployed worker. State unemployment compensation insurance taxes for individual employers vary from state to state according to state laws and the turnover experience of the business.

In order to receive unemployment insurance, the employee must have worked for an employer who has paid, or was required to pay, unemployment compensation taxes. However, certain types of employers are exempt, such as employers for religious, educational, or charitable organizations; employers for small farming operations; employers of family members; and employers who use federal government labor.

While state unemployment insurance law provides temporary payments for those who lose their jobs, if an employee is fired for good cause, the employee is not entitled to unemployment benefits. In the case of *Love v. Heritage House Convalescent Center,* the court found that a nursing assistant was properly denied unemployment benefits because she was terminated for poor work attendance. According to the employee's personnel record, the convalescent center had already shown great tolerance in allowing the employee to continue working as long as it had (*Love v. Heritage House Convalescent Ctr.,* 463 N.E.2d 478, Ind. Ct. App. 1983).

Unemployment compensation was also denied in a case in which a nurse's aide was discharged for leaving a resident unattended and unrestrained on a commode and for using the medication of one patient (a medicated cream) on another patient (*Starks v. Director of Div. of Employment Section,* 462 N.E.2d 1360, Mass. 1984).

Federal Insurance Contribution Act (FICA) of 1935

The **Federal Insurance Contribution Act** is the oldest act relating to compensation. Under FICA, employers are required to contribute to Social Security plans for their employees. There is a severe fine if the payment by the employer is not made on time. This act also requires detailed record keeping documenting the employer's payment. The key to the proper implementation of this act is to hire a trusted office manager.

Workers' Compensation Act

The **Workers' Compensation Act** protects workers and their families from financial problems resulting from employment-related injury, disease, and even death. Under the law, employers typically pay into a fund to help cover costs when an employee is hurt or sustains an injury arising in the course of employment. Examples include a back injury, or a work-related disease, such as carpal tunnel syndrome from improper or prolonged computer keyboard usage.

The goal of workers' compensation is to get the employee back to work as soon as possible. COBRA may allow for a retraining opportunity if the injury results in permanent inability to work in the same job. If there is a health problem within the first three months of employment on a new job, the previous employer may have to pay the workers' compensation, as most of the benefits were paid into the employee's fund by that employer. Some medical practices only handle patients with workers' compensation injuries. Workers' compensation programs are administered at the state level with no federal involvement or mandatory standards.

Under the Workers' Compensation Act, an employee must submit a written notice of the injury to the employer. Generally, an employee will receive only a partial salary, such as two-thirds of salary, as compensation.

Workers' compensation benefits are generally available even if the employee is at fault for his or her injury, but an employee who has violated hospital policy is not eligible to receive benefits. In *Fair v. St. Joseph's Hospital,* the hospital employee was disqualified from receiving compensation because he violated the policy by fighting with a co-worker (*Fair v. St. Joseph's Hosp.,* 437 S.E.2d 875, N.C. App. 1933).

Even if an employee is covered by workers' compensation, the employee may still sue and recover for injuries caused by nonemployees. For example, in a 1994 case in California, a psychiatric nurse sued a psychiatric patient who kicked her in the abdomen, causing injury to her unborn child. The court ruled that the workers' compensation law did not bar this lawsuit (*Agnew-Watson v. County of Alameda,* 36 Cal. Rptr. 2nd 196, CT. App. Cal. 1994).

Employee Retirement Income Security Act (ERISA) of 1974

The **Employee Retirement Income Security Act (ERISA)** regulates employee benefits and pension plans. Prior to the passage of ERISA, widespread abuse of pension plans led to their collapse, leaving retired employees without the pension benefits their companies had promised. ERISA responded to this problem by requiring employers to put aside money that can be used only to pay future benefits. ERISA also guarantees vesting of pension plans.

Vesting refers to a certain point in time; such as after ten years of employment, when an employee has the right to receive benefits from a retirement plan. Under ERISA, employees who stay with a company for ten years are entitled to 50 percent of the employer's retirement plan even if they leave the company and take another job. The employee is entitled to 100 percent of the employer's pension contribution after fifteen years of employment, when he or she becomes fully vested. In some cases in the past, employees had been laid off just before they become vested. ERISA now prohibits this practice.

Family and Medical Leave Act (FMLA) of 1994

The **Family and Medical Leave Act (FMLA)** allows both the mother and father to take a leave of absence of up to twelve weeks, in any twelve-month period, when a baby is born. The employee's job, or an equivalent position, must be available when he or she returns to work. In almost all cases, the leave is without pay. The FMLA also requires employers to provide unpaid leave for up to twelve weeks to employees who request leave for their own or a family member's medical or family-related situation, such as birth, death, or adoption.

The company must maintain the employee's health coverage while the employee is on a family medical leave. The employee must be returned to the original or equivalent position he or she held before going on the leave. In addition, there cannot be any loss of employment benefits that accumulated prior to the start of the leave.

CONSUMER PROTECTION AND COLLECTION PRACTICES

The consumer protection and practices laws serve to protect the consumer from unfair practices. See Table 8.8 ■ for a listing of these laws.

> ▶ Emergency Medical Treatment and Active Labor Act (EMTALA)
> ▶ Fair Credit Reporting Act of 1971
> ▶ Equal Credit Opportunity Act of 1975
> ▶ Truth in Lending Act (Regulation Z) of 1969
> ▶ Fair Debt Collection Practices Act of 1978
> ▶ Federal Wage Garnishment Law of 1970

TABLE 8.8

Protection and Collection Practices

Emergency Medical Treatment and Active Labor Act (EMTALA)

The **Emergency Medical Treatment and Active Labor Act (EMTALA)** is a section of the Consolidated Omnibus Budget Reconciliation Act (COBRA) dealing with **patient dumping,** a slang term for transferring emergency patients from one hospital to another if the patient does not have health insurance or is unable to pay for services.

Patients entering a hospital emergency room must now be stabilized before they can be transferred to another facility. If the patient cannot be stabilized then he or she can be transferred to a regional trauma center without incurring an EMTALA violation. According to this law, if a hospital is reported for patient dumping, the person doing the reporting (the whistleblower) may not be penalized. The government may impose stiff fines and even terminate Medicare agreements if the hospital is determined to have violated EMTALA. In addition, the patient can also sue the hospital. A physician may also be at risk for legal action if he or she misrepresents the patient's condition. However, EMTALA does not apply to health maintenance organizations, private clinics, or private physicians' offices. The practice of patient dumping has significantly diminished since the passage of EMTALA.

Fair Credit Reporting Act of 1971

The **Fair Credit Reporting Act** establishes guidelines for use of an individual's credit information. If a patient has been denied credit based on a poor rating from a credit agency, the patient must be notified of this fact and given the name and address of the reporting agency. The agency must disclose the credit information to the consumer, who may correct and update this information.

Equal Credit Opportunity Act of 1975

The **Equal Credit Opportunity Act** prohibits businesses, including hospitals and medical offices, from granting credit based on the applicant's race or gender—unfair treatment referred to as discrimination. This law mandates that women and minorities must be issued credit if they qualify for it, based on the premise that if credit is given to one person, it should be given to all persons who request it and are qualified.

Truth in Lending Act (Regulation Z) of 1969

The **Truth in Lending Act (Regulation Z)** requires a full written disclosure about interest rates or finance charges concerning the payment of any fee that will be collected in more than four installments. This is also called Regulation Z of the Consumer Protection Act. Installment payments are often used for orthodontia, obstetrical care, and surgical treatment. It is legal to include a finance charge if a patient pays the bill in installments. However, few physicians and dentists require this charge.

Fair Debt Collection Practices Act of 1978

The **Fair Debt Collections Practices Act** prohibits unfair collection practices by creditors (institutions or persons who are owed money). For example, the Federal Communications Commission (FCC) has issued guidelines for the specific times that credit collection phone calls can be made. It also prohibits telephone harassment and threats. Under this law, telephone calls for purposes of collections must be made between the hours of 8:00 A.M. and 9:00 P.M., with no weekend calls (Figure 8.3 ■).

Table 8.9 ■ provides some guidelines for collection efforts.

Using a Collection Agency

Medical offices and hospitals would not be able to remain in business if patients didn't pay their bills for medical care. However, fair collection practices must be honored.

Professional collection agencies are available when all other attempts to collect unpaid bills fail. The account should always be reviewed with the physician or head of the medical practice before turning it over for collection.

Once the patient is told the account is going to a collection agency, it must, by law, go. After the account has been turned over, no further collection attempts can be made by the physician's office or hospital—that would be considered harassment. If the patient should contact the office or hospital after the account has been turned over for collection, the patient should be referred to the collection agency.

MED TIP

Personnel involved in the billing and collections operations of any facility must have a full understanding of the laws regulating the collection process.

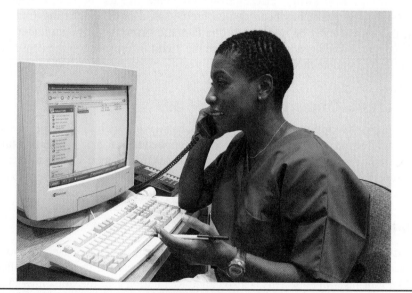

FIGURE 8.3
Collection Calls Are Made Between 8:00 A.M. and 9:00 P.M.

TABLE 8.9

Guidelines for Collection Efforts

1. Establish policies and procedures relating to collections and instruct all staff on these procedures.

2. Have a list of the established fees available for patients and staff.

3. Discuss the fee, and when the fee is due, with the patient prior to treatment.

4. Prepare written material for patients that includes general information about the office, such as office hours and emergency numbers to call when the office or facility is closed. Include information about the billing process and how insurance claims are handled.

5. Request payment, whenever possible, before the patient leaves the office or healthcare facility.

6. Be consistent in all billing practices. This includes sending statements to arrive on the first of each month and sending a follow-up letter on delinquent accounts when they reach a certain date, such as one month overdue.

7. Use care when making telephone collection calls:

   a. Always be courteous when speaking to patients.

   b. Always introduce yourself. Make sure the patient understands the reason for the call. Do not misrepresent yourself by implying you are someone other than who you are.

   c. Make all calls on weekdays between 8:00 A.M. and 9:00 P.M., observing the time difference for patients living in another time zone.

   d. Protect the patient's privacy. Carefully identify the person accepting the telephone call. Do not discuss a delinquent account with anyone except the patient (debtor). Do not leave a message on a telephone answering machine.

   e. Never threaten an action that you do not intend to take. For example, do not tell the patient that the account will be handed over to a collection agency if payment is not received by this afternoon.

   f. Try to establish a payment plan to get a commitment from the patient on when a full or partial payment can be made.

   g. Do not harass, threaten, or intimidate the patient (debtor).

Bankruptcy

When patients become unable to pay their debts, they may file for bankruptcy. Bankruptcy is a legal method for providing some protection to individual **debtors** who owe money by establishing a fair method for distribution of the debtor's assets to all the creditors. If a patient files for bankruptcy, a court-appointed trustee may place the patient's assets in a special fund. The trustee then distributes the funds according to a predetermined method. Once a debtor files for bankruptcy a **creditor,** to whom money is owed, such as a physician who has an outstanding debt owed by the patient, may no longer seek payment from the patient but must instead file a claim in bankruptcy court at a later date.

MED TIP

A creditor who fails to comply with bankruptcy laws, such as by harassing the debtor, can be cited for contempt of court.

Federal Wage Garnishment Law of 1970

Garnishment refers to a court order that requires an employer to pay a portion of an employee's paycheck directly to one of the employee's creditors until the debt is resolved. **The Federal Wage Garnishment Law** restricts the amount of the paycheck that can be used to pay off a debt.

Claims against Estates

When a patient dies, a bill should be sent to the estate of the deceased. It is important to follow up with the collection of bills to prevent the impression that the physician was at fault in the patient's death. There is generally a specific time limit allowed when filing a claim against an estate. The probate department of the superior court in the county that is handling the estate can provide information on the time limits and also the name of the administrator of the estate.

The Statute of Limitations

This statute defines how long a medical practice has to file suit to collect on a past-due account. Because the time limit varies from state to state, an attorney should be consulted to determine the particular state's law. If an aging account is more than three years old, the creditor should investigate the state's statute of limitations before spending time, effort, and money to collect the debt. Because there is a statute of limitations on collecting a debt, it is important to attempt any debt collection as soon as possible.

POINTS TO PONDER

1. Why did the federal government enact laws such as Title VII, the ADA, and COBRA?

2. How do you respond to an illegal interview question?

3. Isn't it important for an employer to know if a potential employee has a disability? Why or why not?

4. Should all healthcare employees be tested for HIV? Why or why not?

5. In your opinion, does the Family and Medical Leave Act of 1994 discriminate against working persons who do *not* have children or elderly parents?

6. Are you entitled to take off a couple of days to re-energize yourself if you do not use up all of your sick days during the year?

DISCUSSION QUESTIONS

1. Identify the principal kinds of illegal discrimination that result in unequal employment opportunities.

2. What amendments to Title VII are discussed within this chapter?

3. What are considered potentialy infectious materials under OSHA guidelines?

4. What regulation assists terminated employees in obtaining extended healthcare coverage?

5. What does the Fair Labor Standards Act of 1938 control?

6. Who is eligible to receive a leave of absence under the Family and Medical Leave Act of 1994?

7. What does ERISA control?

REVIEW CHALLENGE

Short Answer Questions

1. What does the statement "a need to know" mean to you?

2. What do the initials EMTALA stand for and who does this law protect?

3. As a healthcare worker, is it legal for your employer to ask you to provide a urine sample for a drug test? Why or why not?

4. Under what federal regulation(s) are deaf children offered interpreters?

5. Give examples of efficiency and effectiveness. Why is effectiveness more important?

6. What does the term "just cause" mean?

7. What are six illegal interview questions?

8. Under what federal law must an employer provide a healthy and safe work place?

Matching

Match the responses in column B with the correct term in column A.

Column A

_____ 1. creditor
_____ 2. preempt
_____ 3. vesting
_____ 4. discrimination
_____ 5. just cause
_____ 6. employment-at-will
_____ 7. OSHA
_____ 8. ADA
_____ 9. Title VII
_____ 10. debtor

Column B

a. Civil Rights Act of 1964
b. Occupational Safety and Health Act
c. having a legal reason
d. overrule
e. one who owes money to another
f. to whom a debt is owed
g. unfair treatment
h. employee gains the rights to receive benefits
i. Americans with Disabilities Act of 1990
j. employment can be terminated

Multiple Choice

Select the one best answer to the following statements.

1. In most cases, federal laws
   a. are better than state laws.
   b. are not followed as closely as state laws.
   c. preempt state laws.
   d. are used when state laws are not effective.
   e. none of the above.

2. Title VII of the Civil Rights Act of 1964 prohibits discrimination based on
   a. color, race, and national origin.
   b. religion.
   c. gender.
   d. income level and education.
   e. a, b, and c only.

3. The following acts are covered as amendments under Title VII with the exception of the
   a. Pregnancy Discrimination Act of 1978.
   b. Drug-Free Workplace Act of 1988.
   c. Equal Employment Opportunity Act of 1972.
   d. Civil Rights Act of 1991.
   e. Age Discrimination in Employment Act of 1967.

4. The Occupational Safety and Health Act (OSHA) developed standards in 1991 stating that infectious materials include
   a. any unidentified body fluid.
   b. amniotic fluid.
   c. saliva in dental procedures.
   d. cerebrospinal fluid.
   e. all of the above.

5. The most important act covered under compensation and benefits regulations is said to be the
   a. Workers' Compensation Act.
   b. Social Security Act of 1935.
   c. Federal Insurance Contribution Act of 1935.
   d. Fair Labor Standards Act.
   e. Family and Medical Leave Act of 1994.

6. Regulation Z of the Consumer Protection Act is also referred to as
   a. Equal Credit Opportunity Act of 1975.
   b. Fair Credit Reporting Act of 1971.
   c. Truth in Lending Act of 1969.
   d. Employee Retirement Income Security Act of 1974.
   e. Workers' Compensation Act.

7. When making a claim for payment after a patient has died, the claim (or bill) must be
   a. sent in the name of the deceased person to his or her last known address.
   b. sent to the administrator of the estate of the deceased person.
   c. sent to a collection agency with specific instructions to collect the payment from the next of kin.
   d. waived.
   e. none of the above.

8. When using a collection agency to collect outstanding debts (unpaid bills) from a patient,
   a. allow the collection agency to take a tough, aggressive attitude with patients who owe money.
   b. stay closely involved in the process and make frequent follow-up phone calls to the delinquent patient.
   c. it is wise to first threaten the patient that you will send the unpaid account to a collection agency and then give the patient a second chance.
   d. review the delinquent account with the physician or office manager before turning over the account to the agency.
   e. all of the above.

9. ERISA
   a. controls employee benefit plans.
   b. controls employee pension plans.
   c. determines eligibility.
   d. determines vesting.
   e. all of the above.

10. Under the Workers' Compensation Act,
    a. employers must pay into a fund to help cover costs when an employee is hurt.
    b. the previous employer never has to pay for Workmen's Compensation.
    c. Workers' Compensation is only administered at the federal level.
    d. employees may not sue nonemployees.
    e. there is a guarantee of receiving a full salary while on workers' compensation.

DISCUSSION CASES

1. Analyze *"The Case of Janet K. and Epilepsy"* (found at the beginning of the chapter) using the Three-step Ethics Model (Blanchard-Peale model found in Chapter 1).

   a.
   _____
   _____

   b.
   _____
   _____

   c.
   _____
   _____

2. *You and your friend Rob both work as technologists in the Medical Imaging Department of the local community hospital. The department is short staffed and Rob agreed to work extra shifts during the past week to help out. He tells you, "Now I'm taking two days off as sick days. I've earned them and I need the rest."*

   a. Can your friend use his sick days for this purpose?
   _____
   _____

   b. What is your advice to Rob?
   _____
   _____

   c. Do you need to do anything else?
   _____
   _____

3. *Nancy Moore, a registered nurse, is assisting Dr. Brown while he performs a minor surgical procedure. Dr. Brown is known to have a quick temper, and he becomes very angry if a surgical procedure is delayed for any reason. As Nancy is handing a needle with suture thread to Dr. Brown, she feels a slight prick in her sterile gloves. She tells Dr. Brown about this and explains that she will have to be excused from the procedure for a few minutes while she changes gloves. He becomes angry and tells her to "forget about it and help me finish."*

   a. Will it be harmful to anyone if Nancy wears the gloves during the rest of the procedure, as it was just a slight prick and the patient's wound does not appear to be infected?
   _____
   _____

   b. Who is at fault if the patient does develop an infection?
   _____
   _____

c. What recourse does Nancy have if she develops a bloodborne pathogen infection, such as hepatitis, from the small hole in her gloves?

_____

_____

d. Is this an ethical or a legal issue, or both?

_____

_____

e. Are there any federal regulations that might help Nancy in the event of an injury or infection? If so, what are they?

_____

_____

PUT IT INTO PRACTICE

Write a letter of application for a position you may wish to seek upon graduation from your program of study. Submit this letter, along with an updated résumé, to your instructor for comments. Using Table 8.2 as a guide, review the personal information you provided in your cover letter and résumé. Have you given any information that is not required? Are there any gaps in your employment record? If so, why? How will you answer any of the questions in Table 8.2 if you are asked them during an interview?

WEB HUNT

Search the website of the Occupational Safety and Health Administration Act (www.osha.org) to find an article that relates to OSHA or workers' compensation. Summarize the article.

CRITICAL THINKING EXERCISE

What would you do if you observed a colleague, who you know is HIV positive with an open sore, teaching CPR to students?

BIBLIOGRAPHY

Bachman, M. 2001. "Waived Testing: Setting the Record Straight." *PMA*, (May/June), 21–23.

Beaman, N., and L. Fleming-McPhillips. 2007. *Comprehensive medical assisting.* Upper Saddle River, NJ: Pearson/Prentice Hall.

Black's law dictionary. 2009 8th ed. St. Paul, MN: West Publishing.

Brownell, K. 2005. *Weight bias: Nature, consequences, and remedies.* New York: Guilford Publications.

Druy, C., and M. Louis. 2002. "Exploring the Association between Body Weight, Stigma of Obesity and Healthcare Avoidance." *Journal of the American Academy of Nurse Practitioners, 14* (12), 554–561.

Flynn, E. 2000. *Issues in healthcare ethics.* Upper Saddle River, NJ: Prentice Hall.

Lerner, B. (2009). "A Life-changing Case for Doctors in Training." *New York Times,* (March 3), D5 & 7.

Perez-Pena, R. 2006. "City Seeks Action against 39 in Case of 'Nixzmary' Prying." *New York Times* (Sept. 23), B5.

Precourt, G. 2008. "Memo to Employees: Your Health, Our Business." *Notre Dame Business*, (Spring), 14–21.

Puhl, R. 2006. "The Stigma of Obesity." *New England Advance for Nurses* (July 31), 39–40.

Schmalleger, F. 2007. *Criminal justice today.* Upper Saddle River, NJ: Pearson/Prentice Hall.

The Medical Record

Learning Objectives

1. Define the glossary terms.
2. List five purposes of the medical record.
3. List seven requirements for maintaining medical records as recommended by the Joint Commission on Accreditation of Healthcare Organizations.
4. Discuss guidelines for effective charting.
5. Discuss what is meant by timeliness of charting and why it is important in a legal context.
6. Define the Privacy Act of 1974.
7. Describe ways to protect patient confidentiality that relate to the use of fax, copiers, e-mail, and computers.
8. Discuss the time periods for retaining adults' and minors' medical records, fetal heart monitor records, and records of birth, death, and surgical procedures.
9. Explain thirteen guidelines to follow when a subpoena *duces tecum* is in effect.
10. Describe confidentiality obligations using electronic medical record keeping.

Key Terms

Credibility gap
Credible
Disclosed
Doctrine of professional
  discretion
Electronic medical record
  (EMR)

Encryptions
Firewalls
Medical record
Microfiche
Open-record laws
Privileged communication

Public Health Services Act
Subpoenaed
Timeliness of documentation

THE CASE OF ANESHA AND THE LOST MEDICAL RECORD

Anesha's 15-year-old daughter, Robin, is experiencing abdominal pain when exercising during her gym class. After reviewing the results of several tests, Robin's pediatrician still cannot determine the cause of Robin's abdominal pains. He asks Anesha if she had any obstetrical problems when she was pregnant with Robin. Anesha had just read a report in a national newspaper discussing the use of a hormonal treatment to control bleeding that was used on expectant mothers at about the time that Anesha was pregnant with Robin. The report stated that female children could develop serious uterine problems, including cancer, during their adolescence if their mothers were given a particular hormone during their pregnancy that was in use fifteen to twenty years ago. The report went on to state that male children were unaffected. Anesha recalled that her obstetrician, Dr. C., had given her that particular hormone medication to control bleeding during her pregnancy with Robin and also when she was expecting Robin's brother, Sam. Anesha wrote Dr. C. to request her medical record and ask if the doctor had prescribed the hormone treatment during her pregnancy. She received a letter stating that Dr. C. could not recall what he prescribed fifteen or sixteen years previously. The letter also stated that all his records were destroyed in a fire five years ago.

1. What should Anesha tell Robin's pediatrician?

2. What does Robin need to know about her potential for a serious uterine diagnosis?

3. How could this situation have been prevented?

The **medical record** is all of the written documentation relating to a patient. It includes past history information, current diagnosis and treatment, and correspondence relating to the patient. Billing information is often maintained in a separate accounting record. It is important to remember that the medical record is a legal document. Various laws cover the reporting, disclosure, and confidentiality of medical records. Thus, medical record management requires attention to accuracy, confidentiality, and proper filing and storage. Proper management is also necessary because the records may be **subpoenaed,** ordered by the court, during a malpractice case.

Each patient's medical record contains essentially the same categories of material but with information unique to that patient. For example, not every patient has a consultation report from another physician or a surgical report. The format for the medical record reflects the physician's specialty. An obstetrician, for instance, uses a format that includes questions pertaining to the mother's prenatal (before birth) and postnatal (after birth) periods.

PURPOSE OF THE MEDICAL RECORD

Medical records serve multiple purposes. They provide a medical picture and record of the patient from birth to death. The medical record is an important document for the continual management of a patient's healthcare and furnishes documentary evidence of the course of evaluation and treatment. The patient record, which can result from a lifetime of medical visits, can assist the physician in diagnosing, treating, and tracking the patterns of the patient's health. It also provides data and statistics on health matters such as births, deaths, and communicable diseases. A physician can track the ongoing patterns of the patient's health through the medical record (Figure 9.1 ■).

The medical record is invaluable in an ambulatory health care or hospital setting as it provides the base for management of the patient's care, alerts the physicians and staff to patterns and changes in patient responses, and provides data for research and education.

In addition, because this legal document contains an objective, factual record of a patient's medical condition and treatment, either the patient or the physician in a malpractice suit may use this information. Finally, the medical record is a legal document and, as such, should not contain flippant or unprofessional comments such as "The patient is very annoying."

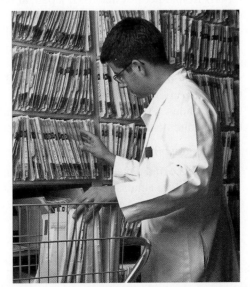

FIGURE 9.1
A Medical Records Filing System

The medical record serves as an important path for communication between medical personnel. In a case previously discussed in Chapter 3, *Norton v. Argonaut Insurance Company,* the medical record played a key role in documenting a medication error. A physician prescribed 2.5 c.c. of Elixir Pediatric Lanoxin, used to treat a heart condition, to be given orally to the baby by the infant's mother while the baby was hospitalized. The doctor increased the baby's Lanoxin dosage to 3.0 c.c. and told the mother about the new dosage. He signed a chart order that read, "Give 3.0 c.c. Lanoxin today for one dose only." The mother gave the baby 3.0 c.c. as she was told to do by the doctor. A nurse, who was not familiar with the fact that the doctor allowed the mother to give the baby her medication, read the doctor's order for 3.0 c.c. of Lanoxin to be given today. She then gave an injection of the drug to the baby not knowing that the mother had already administered the dose orally. This overdose of medication caused the baby's death. In this case, the parents sued the doctor, nurse, and the hospital. In this landmark case, a nurse was held responsible for the infant's death due to injecting a potentially lethal dose of a heart medication without questioning the prescribing physician. The physician's order was unclear because he did not state that the mother would administer the 3.0 c.c. of Lanoxin orally (*Norton v. Argonaut Ins. Co.,* 144 So. 2d 249, La. App. 1962).

CONTENTS OF THE MEDICAL RECORD

The medical record contains both personal information about the patient and medical or clinical notations supplied by the physician and other healthcare professionals caring for the patient. Personal patient information includes full name, address, telephone number, date of birth, marital status, employer, and insurance information. The clinical data or information includes all records of medical examinations, including x-rays, laboratory reports, and consent forms. The medical record will also contain any correspondence between the physician and the patient such as letters of withdrawal and consultation reports from other physicians. If a patient has provided informed consent for a procedure or test that has been explained to him or her, then a record of this explanation and the oral consent must be documented in the medical record.

As a legal document, both the defendant (physician) and plaintiff (patient) in a lawsuit can use the medical record. Because of its importance, some states have passed statutes that define what must be contained in the record. Many of these statutes reflect the accreditation requirements of the Joint Commission on Accreditation of Healthcare Organizations (JCAHO) or Medicare requirements as the minimum standard. Under these requirements, the medical record must include

- Admitting diagnosis.
- Evidence of a physician examination, including a health history, not more than seven days before admission or 48 hours after admission to a hospital.
- Documentation of any complications such as hospital-acquired infections or unfavorable medication reactions.
- Signed consent forms for all treatments and procedures.
- Consultation reports from any other physicians brought in on the case.

▶ All physicians' notes, nurses' notes, treatment reports, medication records, radiology and laboratory reports, and any other information used to monitor the patient.

▶ Discharge summary, with follow-up care noted.

The components of a standard medical record are listed in Table 9.1 ■.

Patient's complete name, address, home and work telephone numbers, social security number, birth date, and marital status	**TABLE 9.1**
Patient's past medical history	**Standard Medical Record**
Dates and times of all medical appointments and treatments	
History of present illness	
Review of symptoms, reason for appointment	
Chief complaints (CC)	
Results of physical examination performed by physician	
Physician's assessment, diagnosis, and recommendations for treatment	
Progress notes from past visits and treatments	
Family medical history	
Personal history	
Medication history with notations of all refill orders	
Treatments	
X-ray reports	
Laboratory test results	
Consultation (referral) reports	
Diagnosis	
Other patient-related correspondence:	
▶ Informed consent documentation, when appropriate	
▶ Signature for release of information	
▶ Copy of living will	
Documentation of all prescriptions and authorization for refill orders	
Documentation of dates when the medical record (or portions) is copied, including to whom it was sent	
Documentation of any missed appointments and the subsequent action taken, such as follow-up telephone calls	
Instructions concerning diet, home care, exercise, and follow-up appointments	
Hospital clinical records will also include:	
▶ Nurses' notes (observations by the nursing staff)	
▶ Operative report	
▶ Delivery record	
▶ Anesthesia reports	
▶ Medication and treatment records	
▶ Social service reports	
▶ Physical therapy notes and reports	
▶ Dietary notes and reports	
▶ Fluid intake and output (I & O) charts	
▶ Discharge summary	

TABLE 9.2 **Guidelines for Charting**	1. Always double check to make sure that you have the correct chart.
	2. Use dark ink, preferably black, and write legibly. Printing is preferred if one's handwriting is difficult to read.
	3. The patient's name and identification number should appear on each page. A stamping device can be used for this purpose.
	4. Every entry must be dated and signed by the person writing the record. If initials are used then the person's entire signature must be either in the medical record or on file in the medical office or institution. No one can sign for anyone else.
	5. Entries should be brief but complete.
	6. Use only accepted medical abbreviations known by the general staff.
	7. Correctly spell all medical terms.
	8. Never erase or use a liquid eraser, or in any way remove information from a medical record.
	9. Never leave spaces for someone to add later charting.
	10. Document all telephone calls and correspondence relating to the patient.
	11. Document all action(s) taken as a result of telephone conversations.
	12. Document all missed appointments.
	13. Document all incidents of noncompliance.
	14. Document all patient education.
	15. Do not record any personal opinions, speculations, or judgments.

MED TIP

Document patient comments such as "I'm all alone" or "I just feel I can't go on." Any comments of this nature should be relayed to the physician because they may indicate an emotional problem in addition to the physical one for which the patient is seeking treatment.

The medical record should never contain irrelevant material that is not related to the patient or the patient's care. For example, information about a hospital staff shortage resulting in the inability to perform a treatment or arguments between staff about the patient's care are not included in the medical record. All healthcare personnel who provide care must document that care or treatment and then sign their name to the documentation. No personnel may sign any name other than their own. In addition, not all healthcare professionals will chart information on a patient's medical record.

Table 9.2 ■ provides guidelines for charting.

Corrections and Alterations

Some medical record errors are unavoidable. These might include errors in spelling, transcription, or inadvertently omitted information or test results. Occasionally, an error occurs when patient information is written in the wrong chart. It is perfectly acceptable to correct these errors as long as this is done properly. All corrections on paper files should be made by drawing a single line through the error, writing the correction above the error, dating the change, and then initialing it. Do not erase or use correction fluid. The original statement or error should *never* be obliterated. Many healthcare professionals will also note in the margin of the record why the change was made, as for example, "incorrect chart." See Figure 9.2 ■ for an example of a corrected chart notation.

Date	Time	Order	Doctor	Administered by
9/9/11	3 pm	Erythromycin ~~500 mg~~ 250 mg BF 9/9	Williams	B. Fremgen RN.

FIGURE 9.2
Example of Corrected Chart Notation

Electronic medical record corrections are handled very differently than the paper record corrections. Each facility, depending on their software program, will have their own guidelines for correcting errors. One example occurs when an addendum or revision must be added after the date of the original entry. For example, in a medical office if a patient is unable to provide a urine sample on the day of his or her exam but brings one in the following day, a CMA or RN can draft a temporary revision or addition to the medical record, such as a test result, along with the notation "revision" and their name. The physician, who is the only authorized person, in this case, to permanently add or change the record, will then go into the program and approve the revision and sign it, making it a permanent part of the record. Therefore, all needed revisions must be brought to the attention of the physician when using this software system. Any time this record is examined the word "revision" will show up. All entries should be double-checked before transmitting the information. The user should sign-off all electronic patient records when not in use.

While it is acceptable to make an immediate correction in a medical record, it should never be altered. In one case, the plaintiff's attorney waited several weeks after the defendant was found not guilty and requested the medical record a second time. He noted that it had been altered after the case was closed. Upon review of the case, the judge ordered punitive damages.

MED TIP

Security is an ever-present concern with electronic medical records. For example, the computer should not be left on when the patient is alone in an exam room. In addition, computer "hackers" can often access and change information that is not protected with tight security systems such as "firewalls."

Falsification of medical records is grounds for criminal indictment. In a New York case, two orthopedic surgeons performed a procedure on a patient that required implanting a prosthetic device into the hip joint. The salesman of the prosthetic device was in the operating room when the patient had to be reopened in order to correct the placement of the device. One of the surgeons left the operating room to return to his office and agreed that the salesman could assist the remaining surgeon. The salesman assisted by removing the prosthesis from the patient and preparing it for the surgeon to re-implant. The surgeon who left the operating room was sued for malpractice because the surgical record did not show that he had been replaced with a nonphysician during the surgery. The hospital and surgical nurse were also indicted for violating a duty imposed on them by the nature of their profession (*People v. Smithtown Gen. Hosp.* 736, 402 N.Y.S.2d 318, Sup. Ct. 1978).

MED TIP

Use only black or blue ink when charting in a medical record. Never use pencil or colored ink pens.

Normal, as well as abnormal or negative, findings should all be noted in the medical record. Some doctors and staff become hurried and only document the abnormal. This can result in a problem if the medical record becomes part of a court record. If a jury does not see a test or procedure documented, then they tend to assume that it was not done no matter how strongly the physician or healthcare provider asserts that it was.

MED TIP

It is almost impossible to hide a change in a medical record as handwriting, type of ink, and paper used can all be detected through scientific testing.

Timeliness of Documentation

Medical records must be accurate and timely. **Timeliness of documentation** means that all entries should be made as they occur or as soon as possible afterward. Federal reimbursement guidelines mandate that all medical records should be completed within 30 days following the patient's discharge from a hospital. The Joint Commission on Accreditation of Healthcare Organizations, an agency that oversees hospital accreditation standards, also has issued guidelines for timeliness in charting.

Late entries into the medical chart mean that, even for a brief period of time, the medical record is incomplete. This can cause a serious problem if the incomplete record is subpoenaed for a malpractice suit. Any entry made into a medical record after a lawsuit is threatened or filed is suspect. Also, if the medical record is not updated promptly, there could be a lapse of memory about what actually occurred.

Completeness of Entries

The medical record may be the most important document in a malpractice suit because it documents the type and amount of patient care that was given. If the medical record is incomplete, the physician or other healthcare provider may be unable to defend allegations of malpractice, even if there was no negligence. For instance, in a 1985 Missouri case, a physician ordered that a patient be turned every two hours. The attending nurses, however, failed to note in the patient's record when they turned her. The patient claimed that she had not been turned as ordered and that this caused her to develop serious bedsores, which led to the amputation of one leg. The nurses presented an expert witness who testified that in some instances nurses become so busy that they place the needs of the patient, such as turning, before the need to document. The court eventually dismissed this case. However, not all such cases are dismissed (*Hurlock v. Park Lane Med. Ctr. Inc.,* 709 S.W.2d 872, Mo. Ct. App. 1985).

In a California case, an appeals court ruled that the physician's inability to provide the patient's medical record created the inference of guilt. (*Thor v. Boska,* 113 Cal. Rptr. 296, Ct. App. 1974.) This is an example of a situation in which the physician may not have been at fault. However, the fact that he was unable to provide any documentation about his treatment of the patient meant that even at the appeals court level, he did not win his case.

Credibility of the Medical Record

According to Webster's dictionary, for something to be **credible** it must be believable or worthy of belief, trustworthy, and reliable. This is asking a lot of brief statements written in a medical record. However, credibility is exactly what is necessary for everyone, including lawyers, to acknowledge that the medical record is an accurate picture of what happened to the patient. A **credibility gap** exists if there is an apparent disparity between what is said or written and the actual facts. This gap results in a failure to accept one's statements as factual, or a person's professed motives as the true ones. For example, if a hospital record concerning a patient's fall from a hospital bed includes an inserted statement such as "siderails were up," a lawyer and jury may believe otherwise. If x-rays or other important medical records are missing, an assumption may be made that this was purposely done to hide something. Even a documented fire or flood can cause a credibility gap to occur such as in the case of Anesha and the Lost Medical Record at the beginning of this chapter.

One physician may be asked by an attorney to review a medical record pertaining to a medical malpractice case of another physician to help determine if there is evidence of malpractice. The second physician will be looking for gaps or other problems with the record such as illegible handwriting, delays in placing x-ray and laboratory reports into the file, altered records, or any contrived or invented documentation. Medical records are frequently examined during Medicaid or Medicare fraud cases in which a physician has falsely claimed payment for services that were never rendered.

> ### MED TIP
>
> Anyone processing medical billing records must be conscientious about the accuracy of names, dates, and services rendered. Careless documentation for claims of insurance payments can result in physicians being brought up on charges of fraud.

OWNERSHIP OF THE MEDICAL RECORD

State statutes may establish who owns the medical records. In most states, the general rule is that the physician or owners of a healthcare facility, such as a hospital or nursing home, own the medical records, but patients have the legal right of **privileged communication** (confidential information told to their physician) and access to their medical records. Therefore, patients must authorize release of their records in writing. Patients also have a right to see their records and to request a copy of those records. Because some records are large and require duplicating time and expense, the physician or institution may charge for this service.

Patients have the right to expect that accurate medical records will be recorded and maintained in a safe manner. In some cases, such as for a patient with mental health problems, it may cause harm to the patient if they read their own records. Under the **doctrine of professional discretion,** a physician may determine, based on his or her best judgment, if the patient with mental or emotional problems should view the medical record.

Because the medical record is a written documentation of the contract established between the physician or healthcare provider and the patient, it must be retained for legal purposes. There is often a need for a healthcare provider, such as hospital personnel and consulting physicians to view a patient's medical record. However, when the need no longer exists, then the right to view the medical record, or access to it, stops.

CONFIDENTIALITY AND THE MEDICAL RECORD

To protect patient confidentiality, medical records should not be released to third parties without the patient's written consent. If an attorney obtains a subpoena for the medical records, only the specific records that are requested, such as the surgical notes, should be copied and sent. For example, the fact that a patient is HIV-positive or has been seen in an emergency room after an auto accident may have no bearing on a malpractice suit relating to a surgical procedure.

> ### MED TIP
>
> Many healthcare facilities require all employees to sign a confidentiality agreement. Failure to honor this agreement can result in dismissal and possible legal action.

Taking photographs or other visual images of patients, such as videotapes, without the proper patient consent is an invasion of the patient's privacy. The patient must sign an authorization form in order for photos and films, such as mammograms and x-rays, to be used or released outside of the medical facility. Guidelines for maintaining patient confidentiality when using a fax machine, copy machine, e-mail, or computer are listed in Table 9.3 ∎.

Fax Machines	TABLE 9.3
1. Send patient information via fax only when absolutely necessary.	Maintaining Patient Confi-dentiality When Using Fax (facsimile) Machines, Copy Machines, or E-mail
2. Verify the fax telephone number of the receiver before sending the fax.	
3. Make sure the intended receiver is there before sending confidential records by fax.	
4. Shred confidential fax papers that are no longer needed. Do not place them in the trash.	
5. Use a fax cover sheet that states "Confidential. Please return if received in error."	
6. Only fax the specific documents requested, not the entire medical record.	
7. Do not leave confidential material unattended on a fax machine.	
8. Ideally the fax machine should be located in a restricted access area.	

Copy Machines

1. Never leave medical records unattended on a copy machine where others may read them.
2. Shred all discarded copies.
3. Be diligent about removing all papers caught in a paper jam.
4. Do not print confidential medical information on a printer that is shared with another department or person.

E-mail

1. Avoid using e-mail to send confidential information.
2. Do not allow other patients or unauthorized staff members to view a computer screen with confidential patient information.
3. Screen savers should be used to prevent confidential patient information being viewed by others.
4. Computer screens should be out of view of the general public.
5. Passwords should be changed on a regular basis and not shared with others.

MED TIP

An *original* version of a medical record should never be sent to a patient. A copy should be made of the original, and the copy sent to a patient who has requested the record in writing. In the case of x-ray film, the physician or institution may allow the original to be sent, with the stipulation that it be returned.

Release of Information

Records should not be released to the patient without the physician's knowledge and permission. The information contained in the record can be upsetting to some patients without the proper explanation. Insurance companies often have a desire to examine the medical records before they issue a reimbursement for a procedure. If the patient personally receives the records, then he or she must sign a release form. Only the specific information that is requested should be sent to the insurance company.

In addition, patients must always sign a release form when they request to have their medical records and films sent to another physician. This often occurs when the primary care physician (PCP) has requested that the patient have a consultation with another physician.

In general, only a patient can authorize the release of his her own medical records. However, there are some exceptions to the rule which include:

▶ Parents of minor children
▶ Legal guardian
▶ An agent (someone the patient selects to act on their behalf in a Health Care Power of Attorney)

Under some circumstances, such as with an emancipated minor, the minor and not the parent must sign the release.

MED TIP

Because the patient does have a legal right to his or her medical record, it is never acceptable to refuse to turn over a copy if the patient has not paid his or her bill.

State hospital licensing regulations typically stipulate that the medical record is the property of the hospital and should not be removed from the premises unless there is a court order. Under the law, access to mental health records is more limited than to general medical records. See Chapter 10 for a further discussion of release of patient information under HIPAA regulations.

MED TIP

Never send the entire medical chart unless it is requested. Send out only the exact material, or portion of the medical record, that is requested.

Privacy Act of 1974

The Privacy Act of 1974 provides private citizens some control over information that the federal government collects about them by limiting the use of information for unnecessary purposes. Under this 1974 law, an agency may maintain only the information that is relevant to its authorized purpose. Additionally, under this law citizens have the right to gain access to their records and to copy any of the records, if necessary. Under the privacy act individuals were given the right to:

▶ Find out what information is collected about them by the government.
▶ See and have a copy of that information.
▶ Correct or amend their information.
▶ Exercise control over disclosure of that information.

The Privacy Act only applies to federal agencies and government contractors. However, hospitals that are operated by the federal government, such as Veterans' Administration hospitals, are bound by the act to make their records available for public disclosure.

It is sometimes necessary for confidential information to be shared without the knowledge or consent of the person. Thus, this law also permits federal agencies to collect, maintain, use, or disseminate any record of identifiable personal information but only in a manner that assures that:

▶ Such action is for a necessary and lawful purpose.

▶ The information is current and accurate for its intended use.

▶ Adequate safeguards are provided to prevent misuse of such information.

▶ The information is used only in those cases where there is an important public policy need that has been determined by a specific statutory authority.

The Health Insurance Portability and Accountability Act (HIPAA) of 1996 is a federal law that affects the entire population. This act is discussed more fully in Chapter 10.

State Open-Record Laws

Some states have freedom of information laws, called **open-record laws,** that grant public access to records maintained by state agencies. However, medical records are generally exempt from this statute, so the public cannot obtain such information. In some cases, though, if the private patient's interest in confidentiality is outweighed by the benefit of disclosure for the public interest, then disclosure is allowed. For example, in the case of *Child Protection Group v. Cline,* the court allowed personal information about a bus driver's psychiatric records to be **disclosed,** or made known, to parents of schoolchildren when there was a concern that he would not be able to drive the school bus safely. (*Child Protection Group v. Cline,* 350 S.E.2d 541, W. Va. 1986.)

Alcohol and Drug Abuse Patient Records

The **Public Health Services Act** protects patients who are receiving treatment for drug and alcohol abuse. Any person or program that releases confidential information relating to these patients is subject to criminal fines. Hospitals maintain a patient registry at their switchboard or front desk, but they cannot divulge that a patient with drug or alcohol abuse problems is even a patient at their facility.

An exception to this disclosure of information law would be if the patient should require emergency care that would necessitate divulging the abuse problem.

RETENTION AND STORAGE OF MEDICAL RECORDS

Each state varies on the length of time for which medical records and documents must be kept. It also varies by state according depending on whether it is the record of a minor or adult. However, most states require that medical records should be stored for ten years from the time of the last entry. Most physicians store medical records permanently because malpractice suits can still be filed within two years from the date that the occurrence or alleged malpractice event became known.

Using the statute of limitations as a guide for retaining records, the medical record of a minor would be kept until the patient reaches the age of maturity plus the period of the statute. As an example, in a state where the age of maturity is 21 and the statute of limitations for torts is two years, the retention period for a newborn's record would be twenty-three years.

MED TIP

Remember that the statute of limitations can be extended for many reasons. It is always better to err on the side of retaining medical records too long, rather than not long enough. Check your own state to determine the statute of limitations for record keeping.

Due to limited storage space, medical records may have to be destroyed after a period of time has elapsed. State laws should always be checked before destroying any records.

The courts take the requirement to retain records seriously. An Illinois appeals court declared that a patient could sue when a hospital failed to retain her x-rays (*Rodgers v. St. Mary's Hospital,* 556 N.E.2d 913, Ill. App. Ct. 1990). In a Florida case, a woman whose husband died during the administration of anesthesia was unable to present expert testimony because her husband's anesthesiology records were missing. The court ruled that she could sue the hospital because it was the hospital's duty to make and maintain medical records (*Bondu v. Gurvich,* 473 So. 2d 1307, Fla. Dist. Ct. App. 1984). Table 9.4 ■ describes time period recommendations for retaining medical records as adopted by the American Health Information Management Association (AHIMA).

TABLE 9.4 **Time Periods for Retaining Medical Records**		
Adult patient records	Ten years after the most recent encounter
Minor's health records	Age of maturity plus statute of limitations
Fetal heart monitor records	Ten years after infant reaches maturity
Medicare and Medicaid records	Five years
Register of birth	Permanently
Register of death	Permanently
Register of surgical procedures	Permanently
Immunization records	Permanently
Chemotherapy records	Permanently

In the event that a physician cannot retain patients' records beyond a ten-year time frame, there are certain considerations for the methods of destruction:

▶ Maintain careful records relating to when a record can be destroyed.

▶ Designate a person to be responsible for deciding, based on established policies, what records to keep and what to purge.

▶ Define which records are kept on-site and which are off-site.

▶ Maintain a log that details which records have been destroyed, as well as when and how this was done.

▶ Provide a method for disposal (e.g., shred, pulp, or incinerate) that destroys all information in the record. Some facilities hire a service that handles the destruction of medical records. This service must abide by HIPAA guidelines. (See Chapter 10 for HIPAA.)

Storage

Records of current patients are usually kept within the physician's office for easy access (Figure 9.3 ■). Older records of former patients do not need to be kept in the office where they will take up valuable space. Physicians often rent storage space. It is important to use a clean, dry warehouse space for storage. If records that are needed in court have been destroyed in a warehouse fire or flood, the court may believe that it was a deliberate attempt by the physician to avoid the truth. Some physicians hire a service to place all

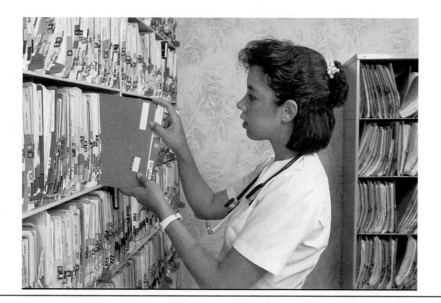

FIGURE 9.3
Medical Records
Storage Unit

their records on **microfiche,** which results in a space-saving, miniaturized film of the medical record.

Electronic Medical Records

The **electronic medical record (EMR)**, in which all patient-related data is computerized into one record, is becoming more widespread in all aspects of health care. Data and patient records can be created, modified, authenticated, stored, and retrieved by the computer. This has made record maintenance and retrieval much more efficient and effective in medical offices, clinics, laboratories, and hospitals. However, it has resulted in increased concerns about patient privacy as so many healthcare professionals may now be able to view a patient record unless precautions are taken. A well-designed computerized system may offer better protection than a "file-drawer" storage system because there are passwords, **encryptions** (scrambling and encoding information before sending it electronically), and the use of **firewalls** (software to prevent unauthorized users) to maintain security.

Legal confidentiality obligations apply to all methods of record keeping. With a computer-based system, it is even more important to be diligent in protecting the patients' rights because generally more people have access to the computerized records. Special safety measures should be taken, such as establishing personal identification and user verification codes for access to records. Computer-based records should be accessed only on a need-to-know basis. Not everyone in a healthcare facility should have authorization to pull up patient records on the computer screen. (Figure 9.4 ■)

Loss of Medical Records

As Anesha's case at the beginning of this chapter indicates, the loss of a medical record can be a frustrating, and even a harmful experience for all those involved. It can even result in a deadly outcome if vital information relating to the patient is gone. Whether a medical record is lost through careless filing of the record or as a result of a deliberate attempt to prevent litigation, it is always preventable. There are many safeguards that a medical office, clinic, and even a hospital can implement to prevent the loss of a record.

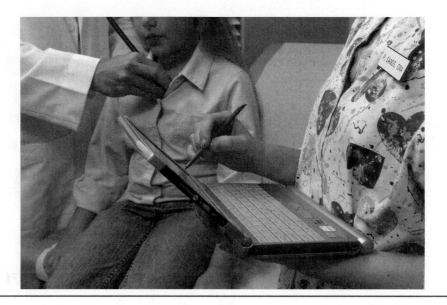

FIGURE 9.4
Medical Assistant Uses a Laptop Computer for Bedside Charting

1. All records removed from files should be listed in a journal. The person to whom the file was given and the date should be recorded.

2. Place some indication in the file cabinet that a file has been removed. Many offices use a color-coded insert to alert personnel about the file removal.

3. If possible, designate one person responsible for maintaining a list of all records removed from files. That person then collects all files and returns them to the proper location.

4. Placing all medical records on microfiche is an excellent way to safeguard against record loss. The microfiche can be "backed up" with a duplicate film that is kept in a safe, fireproof area.

Juries tend to be unsympathetic in a court case that revolves around a lost medical document or record. For example, during the discovery phase in the case of *Keene v. Brigham & Women's Hospital,* the plaintiff was told that the hospital had lost his medical records. A default judgment for the plaintiff was entered at the Appeals Court level and upheld at the Supreme Court level. The courts maintained that without the medical record containing evidence relating to the medical malpractice claim against the hospital, it was impossible to make a determination of guilt or innocence of the defendant (*Keene v. Brigham & Women's Hosp., Inc.* 439 Mass. 223, 2003).

REPORTING AND DISCLOSURE REQUIREMENTS

State laws require the disclosure of some confidential medical record information without the patient's consent. These items are discussed in Chapter 7 under public duties of the physician.

MED TIP

Laws regarding medical records vary from state to state. Healthcare professionals who have any involvement with the medical record should learn what the statutes in their own state require.

USE OF THE MEDICAL RECORD IN COURT

Improper Disclosure

Healthcare providers and institutions such as hospitals and clinics may face civil and criminal liability for releasing medical records without the proper patient authorization. Private citizens can institute a civil lawsuit to recover damages if their records are released inappropriately. Wisconsin statutes provide for compensatory as well as punitive damages for improper disclosure (*Wis. Stat.* § 252.15(8)). Many of the cases that have been tried for improper disclosure relate to HIV and AIDS patients. While disclosure of a patient's HIV and AIDS status to the health department is required by state statute, disclosure to any other person or organization is not allowed.

Subpoena *Duces Tecum*

A subpoena *duces tecum* is a written order requiring a person to appear in court, give testimony, and bring the particular records, files, books, or information that are described in the subpoena. The court issues a subpoena for records that document patient care and, in some instances, billing and insurance records. The purpose of issuing a subpoena for a patient's medical record is to receive written evidence of the patient's medical condition and the care that was received. All copying costs associated with subpoenaed records must be borne by the attorney requesting the subpoena.

MED TIP

Ordinarily, a medical record cannot be sent to anyone without consent in writing from the patient and the physician's approval. One exception to this is when a record is subpoenaed.

A local sheriff or federal marshal often serves a subpoena, but many state statutes allow anyone over the age of 18 to serve a subpoena. The subpoena may be served either by certified mail or in person, depending on the state requirement.

In general, only the person who is named on the subpoena can accept it. The subpoena can then be said to "have been served." In some cases "a conservator of the record," such as a medical records administrator, is authorized to accept a subpoena on behalf of a healthcare facility or a physician. Before accepting a subpoena, the person accepting the subpoena must make sure to check that the name of the attorney and the court case number are on the subpoena. In addition, they must check to make sure that the physician named on the subpoena saw the patient.

When a record, such as a medical file or chart, is subpoenaed, only the parts of the record requested should be copied and provided to the requesting attorney. Unless the original document is subpoenaed, a certified photocopy may be sent. If the original record is subpoenaed, a photocopy is marked COPY and placed in the file along with a note about the location of the original copy. Until the original is returned, a receipt for the subpoenaed record should be placed in the file, and the patient or the patient's attorney should be notified that the record has been subpoenaed. Any notice relating to subpoenaed records should be sent to the patient by certified mail.

If a medical record has been subpoenaed, or requested by the court, certain guidelines should be followed.

1. Notify the physician that a subpoena has been received. In most cases, a subpoena has to be personally served to the person named on the document. In the case of an institution, such as a hospital, a "custodian of the record" such as a hospital records administrator will be appointed to receive a subpoena for hospital medical records.

2. Notify the patient that his or her record has been subpoenaed. If the patient is represented by an attorney and suing the physician, then the physician and his or her staff cannot contact the patient except via the attorney.

3. Notify the physician's attorney that a subpoena has been received.

4. Verify that all the information on the subpoena is correct. Pay particular attention to identification numbers such as the Social Security number. In some cases, patients may have the same name, and a subpoena is sent to a physician in error.

5. Carefully make sure that the requesting attorney's name and phone number as well as the court case (docket) number are listed on the subpoena.

6. Review the records to make sure that all the records requested are available. No attempt should be made to alter, delete, or add any information to the record.

7. Make sure that a copy of the medical record is acceptable. In some cases, only the original record will be accepted. Most physicians do not want their original records to leave their possession.

8. Photocopy the original record and number all the pages. Place the total number of pages on the front of the file folder. Prepare a cover list of the contents and place that in the file folder along with the medical documents.

9. Turn over only the specific materials that have been requested.

10. After the medical record materials relating to the subpoena have been compiled, lock the file in a secure place.

11. Turn the records directly over to the judge on the due date. The materials should not be left with a clerk or receptionist.

12. The healthcare professional who takes the records to court should be prepared to be sworn in to make the records admissible as evidence.

13. Check with the court to make sure that the trial date is the same as the date listed on the subpoena.

POINTS TO PONDER

1. Do you agree with the statement, "If it's not documented, it wasn't done?" Why or why not?

2. In order to protect your physician/employer, should you "hide" to avoid receiving a subpoena *duces tecum*? Why or why not?

3. As a healthcare professional, are you able to read the medical record of a person you know? Why or why not?

4. Would it be helpful to other healthcare professionals who will be using the same patient's medical record to document that patient's poor attitude by including a statement such as "bad attitude?" Why or why not?

5. Can you be liable if you or your staff lose a patient's medical record?

6. A patient requests her physician's office to change her diagnosis in her medical record from R/O (rule out) bladder infection to "bladder infection," because her insurance will not pay for an R/O diagnosis. Should the record be changed?

DISCUSSION QUESTIONS

1. What is the significance of the medical record for the physician? For the healthcare professional? For the patient?

2. What laws affect patient privacy issues?
3. Who owns the medical chart?

REVIEW CHALLENGE

Short Answer Questions

1. How long should a medical record be kept for a one-year-old child who resides in a state with a statute of limitations of two years for a tort offense?

2. What does a subpoena *duces tecum* request the subpoenaed person to provide?

3. Exactly what does "timeliness in documentation" mean?

4. What are some of the precautions to follow when using electronic medical records?

5. What would you say to a patient who demands his x-ray and says "It's my x-ray. I paid for it?"

6. What is the doctrine of professional discretion?

7. What are some examples of a "custodian of the record?"

8. Who can serve a subpoena?

9. Explain the precautions that must be taken when faxing medical records.

10. Explain the precautions that must be taken when using a computer in a medical setting.

Matching

Match the responses in column B with the correct term in column A.

Column A
1. subpoenaed
2. credible
3. disclosed
4. chronological record
5. falsification of records
6. subpoena *duces tecum*
7. EMR
8. timeliness
9. Privacy Act of 1974
10. JCAHO

Column B
a. made known
b. provides control over release of information
c. electronic medical record
d. when something has been requested by the court
e. in the order of occurrence
f. Joint Commission on Accreditation of Healthcare Organizations
g. reliable
h. grounds for criminal indictment
i. no late entries on medical chart
j. written order to bring materials to court

Multiple Choice

Select the one best answer to the following statements.

1. Medicare and Medicaid records should be retained for

    a. one year.
    b. five years.
    c. ten years.
    d. for the lifetime of the patient.
    e. for an indefinite period of time.

2. The contents of the medical record include all of the following except

    a. past medical problems.
    b. informed consent documentation.
    c. patient's income level.
    d. family medical history.
    e. a and b only.

3. Medical record entries should be made

    a. within 60 days of the patient's discharge.
    b. at the physician's discretion.
    c. after the patient gives consent.
    d. as soon as possible.
    e. ten days after the procedure.

4. The patient

    a. has the legal right of privileged communication.
    b. owns the medical record.
    c. cannot have any portion of the medical record.
    d. a and c only.
    e. a, b, and c.

5. When correcting a written medical error, one should

    a. use a professional brand of error correction fluid to make the correction.
    b. erase the error and make the correction.
    c. draw a line through the error, write the correction above the error, and initial the change.
    d. never make any corrections on the medical record.
    e. none of the above.

6. The medical record is legally owned by the

    a. patient.
    b. physician.
    c. state.
    d. lawyer.
    e. no one.

7. Medical records

    a. provide a record from birth to death.
    b. provide statistics on health matters.
    c. are legal documents.
    d. a and c only.
    e. a, b, and c.

8. All of the following are guidelines to use when sending medical records by fax except

    a. make sure there is a receiver waiting for the fax.
    b. use a cover sheet marked "confidential."
    c. send the entire medical record via fax.
    d. do not place the original fax in a trash container.
    e. all of the above are correct.

9. An exception to the open-record laws in some states is/are

    a. psychiatric history.
    b. confidential medical record information such as HIV test results.
    c. safety and criminal records of persons involved in the education of children.
    d. all of the above.
    e. none of the above.

10. The records of all adult patients should be kept a minimum of

    a. two years.
    b. five years.
    c. ten years.
    d. twenty years.
    e. permanently.

DISCUSSION CASES

1. *Mary Smith has been a patient of Dr. Williams from 1985 to the present time. During that time, she has had three children and been treated for a variety of conditions, including depression in 1986 and herpes in 1990. Mary and her husband, George, have filed for divorce. George wants custody of the children and is claiming that Mary has a medical condition that makes her an unfit mother. An attorney, acting on George's behalf in the divorce proceedings, has obtained a subpoena for Mary's medical records for the years 1995 to the present. Dr. Williams' assistant, who is a medical records technician, copies Mary's entire medical record from 1985 to the present and sends it to the attorney.*

   a. What negative effects for Mary might this error cause?

   _____

   _____

   b. Is there a violation of confidentiality? Why or why not?

   _____

   _____

   c. Do you believe that this is a common or uncommon error?

   _____

   _____

   d. Was it appropriate for the assistant to make a copy of any part of Mary's medical record?

   _____

   _____

2. *Peter B. is admitted to a local hospital emergency room (ER) suffering from an anxiety attack. He tells the ER physician that he is anxious about a job promotion for which he is being consid-ered. Peter's secretary is worried about him and asks her father, Dr. K., who is on the medical staff at the hospital, to go to the ER and see how Peter is doing. Dr. K., who is often in the ER, knows all the staff and they willingly give him Peter's chart when he asks for it. Dr. K. calls his daughter to tell her that Peter is being treated for anxiety with an anti-depressant drug and will probably be discharged. She relays this encouraging message to Peter's boss. Peter does not receive the promotion.*

   a. Will it be an easy matter for Peter to prove that the ER staff caused Peter to lose his promotion? Explain your answer.

   _____

   _____

   b. What precautions can be taken to avoid giving confidential information to medical personnel who have no need to see it?

   _____

   _____

   c. In your opinion, should a diagnosis of anxiety be a concern for an employer? Why or why not?

   _____

   _____

3. *Demi Daniels calls to ask you to change her diagnosis in her medical record from R/O (rule out) bladder infection to "bladder infection" because her insurance will not pay for a R/O diagnosis. In fact, she tested negative for an infection, but the physician placed her on antibiotics anyway.*

    a. What do you do?

    _____

    _____

    b. Is this a legal question? Why or why not?

    _____

    _____

    c. Is this an ethical question? Why or why not?

    _____

    _____

    d. What could happen to the physician you work for if you make a mistake?

    _____

    _____

PUT IT INTO PRACTICE

Request a copy of your medical record from your primary care physician (PCP). Examine the contents to determine how well they document your medical history.

WEB HUNT

Using the website of the American Health Information Management Association (www.ahima.org), provide a description of the organization. Go into the patient resource center of the site and summarize the statement concerning who owns the medical record.

CRITICAL THINKING EXERCISE

What would you do if you saw a nurse making a change in a patient's medical chart after receiving a subpoena *duces tecum* for that medical record.

BIBLIOGRAPHY

Beaman, N., and L. Fleming-McPhillips. 2007. *Comprehensive medical assisting.* Upper Saddle River, NJ: Pearson/ Prentice Hall.

Black, H. 2009. *Black's law dictionary.* 8th ed. St. Paul, MN: West Publishing Co.

Hartley, C., & E. Jones. 2004. *HIPAA plain and simple: A compliance guide for health care professionals.* Chicago: A.M.A. Press.

Joint Commission on Accreditation of Healthcare Organizations. 2010. *Comprehensive accreditation manual for hospitals.* Chicago: JCAHO.

Roach, W. 2001. *Medical records and the law.* Gaithersburg, MD: Aspen Publishers.

Taber's cyclopedic medical dictionary. 2009. 21st. ed. Philadelphia: F. A. Davis.

Patient Confidentiality and HIPAA

10

Learning Objectives

1. Define the glossary terms.
2. Identify the problems associated with patient confidentiality.
3. Discuss the purpose of the Health Insurance Portability and Accountability Act (HIPAA) of 1996.
4. Describe the information to which the Privacy Rule refers and how it applies to your profession.
5. List which entities are affected by HIPAA.
6. Discuss the penalties for noncompliance with HIPAA.
7. List the patients' rights under the Privacy Standards.
8. Discuss the ethical issues concerning information technology.

Key Terms

Clearinghouse
Covered entities
Covered transactions
Deidentifying
Employer Identification Number (EIN)
Employer Identifier Standard
Health Insurance Portability and Accountability Act of 1996 (HIPAA)

Healthcare Integrity and Protection Data Bank (HIPDB)
Healthcare plan
HIPAA-defined permission
Medical informatics
Minimum necessary standard
Notice of Privacy Practices (NPP)
Office of Civil Rights (OCR)
Permission

Privacy Rule
Protected Health Information (PHI)
Sanctions
State's preemption
Telemedicine
Treatment, payment, and healthcare operations (TPO)
Wireless Local Area Networks (WLANs)

THE CASE OF THE NEW MINISTER

Dawn is an ordained minister in a little church located in a small Midwest community. She has had to overcome some discrimination as the first female clergy member in the town. However, Dawn feels that her church congregation and other members of the community have finally started to accept her in this new role. Dawn was recently diagnosed with irritable bowel syndrome by a gastroenterologist in the next town. He performed a colonoscopy on Dawn to rule out cancer of the bowel and found nothing more than a few benign polyps, which he removed. He told Dawn that he wanted her to start taking amitriptyline for three months to see if that would solve her irritable bowel problem. He said that he had success using this antidepressant, also known as Elavil, to treat irritable bowel syndrome. He said he would call the prescription into Dawn's local pharmacy.

When Dawn went in to pick up her prescription, she met two members of her congregation who were also picking up their prescriptions. The pharmacist leaned over the front counter and said to Dawn, "Why are you taking this antidepressant?"

1. What rights of Dawn's were violated?

2. Were any laws broken by the pharmacist's statement? If so, what are they?

3. How could Dawn's reputation suffer from this brief comment by the pharmacist?

atients have two major expectations when they visit a physician's office or other medical facility: quality care and confidentiality. They have a right to expect both. However, with the advent of modern technology, including the Internet, e-mail, fax machines, and computers, the number of people who have access to patient information has increased at a rapid rate. In order to address the concern for patients' privacy, especially via electronic transmissions, Congress mandated that the Health Insurance Portability and Accountability Act of 1996 (HIPAA) enforce its privacy provision by April 14, 2003. This law, while somewhat complicated and expensive for physicians to implement, has meant more careful attention to issues of patient privacy.

CONFIDENTIALITY

One version of the Hippocratic Oath states, "What I see or hear in the course of the treatment . . . , which on no account must be spread abroad, I will keep to myself. . . ." Historically, physicians were expected to maintain all confidences concerning their patients, and patients took this confidentiality for granted. However, the image of one patient sharing his or her medical information with only one physician is no longer applicable in today's modern world. A dozen or more physicians may be involved in a patient's care along with multiple institutions, including hospitals, MRI testing centers, rehabilitation centers, and skilled-nursing facilities. Today, there is widespread use of computerized record keeping and transmission of medical records. For example, information needs to be transmitted to third-party providers, such as insurance companies, to arrange for payment of the patient's medical services.

Modern medicine and technology have meant that patient privacy issues have become of paramount concern among patients, medical professionals, and ethicists. In many cases, patients have become fearful of admitting to what could be embarrassing information, such as past drug use, abortions, homosexuality, and mental health problems. When patients fail to convey this information to their physicians, it creates a difficult environment for the physicians who are treating the patients without benefit of complete medical information (Figure 10.1 ■).

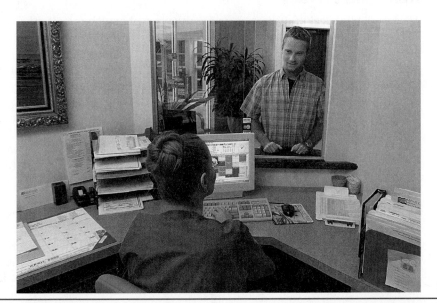

FIGURE 10.1
Computer Screen
Hidden from Patient View

Confidentiality about sensitive information is necessary to preserve the patient's dignity. However, in order to receive payment from third-party payers such as insurance companies, Medicare, and Medicaid, the patient's diagnosis may have to be revealed, no matter how embarrassing it is for the patient. But patients want to be assured that the information relayed about them to a third party is limited to just the minimum amount necessary in order to carry out the request. In addition, patients expect to be told when information about them is being relayed to a third party such as an insurance company.

MED TIP

Personal and confidential information about patients should be limited to conveying it to the absolute minimum number of healthcare employees.

Our Right to Privacy

U.S. Supreme Court Justice Louis Brandeis defined our right to privacy as ". . . the right most valued by civilized men." While we realize that much has changed since 1928 when Justice Brandeis wrote these words, we still believe that this is a precious right that needs to be protected. Our right to privacy is not protected specifically by the Bill of Rights or any portion of the Constitution. However, many legal scholars believe that the right to privacy is found in some of the constitutional amendments, such as the First, Fourth, Fifth, Ninth, and Fourteenth Amendments.

There are numerous court cases, creating case law, which defend our constitutional rights to privacy. These decisions have then become precedent for future cases. Unfortunately, new technology, especially computer data banks, since Justice Brandeis, has allowed personal patient information to become public. For example, testing for the presence of drugs and alcohol in some business areas such as transportation and private industry may infringe on individual rights.

AIDS and Privacy

There is a great deal of discussion and controversy about the role of privacy for patients who have AIDS. AIDS is not only a threat to the homosexual population, but also to pregnant women, children, and heterosexual couples. Because this disease is transmitted through direct sexual contact including rape, as well as through contaminated needles and the accidental use of infected blood products, it is now apparent the public needs information to protect themselves. This information needs to be carefully communicated in order to protect the privacy rights of the infected individuals. Tennis champion Arthur Ashe, who contracted AIDS through a contaminated blood transfusion, wrote that, "keeping my AIDS status private enabled me to control my life. 'Going public' with a disease such as AIDS is akin to telling the world in 1900 that you had leprosy." Before his death, he asked "To what extent is my private life not my own?"

Republican Representative Susan Molinari of New York promoted legislation to compel all those who are accused of sex crimes to be tested for AIDS. These test results would then be told to the victim as well as the court. Many states have passed laws to this effect. However, there are many opponents to this type of legislation; they believe it to be "an extraordinary intrusion on the accused's right to privacy." They believe that "the mere ordering of such a test would . . . make a fair hearing difficult if not impossible."

Representative Molinari expresses concern that a victim might avoid becoming pregnant so as not to infect her baby. In fact, babies with AIDS have a very poor prognosis. Many healthcare professionals are caught in the middle of the dilemma about a concern for the patient's privacy and a concern for the victim's future health.

Another concern relates to healthcare professionals who are infected with AIDS. The public has voiced their opinion that it should be illegal for healthcare professionals, such as physicians and dentists, to withhold this information from their patients. On the other hand, many doctors believe that this is unnecessary because they believe that if they become infected they are competent to take any necessary precautions to prevent the spread of AIDS.

The medical community has been conscientious about having patients sign an approval form granting permission for the release of their medical records. See Figure 10.2 ■ for a copy of an approval form for release of medical information. However, patients' confidentiality and privacy have become more difficult with the advent of technologies such as fax transmission, the Internet, and computers in every medical office. Unfortunately, the creation of new laws has become necessary as a result of the unethical violation of patients' privacy.

MED TIP

Always keep in mind that computer screens should never be visible to patients or visitors.

WINDY CITY CLINIC
Beth Williams, M.D.
123 Michigan Avenue
Chicago, IL 60610
(312) 123-1234

RECORDS RELEASE   Date _____

To _____
                               Doctor

_____
                               Address

I hereby authorize and request you to release

to _____
                               Doctor

_____
                               Address

all medical records in your possession concerning any
examination, diagnosis, and/or treatment rendered to me
during the period from _____ to _____

_____
          Signature of patient or closest relative

_____
                          Relationship

_____   _____
   Signature of witness   Address

FIGURE 10.2
**Copy of an Approved
Form for Release
of Medical Information**

HEALTH INSURANCE PORTABILITY AND ACCOUNTABILITY ACT (HIPAA) OF 1996

The **Health Insurance Portability and Accountability Act (HIPAA)**, signed into law on August 21, 1996, regulates the privacy of patient health information. This law was an effort to reduce costs of healthcare and streamline the fragmented and complicated healthcare system. HIPAA is a sweeping reform law that affects virtually everyone in the U.S. healthcare system—patients, providers, payers, and intermediaries such as pharmacies and medical device companies. The four objectives are to

▶ Improve the portability of health insurance.

▶ Combat fraud, abuse, and waste in healthcare.

▶ Promote the expanded use of medical savings accounts.

▶ Simplify the administration of health insurance.

Title II, Administrative Simplification, of the law is the section of HIPAA that affects most healthcare providers, insurance companies, and clearinghouses. Within this law, the Title II provisions were meant to make it easier and cheaper to electronically transmit health information. However, Congress realized that widespread electronic transmission of a patient's health information could affect a patient's privacy. Subsequently, Congress mandated that the Department of Health and Human Services (HHS) was responsible for developing detailed privacy standards. The overall objectives were to:

▶ Improve efficiency and effectiveness of the healthcare system via electronic exchange of administrative and financial information.

▶ Protect security and privacy of this stored patient medical information.

▶ Reduce high transaction costs in healthcare, which include paper-based transactions, multiple healthcare data formats, misuse, errors, and the loss of healthcare records.

The **Privacy Rule** went into effect on April 14, 2001, and required that all "covered entities" must be in compliance with the privacy, security, and electronic-data provisions by April 14, 2003. These rules are meant to ensure:

▶ Standardization of electronic patient health records; administrative and financial data, including healthcare claims, healthcare payments and remittance advice; healthcare claims status; enrollment and unenrollment in a healthcare plan; eligibility in a healthcare plan; and healthcare premium payments.

▶ Unique identifying codes for all healthcare providers, healthcare plans, employers, and individuals.

▶ Security of electronic health information with standards protecting the confidentiality and integrity of individually identifiable health information, past, present, or future.

MED TIP

Many of the privacy provisions under HIPAA have caused confusion for the medical community. The original document began as a 337-word guideline, but the final regulation expanded to 101,000 words, or more than 500 pages.

The costs associated with compliance with HIPAA can be extremely high depending on the size of the organization. Blue Cross estimates that the cost of complying with the privacy law would be several billion dollars over a five-year period. This was needed to cover new staffing, computer software, and expanded paperwork.

The Privacy Rule

While it is true that the Privacy Rule is concerned with confidentiality, that is not the basis for this rule. As medical records expanded into electronic format and were transmitted electronically, it became critical to protect patient privacy.

Most laws will permit certain practices unless there is a specific provision or rule *against* doing it. However HIPAA is just the opposite. You can only use and disclose patient information if there is a reason for each disclosure. The basis of the Privacy Rule is that a **permission,** which is a reason for each use and disclosure of patient information, must be identified. For example, permissions or reasons include disclosure to the patient, required disclosures, and payment for treatment.

The Privacy Rule applies to **Protected Health Information (PHI)**, which refers to any individually identifiable information that relates to all past, present, and future physical or mental conditions or the provision of healthcare to an individual. For example, information such as a patient's name, age, gender, Social Security number, zip code, e-mail, and medical diagnosis are all PHI. This information can be oral or recorded in any form or medium, such as with electronic transmission.

HIPAA requires the covered entities to limit the disclosures to only the *minimum* information necessary to carry out the medical treatment. Under HIPAA, this information can be conveyed to vendors, such as health insurance carriers, if they have obtained a written assurance (contract) from the vendor that the information will be protected. These standards to protect the PHI are in effect even if the patient is deceased. See a listing of the five forms required by HIPAA to protect a patient's privacy in Table 10.1 ■.

Under HIPAA, patients must grant written consent or permission to disclose their PHI for treatment, payment, and other healthcare reasons. A **Notice of Privacy Practices (NPP)**, a legal, written statement which details the provider's privacy practices, must be distributed to every patient. The patient is requested to read the document and then sign it. This signed form, or acknowledgment, is then placed into the patient's medical record. See Table 10.2 ■ for recommendations if a patient refuses to sign the NPP.

Patients have six rights under HIPAA that are put in writing in the Notice of Privacy. They are listed in Table 10.3 ■.

1. The privacy notice
2. Acknowledgment that the notice was received
3. Authorization, or consent, from the patient to provide information to others
4. An agreement reached with a healthcare professional's business associates
5. A trading partner agreement

TABLE 10.1

Five Forms Required to Protect Patient's Privacy

▶ Indicate the patient's decision and date on an acknowledgment form or log.
▶ Include the reason for the patient's decision, if known.
▶ Place a copy of this documented unsigned acknowledgment form in the patient's record.
▶ Assure the patient that a refusal to sign the NPP does not mean that he or she cannot exercise their rights.
▶ No physician or institution can refuse to treat the patient based solely on refusal to sign the NPP.
▶ The patient may still request a copy of the NPP even if he or she refuses to sign it.

TABLE 10.2

What to Do If the Patient Refuses to Sign the NPP

TABLE 10.3 **Patient Rights Under HIPAA**	1. Access to and right to copy medical records 2. Requests to have an amendment (or change) made to a medical record 3. Request for an accounting of disclosures 4. Request to be contacted at an alternate location 5. Request for further restrictions on who has access to the medical record 6. Right to file a complaint

MED TIP

A notice should be posted in the reception area of all healthcare providers explaining the HIPAA policy on confidentiality.

Release of Information and Consent

Under HIPAA regulations patients have the right to know how, when, and why their medical information is used (Figure 10.3 ■). They also have the right to some control over the content of the precise information that is disclosed. However, providers can refuse to provide treatment if a patient refuses to sign a consent form. There are three main exceptions to providing consent. One is during an emergency situation, and even then written consent must be obtained as soon as possible after the patient receives treatment. A second exception occurs if there is a language barrier without an interpreter, and then consent may have to be implied. The third exception occurs when treating prison inmates.

Who Are Affected?

Public health authorities, healthcare clearinghouses, and self-insured employers, as well as life insurers, information systems vendors, various service organizations, and universities are all included under HIPAA. These organizations are referred to as **covered entities.** A healthcare **clearinghouse** is a private or public entity that processes or facilitates the

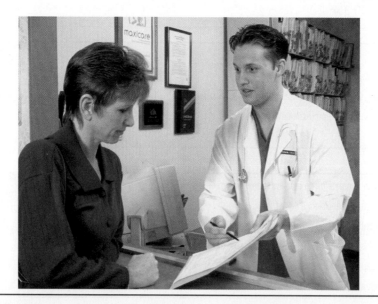

FIGURE 10.3
Healthcare Professional Explaining HIPAA Document to Patient

		TABLE 10.4
▶ Physician practices	▶ Pharmacies and pharmaceutical companies	**Covered Entities Under HIPAA**
▶ Hospitals, including academic medical centers	▶ Medical device companies	
▶ Skilled-nursing facilities	▶ Physical therapists	
▶ Laboratories	▶ Podiatrists	
▶ Dental practices	▶ Chiropractors	
▶ Home health agencies	▶ Osteopaths	
▶ Hospices	▶ Health plans (payers)	
▶ Private insurers	▶ Healthcare clearinghouses	
▶ Ambulance companies	▶ Comprehensive outpatient rehabilitation centers	
▶ Clinical laboratories		

processing of nonstandard electronic transactions into HIPAA transactions. Thus, a clearinghouse may also refer to a billing service. See Table 10.4 ■ for a listing of covered entities under HIPAA.

In other words, if a provider, such as a physical therapist, submits a bill or receives payment for healthcare or treatment, this healthcare professional would most likely be considered to be a covered entity under HIPAA.

MED TIP

Note that patients are not included as covered entities.

Under HIPAA, a **healthcare plan** is an individual or a group plan that provides or pays for medical care. Healthcare plans include group health plans, health maintenance organizations (HMOs), the Medicare program parts A and B, the Medicaid program, and employee welfare benefit plans. Thus, there are few, if any, healthcare providers that are not affected by this law.

Treatment, payment, and healthcare operations, also referred to as TPO, the term used to indicate that a healthcare provider is qualified to provide care or *treatment*, may reveal a patient's PHI in order to obtain *payment* for healthcare, and can provide functions or *healthcare operations* such as quality assurance.

Covered Transactions
There are certain types of electronic transactions for the transmission of healthcare information that are mandated under HIPAA regulations. These are called **covered transactions** between two covered entities and they include the following:

▶ A physician or healthcare provider submitting an electronic claim to an insurance company or healthcare plan

▶ A physician sending any protected health information (PHI) to another physician

▶ A physician sending any protected health information (PHI) to a billing service he or she uses

---
MED TIP

Remember that because patients are not included as covered entities, they can send electronic requests (e-mail) to their physician requesting information about their own records. However, many physicians are reluctant to send information via e-mail to their patients due to privacy concerns.

Denial of the Request for Privacy

There are extraordinary circumstances in which a request for a patient's medical and personal information must be denied in order to protect the patient. One example occurs with nursing homes, because some of their patients may be confused. They often have no family members who are responsible for their care and, thus, the nursing home administration becomes the responsible party. If there is a concern that the patient's healthcare information may be misused, then the nursing home may refuse to allow access.

In addition, certain businesses and individuals, such as employers who sponsor health plans, lawyers, accountants, consultants, and other professionals working for the covered entities, are affected by HIPAA in an indirect manner. The covered entity must make sure that the businesses or business associates it works with, comply with the Privacy Rule. There are severe penalties for violations for both the covered entity and the indirect supplier.

State's Preemption

There are some situations in which a state's privacy laws are stricter than the privacy standards established by HIPAA. In this case the state's laws would take precedence over the federal HIPAA regulation. This is referred to as a **state's preemption.** There are situations when state laws will require the release of information for the good of society. For example, when a state law requires a disclosure, such as reporting an infectious disease outbreak to the public health authorities, the federal privacy regulations would not preempt the state law.

Unique Identifiers for Healthcare Providers

In the past, healthcare organizations used multiple identification formats when doing business with each other. This resulted in confusion and errors. Standard identifiers are now being used in an attempt to reduce these problems. The **Employer Identifier Standard,** which was published in 2002, uses an employer's tax ID number or their **Employer Identification Number (EIN)** as the standard code number for all electronic transmissions.

An individual's Social Security number is still used for insurance identification purposes, as most Americans have a Social Security number and identification card. HIPAA has added the EIN for purposes of electronic transmission by healthcare providers.

Can Protected Health Information (PHI) Be Deidentified?

There are many reasons for obtaining health information in which the patient does not need to be identified. For instance, health statistics relating to communicable diseases can be obtained by **deidentifying,** or removing descriptive information about the patient. See Table 10.5 ■ for a listing of information that must be removed to deidentify PHI.

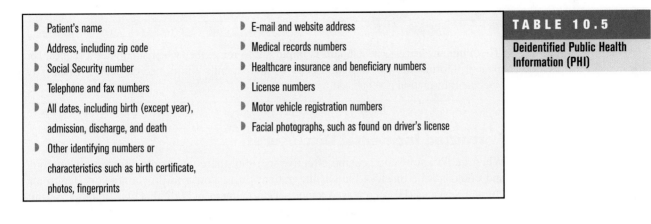

▶ Patient's name	▶ E-mail and website address
▶ Address, including zip code	▶ Medical records numbers
▶ Social Security number	▶ Healthcare insurance and beneficiary numbers
▶ Telephone and fax numbers	▶ License numbers
▶ All dates, including birth (except year), admission, discharge, and death	▶ Motor vehicle registration numbers
▶ Other identifying numbers or characteristics such as birth certificate, photos, fingerprints	▶ Facial photographs, such as found on driver's license

TABLE 10.5

Deidentified Public Health Information (PHI)

What Are the Obligations to the Patient under HIPAA?

The healthcare provider, such as a physician, has several confidentiality obligations to the patient. These include the obligation to obtain patient consent and authorization for any disclosures of medical information and permitting patient access to medical information. In addition, the provider must obtain patient authorization prior to disclosing PHI for purposes other than medical treatment, such as payment collection or a disclosure of psychotherapy notes.

The provider has a requirement to provide only the **minimum necessary standard** information for any disclosure about the patient. This standard means that the provider must make a reasonable effort to limit the disclosure of patient information to only the *minimum* that is necessary to accomplish the purpose of the request. The minimum necessary standard does not apply when a provider is submitting information to the patient, the HHS, or another provider, such as a physician or hospital, for the purpose of treatment (Figure 10.4 ■).

The minimum necessary standard requirements do not apply to any health information disclosures that are required by law. For example, a physician, as a covered entity, is still required to disclose PHI that is requested in a subpoena.

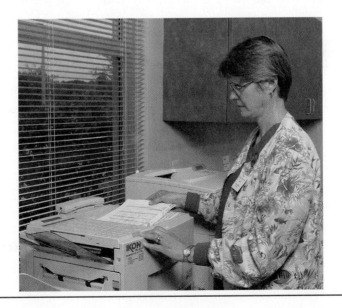

FIGURE 10.4
Only the Minimum of Information That Is Needed Can Be Sent to Another Provider

---

MED TIP

The minimum necessary standard is important to remember when supplying a request for patient information. Never send a copy of the patient's entire medical record when only *specific* information is requested.

Permitted Incidental Disclosures

When the Privacy Rule became effective in 1996, there was confusion as to what could and could not be disclosed about the patient. In response to this confusion Health and Human Services (HHS) released a guidance document in 2002 that clarified the "permitted incidental disclosures." See Table 10.6 ■ for examples of permitted disclosures.

What Are the Penalties for Noncompliance with HIPAA?

Noncompliance with HIPAA can result in serious penalties for healthcare providers such as physicians and hospitals. The penalties for violating HIPAA range from civil penalties of up to $100 per person per incident for minor improper disclosures of health information, and up to $25,000 for multiple violations of the same standard in a calendar year. Federal criminal liability for improper disclosure of information or for obtaining information under false pretenses carries **sanctions** (fines) of up to $50,000 and one year in prison. The liability for obtaining protected health information under false pretenses with the intent to sell, transfer, or use the information for personal gain or for a malicious action, such as Medicare fraud, carries penalties of up to $250,000 and/or up to ten years in prison. Severe penalties are in effect if lax security allows health information to be stolen. There is also a risk of a class action suit as well as public relations damage to the institution's or physician's image.

Healthcare fraud, especially relating to the Medicare and Medicaid programs, has been increasing during the past decade. Fraud alerts issued by the Inspector General's Office of the Department of Health and Human Services (HHS) concerning suspicious practices can alert providers and the public to the potential for medical privacy abuse.

TABLE 10.6 **Permitted Incidental Disclosures**	▶ Healthcare staff at a nursing station can coordinate patient care if they speak in a low voice. ▶ Nurses and other staff members can talk to a patient by phone or discuss the treatment of a patient with another provider if the discussions are conducted in low voices and away from listeners. ▶ Laboratory results can be discussed with patients or other healthcare professionals in a treatment area if privacy precautions are taken. ▶ A message can be left for a patient on an answering machine or with family members, but the amount of information must be limited for just the purpose of the call. ▶ Patients can be asked to sign in and be called by name in the waiting room, but they should not sign the reason for their visit. ▶ The patient's name can be announced in the waiting room or use a public address system to come to a particular location. ▶ A lighted x-ray board can be used in a nursing station if it is not publicly visible. ▶ Patient charts can be placed outside of exam rooms if reasonable precautions are used. The charts should be placed with the name faced to the wall or a cover concealing the chart.

Another provision under HIPAA is the establishment of the **Healthcare Integrity and Protection Data Bank (HIPDB)**. This is a national data bank that collects reports and disclosures of actions taken against healthcare practitioners, providers, and vendors for noncompliance and fraudulent activities. This extensive data bank is not available to the general public, but can be accessed by federal and state government agencies and various health plans.

What Are the Patients' Rights Under the Privacy Standards?

Patients have many rights under HIPAA. Healthcare providers have the additional responsibility of alerting patients to their own rights under this law. See Table 10.7 ■ for patients' rights under the Privacy Standards.

HIPAA-Defined Permissions

HIPAA defines eleven areas in which permission must be granted in order to use or disclose patient health information (PHI). **HIPAA-defined permission** is based on the reason for knowing, or use of, the information. Only two disclosures are *required* by HIPAA: for Health and Human Services (HHS) requests and to honor patient requests. All eleven permissions are described in Table 10.8 ■.

TABLE 10.7

Patients' Rights Under the Privacy Standards

- A copy of the privacy notice from the healthcare provider
- Access to their medical records and the right to restrict access by others, request changes, and learn how their records have been accessed
- Ask the provider to limit the way in which healthcare information is shared and to keep disclosures to the minimum needed for treatment and business operations
- Ask to whom the healthcare information was given
- Ask to be contacted in a special way, such as by mail or at work
- Ask to be contacted in a place other than home or work
- Examine and copy the health information the provider has recorded
- Complain to the covered entity and the Department of Health and Human Services if the patient believes there is a violation of his or her privacy

TABLE 10.8

HIPAA-Defined Permissions

Disclosure	Condition
1. Required disclosures	a. Health and Human Services (HHS) can view accounts, records, and other financial documents b. Patient requests to view own records
2. Valid patient authorization	a. Allows for PHI to be disclosed
3. Patient requests for disclosure	a. May view own records b. May discuss treatment and medical condition with physician
4. For use in treatment of patients, payment, or other healthcare operations (TPO).	
5. For the treatment, payment, and healthcare operations (TPO) of other covered entities	a. Patient's written permission is needed for other covered entities, such as attorneys and insurance plans, to have access to PHI covered entities

TABLE 10.8	Disclosure	Condition
HIPAA-Defined Permissions (*Continued*)	6. For patient representatives such as family	a. Must present a legal document, such as Medical Power of Attorney, before granting access to PHI by family or friend
	7. Qualified disaster relief organizations	a. Used to provide notification regarding disaster relief b. May be provided unless patient objects
	8. Incidental disclosures about patients without their authorization	a. Nurses and healthcare professionals may discuss patient cases when they are out of the hearing distance of others. b. Healthcare professionals may discuss laboratory results with patients and others if they are out of the hearing distance of others. c. Healthcare professionals may leave limited telephone messages for patients; it is always preferable to ask the patient if this is acceptable. d. May call a patient by name in a waiting room or over a public address system e. May leave patient chart outside an exam room if the patient's identity is not visible
	9. For public purposes	a. When the PHI disclosure is required by law such as with a request by the court b. Public health departments are authorized to collect data relating to communicable diseases, births, and deaths. c. In all cases of abuse or neglect d. Disclosure necessary to prevent serious harm, such as when a patient threatens another person or makes a suicide threat; healthcare professionals must notify the patient that this disclosure has been made. e. Food and Drug Administration (FDA) can collect PHI relating to safety of drugs and products. f. PHI may be disclosed in order to notify people at risk of a communicable disease. g. May release PHI in case of subpoena; consult with privacy official to determine specific criteria that apply h. Law enforcement has the right to PHI in cases of abuse, neglect, gunshot wounds, suspicious death, identifying a suspect, or medical emergency. i. Coroners and funeral directors may receive PHI in order to perform their functions. j. Organ and tissue donation agencies may receive PHI to facilitate the donation process. k. Researchers may receive PHI under certain conditions; consult with privacy officer. l. State Worker's Compensation programs may need PHI. m. Government agencies and facilities, such as prisons and the military, may receive PHI under certain conditions.
	10. When deidentification has occurred (ie., when patient identifiers have been removed)	

Disclosure	Condition
11. In a limited data set in which certain identifiers, such as patient's, relative's, and employer's names have been removed, patients do not have the right to access	a. Psychotherapy notes b. Certain laboratory tests, under the Clinical Laboratory Improvement Act of 1988 (CLIA) may only be given to person who authorized the test—usually a physician. c. If they are prison inmates d. Certain research projects in which the limited access has been granted in advance e. If the PHI is part of a government record f. If the PHI was obtained under a promise of confidentiality

TABLE 10.8

HIPAA-Defined Permissions (*Continued*)

Special Rules Relating to Research

HIPAA regulations also relate to medical information that is compiled and used for research purposes. Providers and other covered entities that wish to use individually identifiable patient information that is related to treatment, such as for cancer patients, must perform a very detailed authorization form. The researchers must obtain

- A patient authorization that complies with the rules set by HIPAA, or
- A waiver of authorization from a privacy board or an Institutional Review Board, such as is found in a teaching hospital or university. The waiver must include extensive documentation as required by HIPAA.

This regulation also covers information used for research from deceased patient records.

Problems Relating to Implementation of HIPAA's Privacy Rules

HIPAA is an often misunderstood law. New studies are finding that some healthcare providers are being too overzealous in applying this law, leaving family members, caregivers, public health personnel, and law enforcement officers without necessary information to care for the patients. This results in frustration and delays in treatment of patients. HIPAA was passed by Congress in 1996 to allow patient's easier access to their medical records, while limiting this access to others. Unfortunately, this has not always happened.

HIPAA regulations have made many healthcare agencies, such as hospitals, reluctant to release any information about their patients due to fear of civil or criminal penalties under HIPAA. This is particularly true when a patient refuses to be listed on the hospital's patient directory. In certain situations, some healthcare providers, trying to avoid any error under HIPAA by disclosing PHI inappropriately, refuse to provide medical records to anyone except the patient. For instance, state workers' compensation programs, which are exempted under HIPAA, have difficulty receiving the medical information they require in order to provide financial assistance for the patient.

Reports of problems with accessing patient information have been filed by nonmedical persons. For example, human resource departments often require medical information in order to administer the Family and Medical Leave Act (FMLA), facilitate return-to-work policies, assist in Americans with Disabilities Act (ADA) accommodation discussions, and obtain results from drug testing. In addition, lawyers working with workers' compensation claims, medical malpractice, and personal injury litigation need access to medical records. And members of the clergy complain that the privacy rules keep them from visiting the sick members of their congregations when they are hospitalized. They complain that the law is being too narrowly interpreted.

Police are also confronting problems as a result of HIPAA. The law requires hospitals to report to the police when a patient comes in with a gunshot wound or there is a suspected case of child abuse or neglect. According to some police officials, compliance with HIPAA is slowing police investigations and even impeding the prosecution of crimes. Police officers complain that they are being denied access to anyone, including crime victims and persons previously reported as missing, who have opted not to be listed in hospital directories. Although HIPAA makes exceptions for criminal investigations, some hospitals, concerned with violating the law, err on the side of caution and refuse to release any information. Under HIPAA, hospitals must allow police to interview patients and must provide information about their condition when a serious crime has been committed.

There have been serious problems occurring as a result of improperly interpreting the requirements of HIPAA. For example, Charlie, a mental patient in Chicago, was released from the hospital into the care of his friend to recuperate. Within a week Charlie was dead after jumping to his death from his friend's balcony. The friend did not know that Charlie was suicidal when he was admitted to the hospital after he had attempted to take his own life. The hospital did not release that information to the friend since they believed they could not under HIPAA regulations. The friend said he would have monitored Charlie better if he had only been told about his condition.

In another case, a California mother was unable to get the hospital to produce a key medical record documenting her son's blood pressure in his final hours. The young man had died from an overdose just hours after she was told that he was stable. The record finally arrived six years later and indicated that her son had been in mortal danger for several hours while awaiting care. The medical record arrived too late under state law to file a civil lawsuit. Disputes over an inability to receive records by designated family members has become a common complaint.

In another situation, a heart patient was transferred from one hospital to another in order to receive heart surgery. The first hospital refused to release the patient's laboratory records because they believed it would be a violation under HIPAA.

Educational facilities are coping with the task of gaining access to information about the mental stability of their students after the horrendous killing of 32 students and faculty at Virginia Tech. Many mental health professionals believe their patients' records are protected from disclosure under HIPAA. However, other experts believe that information about mentally disturbed students, who indicate that they would use harmful behavior against others, should be made known to the authorities.

MED TIP

A violation of HIPAA, a federal law, is a criminal offense. Therefore, fear of violating this law has caused an overreaction to it among many healthcare professionals. According to Dr. William Kobler, former president of the Illinois State Medical Association, physicians have become excessively cautious about releasing patient information out of fear that they will be slapped with a large fine.

Misconceptions about HIPAA

The Department of Health and Human Services (HHS) states that the law requires "reasonable safeguards" be taken in order to protect patient privacy. The privacy provision applies to physicians, pharmacists, and insurers. It was originally intended to protect computerized medical records and billing and to allow patients easier access to their own medical records. However, the purpose has been interpreted much more broadly.

According to the HHS, many misconceptions about HIPAA are slowly being cleared up. The privacy law

▶ Does not prevent physicians or hospitals from sharing patient information with other physicians or hospitals in order to treat patients.

▶ Does not prevent hospitals from disclosing names of patients to clergy or from keeping patient directories. It does not require that patients sign in to be included in the hospital directory of patients, only that they can opt out and not be included.

▶ Allows hospitals or physicians to share information with the patient's spouse, family members, friends, or anyone whom the patient has identified as involved in their care.

▶ Does not apply to most police or fire departments. The hospital may release names and information about homicides, accident victims, and other incidents. However, HIPAA does limit the information that emergency medical technicians (EMTs) may disclose.

Office personnel, acting on behalf of physicians and dentists, can still send out reminders about appointments and leave messages on patients' answering machines.

MED TIP

The HIPAA law, as currently written, prohibits patients/consumers from suing over privacy violations. Instead, patient/consumers must register their complaints with the government agency, Health and Human Services. (www.hhs.gov/ocr/hipaa or www.hipaadvisory.com)

Recommendations

Following are some practical recommendations for physicians and physician groups to follow when implementing HIPAA:

▶ Appoint and train a privacy officer to receive complaints and provide information concerning the provider's privacy notice materials.

▶ Conduct an internal assessment of existing policies, procedures, and practices for collecting and handling medical records and patient information to determine where the deficiencies in privacy may occur.

▶ Enter into written agreements with all nonemployee service providers who may have access to PHI.

▶ Adopt procedures for handling patient requests.

▶ Implement a notice of privacy practices.

▶ Revise employee manuals regarding HIPAA standards. These personnel policies must reflect the organization's handling of employees who use or disclose PHI in violation of HIPAA. The **Office of Civil Rights (OCR)** would likely ask for a copy of these policies during an investigation of violations.

▶ Train all employees on policies and procedures regarding HIPAA.

▶ Retain signed authorizations, copies of notices of privacy practices, and any agreements with patients restricting disclosure of PHI. This documentation should be retained for a period of six years from the date they were created or the date when they were last in effect.

▸ Implement and enforce sanctions (penalties) for violations of provider policies and procedures.

▸ Establish a complaint process for noncompliance with the privacy regulation.

See Table 10.9 ■ for a list of precautions relating to HIPAA.

ETHICAL CONCERNS WITH INFORMATION TECHNOLOGY (INFORMATICS)

Wireless local area networks (WLANs) are used by physicians and nurses to access patient records from central databases while they are conducting patient rounds (bedside visits), adding observations and patient assessments to the databases, checking on medications, and completing a variety of other functions. The use of wireless networks by healthcare professionals presents ethical challenges and dilemmas. There can be a trade-off between quick access to the patient's medical records and the security of those records. Decisions relating to the use of WLANs must take into account the impact they have on the patient's privacy as mandated by HIPAA. HIPAA requires that there be safeguards in place to protect the privacy of electronic and nonelectronic protected health information. The HIPAA security rules that were issued in final form on February 20, 2003, apply to PHI in *electronic* form only.

> ## MED TIP
> Because the amount of medical information available is said to double every five years, computerized systems have become indispensable.

TABLE 10.9 **Precautions Relating to HIPAA**	▸ You need to use a fax cover sheet to fax anything with Protected Health Information (PHI). ▸ When conferencing about a patient, you should not be in a place where others can hear you. ▸ Do not leave laptops or desktops unattended with patient information on the screen. ▸ Do not give out your computer password to anyone. Change passwords frequently. ▸ Do not let someone else use your computer when you are already signed on. ▸ Have anti-virus software, robust firewalls, and screensavers installed in all computers. ▸ An organization can be fined each time it breaks the rule, up to $25,000 a year. ▸ An individual person can be fined or sent to prison.

Medical informatics is the application of communication and information to medical practice, research, and education. Many hospitals and healthcare institutions are able to link together diverse areas such as pharmacy, laboratory, administrative, and medical records through the use of informatics. For example, many hospital pharmacies have implemented a fully computerized medication ordering system to lower the incidence of medication errors due to the inability to correctly interpret handwritten orders.

Telemedicine, or the use of communication and information technologies to provide healthcare services to people at a distance, is seen as the future of medicine. Modern technology has the ability to provide health services for homebound and rural patients via telephone, fax, Internet, and even real-time television. All of these methods have been used to provide continuing medical education for the past decade.

Some of these methods for treatment are still in the developmental stage. For example, Virginia Mason Medical Center, a large multispecialty group practice in Seattle, has telemedicine sites in rural Washington and Alaska. This center uses telemedicine to consult on diagnosis and treatment, transmit radiological studies, and conduct presurgical and postsurgical exams. It has telemedicine projects in radiology, cardiology, neurology/neurosurgery, psychiatry, dermatology, oncology, rheumatology, and rehabilitation medicine.

Health Partners, a Minneapolis-based health plan, uses a 24-hour two-way video conferencing method to link the nurses with the home care patients. Ordinary phone lines are used in this system. The nurses are able to inspect wound care and healing over this video link.

A multitude of medical information is currently available over the Internet—in varying degrees of usefulness. Healthcare consumers can use the Internet to research their disease and treatment options. Many healthcare plans and institutions have their own websites with current information about services and medical information (see Appendix B for a listing of useful medical websites).

Telemedicine raises legal issues, such as concerns about practicing medicine across state lines, that must be addressed. Physician reimbursement for these types of consultations is uncertain. Also, the credentials of the person giving medical advice over the Internet are open to both legal and ethical discussion.

Informatics presents a multitude of ethical issues, especially with the use of the Internet by physicians and patients. Healthcare providers have expressed concern about security when patient data, such as that contained in medical records, is transmitted via the Internet. A report on confidentiality and security issues by the Computer Based Patient Record Institute, based in Schaumburg, Illinois, states, "Breaches of confidentiality can lead to loss of employment and housing, health and life insurance problems, and social stigma. . . . Formal information security programs must be established by each organization entrusted with healthcare information."

POINTS TO PONDER

1. Will it be possible to balance the wealth of medical information available to the patient via the Internet with the loss of a personal relationship between the patient and caregiver?

2. How can a patient's PHI be maintained when medical information is being faxed from one location to another?

3. Is the high cost of implementing HIPAA in a small medical practice worth the expense?

4. In your opinion, will HIPAA make it more or less difficult for public services such as police, fire, and ambulance services to administer to patients? Explain your answer.

DISCUSSION QUESTIONS

1. Why has patient confidentiality become more difficult in the present healthcare environment?

2. Why is the implementation of the new Privacy Rule so expensive?

3. Should family members, and even friends, have access to a patient's medical record? Why or why not?

4. Should patients be treated via the Internet? Why or why not?

REVIEW CHALLENGE

Short Answer Questions

1. What is the Privacy Rule and why is it important?

   _____

   _____

2. What is a covered transaction? Give an example of one.

   _____

   _____

3. What are some examples of forms of identity that must be deidentified when health statistics are obtained?

   _____

   _____

4. What are some of the misconceptions about HIPAA?

   _____

   _____

5. What are some of the benefits of telemedicine?

   _____

   _____

6. What might be some of the ethical concerns with WLANs?

   _____

   _____

7. What are some privacy precautions to use when taking care of patients?

   _____

   _____

8. Who should a patient contact if he or she wishes to register a complaint about a potential privacy violation?

   _____

   _____

9. What does "minimum necessary standard" mean and why is it important?

   _____

   _____

10. Explain the quote from Justice Brandeis, found in this chapter, relating to our right to privacy.

    _____

    _____

Matching

Match responses in column B with the correct term in column A.

Column A

_____   1. privacy rule
_____   2. WLANs
_____   3. HIPAA
_____   4. EIN
_____   5. clearinghouse
_____   6. healthcare plan
_____   7. PHI
_____   8. telemedicine
_____   9. employer identifier standard
_____   10. HHS

Column B

a. number assigned to an employer
b. individually identifiable information
c. wireless systems to send and receive data
d. based on employer's tax ID or on their EIN
e. all covered entities must be in compliance
f. Department of Health and Human Services
g. a billing service
h. use of information technologies to treat people at a distance
i. Health Insurance Portability and Accountability Act of 1996
j. individual or group that provides or pays for medical care

Multiple Choice

Select the one best answer to the following statements.

1. The Privacy Rule is meant to ensure

   a. standardization of health data.
   b. standardization of financial data.
   c. standardization of medical care.
   d. a and b only.
   e. a, b, and c.

2. An example of a clearinghouse is

   a. PHI.
   b. a skilled nursing facility.
   c. a billing service.
   d. a government regulation.
   e. EIN.

3. The government organization that investigates a violation of a patient's medical privacy is called

   a. OSHA.
   b. OCR.
   c. PHI.
   d. HIPAA.
   e. none of the above.

4. A network of wireless communication systems used to access patient records is

   a. HIPAA.
   b. PHI.
   c. WLANs.
   d. EIN.
   e. ADA.

5. The privacy law

   a. prevents hospitals from sharing medical information with other facilities.
   b. prevents hospitals from sharing registered patient names with the clergy.
   c. does not apply to most police and fire departments.
   d. allows unlimited information to be shared by EMTs.
   e. none of the above.

6. A violation of HIPAA

   a. is a criminal offense.
   b. does not carry any financial penalty at present.
   c. is not reportable.
   d. does not affect a physician's reputation, as it is just a document.
   e. may have a fine of under $100 for all offenses.

7. When implementing HIPAA, physicians and physician groups should

   a. hire a privacy officer.
   b. implement a notice of privacy practices.
   c. retain signed authorizations for at least six years.
   d. enter into written agreements with nonemployee service providers.
   e. all of the above.

8. Covered entities include all of the following except

   a. hospice programs.
   b. medical device companies.
   c. clinical laboratories.
   d. police departments.
   e. skilled-nursing facilities.

9. Patients' rights under HIPAA include the ability to

   a. examine their medical record.
   b. have a full copy of their medical record.
   c. complain to the HHS if they believe there is a violation of privacy.
   d. a and c only.
   e. a, b, and c.

10. When patient information is requested via a subpoena, you must

   a. comply and send the entire record immediately.
   b. provide only the minimum necessary standard even if more is requested in the subpoena.
   c. provide all PHI that is requested in the subpoena.
   d. provide PHI only with the consent of the patient.
   e. none of the above are correct.

DISCUSSION CASES

1. Mary Smith has just reported for duty and is reviewing the patients she will have during the evening shift. One of them, Ida Monroe, is on isolation for an infectious disease. Dr. Jerome comes into the nursing station around 9:00 p.m. after making hospital rounds to see his patients. He tells Mary that he noticed that one of his neighbors, Ida Monroe, is a patient, and he would like to review her medical chart. Mary starts to give him the chart and then realizes that Dr. Jerome is not Ida's physician. Dr. Jerome says not to worry about that, as he has taken care of the rest of Ida's family for years and is sure that Ida will want him to consult on her case. When Mary hesitates to give him the chart, Dr. Jerome says that he will report her to her nursing supervisor. He walks over to pick up the chart.

   a. Should Mary give Ida's medical chart to Dr. Jerome? Why or why not?

   _____

   _____

   b. What should Mary say to Dr. Jerome?

   _____

   _____

   c. What should Mary do if Dr. Jerome continues to insist on seeing Ida's chart?

   _____

   _____

   d. What ethical principles are involved in this case?

   _____

   _____

   e. What legal regulations are involved in this case?

   _____

   _____

2. You are a CMA working in the office of a physician who performs major surgical procedures on hospitalized patients. A patient, who is the father of a friend of yours, comes in for a pre-surgery exam. You happen to know that this man is an alcoholic. You also know that the surgeon you work for does not like to perform surgery on alcoholic patients as he believes they have difficulty healing and often have excessive bleeding after surgery. You wish to tell the surgeon about the man's drinking problem, but you are afraid that it would be a HIPPA violation.

   a. What do you do?

   _____

   _____

   b. Is this a legal and/or ethical problem?

   _____

   _____

   c. Should you discuss your concerns with your friend?

   _____

   _____

d. What is your first responsibility?

_____

_____

3. *An elderly patient has approached you in the medical office where you work. He is very distressed at having to read and sign a HIPAA document. He asks you the following questions. What do you say?*

    a. "Why am I getting so many of these privacy notices every time I go into a medical office or hospital? Why can't you use one that I already signed before for another doctor?"

_____

_____

    b. "Can I see my medical record?"

_____

_____

    c. "I live with my daughter. Can she see my medical record if she asks for it?"

_____

_____

    d. "I want to file a complaint. Where can I do that?"

_____

_____

PUT IT INTO PRACTICE

Request a copy of a notice of privacy from your physician's office. What does this notice state about filing a complaint?

WEB HUNT

Look under the official government website relating to HIPAA, (www.hhs.gov/ocr/hipaa), to find the answers to frequently asked questions about HIPAA. Describe five questions and answers that you believe all healthcare professionals should know.

CRITICAL THINKING EXERCISE

What would you do if, as part of your job in handling the office mail, you came across a consultation report from a psychiatrist about one of your family members?

BIBLIOGRAPHY

Associated Press. 2004. "Privacy Keeps Clergy from Sick." *Hartford Courant* (April, 12), B2.

Davis, R. 2008. "Across USA, Anxiety over Access to Patient Records" *USA Today* (April 29), 12.

Graham, J. 2004. "Privacy Law a Bitter Pill." *Chicago Tribune* (April 13), 1, 16.

Gross, J. 2007. "Keeping Patients' Details Private, Even from Kin." *New York Times* (July 3), 1, 12.

Hall, R. 2000. *An introduction to healthcare organizational ethics.* Oxford, England: Oxford University Press.

Hartley, C., and E. Jones. 2004. *HIPAA plain & simple: A compliance guide for healthcare professionals.* Chicago: AMA Press.

Heath, B., D. Leinwald, and A. Gomez. 2007. "Police: No Known Link of Cho, Victims." *USA Today* (April 20), 4A.

Keefe, S. 2006. "Telemonitoring in Home Care." *Advance for Nurses* (June 19), 27–28.

Nakashima, E. 2008. "Health Records on Demand." *Hartford Courant* (August 4), A3.

Parker, L. 2003. "Medical-privacy Law Creates Wide Confusion." *USA Today* (October 17), 1, 2.

Reynolds, B. 2003. "Are You Hip to HIPAA, the New Health Care Privacy Laws?" *New Milford Spectrum* (August 8), S 14.

Schiff, M. 2003. *HIPAA: The questions you didn't know to ask.* Upper Saddle River, NJ: Prentice Hall.

Somma, A. 2003. "Privacy Rules Stymie Police." *Hartford Courant* (August 7), 1, 10.

Steinhauer, J. 2008. "California Hospital Faces Sanctions after Workers Looked at Patient Records." *New York Times* (April 8), 16.

Ethical and Bioethical Issues in Medicine

11

Learning Objectives

1. Define the glossary terms.
2. List and discuss at least ten bioethical issues the modern physician and healthcare professional face.
3. Describe how an ethical decision-making model, such as the Seven-Step Decision Model, can be used when confronted with difficult ethical dilemmas.
4. Discuss ethical issues relating to genetic testing.
5. Describe the advances in human stem cell research.
6. Summarize the ethical issues of organ transplantation.
7. Discuss the importance of codes of ethics such as the Nuremberg Code.

Key Terms

Alleges
Censure
Chromosomes
Clone
Control group
Double-blind test
Euthanasia
Expulsion
Gene markers
Gene therapy

Harvested
Human genome
Human Genome Project
Institutional Review Board
  (IRB)
National Organ Transplant
  Law of 1984
Nontherapeutic research
Placebo group
Posthumous

Revocation
Social utility method
  of allocation
Stem cells
Therapeutic research
United Network for Organ
  Sharing (UNOS)

THE CASE OF THE TUSKEGEE SYPHILIS RESEARCH STUDY

Historical Case

In 1929, the United States Health Service worked with state and local departments of health in six states to find a method to control venereal disease. The statistical reports that were conducted between 1930 and 1932 demonstrated a high rate of syphilis in Macon County, Alabama, where over 84 percent of the population were black and 40 percent of the men were infected with syphilis. The methods used for treating this disease consisted of the injection of mercury and other toxic chemicals. Some men recovered with this treatment; others were made even more ill; and in some cases in which no treatment was given, the patient was able to live for several decades.

After funding to treat the disease ran out during the Depression, the researchers conducting the Tuskegee Study attempted to discover how severe this disease was if left untreated. For this study, the U.S. Public Health Service selected 600 men. Of these 600 research subjects, 400 of the men had syphilis and the other 200 nonsyphilitic men became the **control group** of research subjects who received no treatment. The infected patients were not told about the purpose or nature of the research. In fact, the researchers would refer to procedures such as spinal taps as "treatments" to induce patient participation. When some of the men in the control group developed syphilis over the course of the study, they were transferred into the research group without ever being told they had the disease. No treatment was ever given to any of the men to fight the disease.

In the early 1940s, penicillin was found to be effective against syphilis. The Tuskegee Project could have been discontinued at this time, as there was no longer any need to study the course of this disease without treatment. However, the research project did continue. The researchers were able to track the men and make sure they did not receive antibiotics for any condition including syphilis. In the 1960s, a researcher working for the U.S. Public Health Service tried to put an end to the project, which was now being conducted by the Centers for Disease Control (CDC) in Atlanta. When he was unsuccessful, he notified the press and ultimately the project was stopped. The public was outraged that poor black men had been subjected to a research project without their consent and denied treatment for a treatable disease in an attempt to gain what was seen as useless information. In 1973, the surviving patients received an out-of-court settlement of $37,500 for the infected men and $16,000 for the men in the control group. The families of men who had died also received compensation of $15,000 for the infected men and $5,000 for the uninfected men.

In 1997, President Clinton offered a public apology to the men, including one 100-year-old survivor, who were involved in this study. The last remaining survivor of this study died in 2004.

This was never a secret project. This project had been well publicized in medical journals. The people who read about the study did nothing to stop it.

(Summarized from G. Pence. *Classic Cases in Medical Ethics.* New York: McGraw Hill, 1990.)

Healthcare ethics, bioethics, and medical law are intertwined out of necessity. When ethical principles are violated, a civil lawsuit often follows. As we have explained throughout this book, ethics, that branch of philosophy relating to morals or moral principles, involves the examination of human character and conduct, the distinction between right and wrong, and a person's moral duty and obligations to the community.

Introduction

Ethics, as discussed in the healthcare professions, is applied ethics. In other words, while theoretical concepts involving ethics are important for the student to know, the basis for study involves *applying* one's moral and value system to a career in healthcare.

Ethics involves more than just common sense, which is an approach for making decisions that most people in society use. Ethics goes way beyond common sense: It requires a critical-thinking approach that examines important considerations such as fairness for all consumers, the impact of the decision on society, and the future implications of the decision.

MED TIP

The dignity of the individual, whether it is the patient, employee, or physician must always be of paramount concern when discussing ethics and bioethics.

Bioethics concerns ethical issues discussed in the context of advanced medical technology. The somewhat new field of bioethics requires the healthcare professional to ask whether a practice such as gene therapy or cloning can be morally justified. In addition, physicians must ask themselves if these practices are compatible with the character traits of a good physician.

MED TIP

Remember that, as discussed in Chapter 1, an illegal act, or one that is against the law, is almost always unethical. However, an unethical act may not be illegal. For instance, providing medical treatment, such as an organ transplant, to a celebrity and denying the same treatment for an indigent "street person," while legal, is clearly unethical.

EARLY HISTORY

Ethics has been a part of the medical profession since the beginning of medical practice. In 400 B.C., Hippocrates, a Greek physician referred to as "the father of medicine," wrote a statement of principles for his medical students to follow that is still important in medicine (see Figure 11.1 ■). Called the Hippocratic Oath, the code reminds students of the importance of their profession, the need to teach others, and the obligation to never knowingly harm a patient or divulge a confidence. The principles stated in the oath are found today in many of the professional codes of ethics, such as that of the American Medical Association (AMA). The Hippocratic Oath is found in Appendix A.

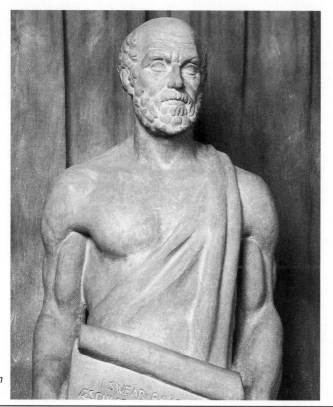

FIGURE 11.1
An Artist's Interpretation of Hippocrates
(Brian Warling/International Museum of Surgical Science, Chicago, IL.)

ETHICAL STANDARDS AND BEHAVIOR

Ethical behavior, according to the AMA, refers to moral principles or practices, the customs of the medical profession, and matters of medical policy. Unethical behavior would be any action that does not follow these ethical standards. For example, it is unethical for physicians to decline to accept patients due to their race or color.

A physician who is accused of unethical behavior or conduct in violation of these standards can be issued a warning or **censure** (criticism) by the AMA. The AMA Board of Examiners may recommend the **expulsion** (being forced out) or suspension of a physician from membership in the medical association. Expulsion is a severe penalty because it limits the physician's ability to practice medicine. Even if the AMA censors its members, it does not have authority to bring legal action against the physician for unethical behavior. However, not all physicians belong to the AMA.

If someone **alleges,** or declares without proof, that a physician has committed a criminal act, the AMA is required to report it to the state licensing board or governmental agency. Violation of the law, followed by a conviction for the crime, may result in a fine, imprisonment, or **revocation** (taking away) of the physician's license.

MED TIP
The loss of a physician's license, as required by law in serious cases of fraud, will usually mean the loss of the physician's reputation.

CODES OF ETHICS

People's behavior must match their set of values. For example, it is not enough to believe that patient confidentiality is important if one then freely discusses a patient's personal information with a co-worker or friend. In this case, the healthcare professional's values and behavior are at odds. Professional organizations have developed codes of ethics that summarize the basic principles and behavior that are expected of all practitioners in that discipline. These codes, also known as statements of intent, are meant to govern the conduct of members of a given profession, such as medicine.

Some codes of ethics were developed as a direct response to atrocities that occurred during wartime, especially in response to the medical experimentation in Nazi concentration camps during World War II (WWII). Public awareness of the ethical and legal problems associated with medical research, such as experimenting on human subjects, gained prominence in the post–WWII trials at Nuremberg, Germany. In these trials, more than twenty-five Nazi medical personnel were accused of committing war crimes against involuntary human subjects. The most infamous experimenter, Josef Mengele, was also known as the "angel of death." What became known as the Nuremberg Code developed after these trials made public what the Nazis had done under the guise of medical research. This code became a forerunner for the subsequent codes and guidelines that were adopted by medical and research organizations and agencies. The Nuremberg Code reminds us that basic ethical principles must be followed when conducting medical research, or any research involving human beings. The Nuremberg Code is found in Appendix A.

Due to advances in medical science and technology, and changes in the medical profession, physicians have developed modern codes of ethics that serve as a moral guide for healthcare professionals. The AMA has taken a leadership role in setting standards for the ethical behavior of physicians in the United States. The first Code of Ethics of the AMA was formed in 1847, shortly after the organization was founded.

American Medical Association (AMA) Principles of Medical Ethics

The AMA Principles of Medical Ethics—which appear in Chapter 5—discuss human dignity, honesty, responsibility to society, confidentiality, the need for continued study, patient autonomy, a responsibility of the physician to improve the community, a responsibility to the patient, and access to medical care.

MED TIP

Every healthcare professional who interacts with patients, such as medical receptionists, medical assistants, nurses, physician assistants, and pharmacy technicians must be familiar with the Principles of the AMA. For example, just as physicians cannot refuse to treat patients based on race or color, neither can their staff. Their behavior can reflect either negatively or positively on their employer/physician.

Judicial Council Opinions of the AMA

The Council on Ethical and Judicial Affairs of the AMA is comprised of nine members who interpret the Principles of Medical Ethics. The council's interpretation or clarification is then published for AMA members. All members of the medical team are expected to cooperate with the physician in upholding these principles. A few of the opinions of the Council on Ethical and Judicial Affairs are adapted and summarized in Table 11.1 ■.

TABLE 11.1	Issue	Opinion
Summary of Opinions of the Council on Ethical and Judicial Affairs of the AMA	Abuse	Physicians who are likely to detect abuse in the course of their work have an obligation to familiarize themselves with protocols for diagnosing and treating abuse and with community resources for battered women, children, and elderly persons. If it were not reported, it might mean further abuse or even death for the victim.
	Accepting patients	A physician may decline to accept a patient if the medical condition of the patient is not within the area of the physician's expertise and practice. However, a physician may not decline a patient due to race, color, religion, national origin, or any other basis for discrimination.
	Allocations of health resources	Physicians have a duty to do what they can for the benefit of the individual patient. Physicians have a responsibility to participate and to contribute their professional expertise in order to safeguard the interests of patients in decisions made at the societal level regarding the allocation or rationing of health resources. The treating physician must remain a patient advocate and, therefore, should not make allocation decisions.
	Confidential care of minors	Physicians who treat minors have an ethical duty to promote the autonomy of minor patients by involving them in the medical decision-making process to a degree equal with their abilities.
	Euthanasia	Euthanasia is the administration of a lethal agent by another person to cause the patient's death and thereby relieve the patient's suffering. Instead of engaging in euthanasia, physicians must aggressively respond to the needs of patients at the end of life. Patients should not be abandoned once it is determined that a cure is impossible.
	Fee splitting	The practice of a physician accepting payment from another physician for the referral of a patient is known as fee splitting and is considered unethical.
	Financial incentives for organ donation	The voluntary donation of organs in appropriate circumstances is to be encouraged. However, it is not ethical to participate in a procedure to enable a donor to receive payment, other than for the reimbursement of expenses necessarily incurred in connection with the removal of any of the donor's nonrenewable organs. In addition, when death of the donor has occurred it must be decided by a physician other than the donor patient's physician.
	Gene therapy	The Council's position is that gene therapy, the replacement of a defective or malfunctioning gene, is acceptable as long as it is used for therapeutic purposes and not for altering human traits.
	Ghost surgery	A surgeon cannot substitute another surgeon to perform a procedure without the consent of the patient.
	HIV testing	Physicians should ensure that HIV testing is conducted in a way that respects patient autonomy and assures patient confidentiality as much as possible.
	Mandatory parental consent to abortion	Physicians should ascertain the law in their state on parental involvement in abortion to ensure that their procedures are consistent with their legal obligations.
	Physician-assisted suicide	Instead of assisting patients in committing suicide, physicians must aggressively respond to the patient at the end of life.
	Quality of life	In making decisions for the treatment of seriously disabled newborns or of other persons who are severely disabled by injury or illness, the primary consideration should be what is best for the individual patient and not the avoidance of a burden to the family or to society.
	Withholding or withdrawing life-prolonging treatment	Patients must be able to make decisions concerning their lives. Physicians are committed to saving lives and relieving suffering. When these two objectives are in conflict, the wishes of the patient must be given preference.

Adapted from the American Medical Association, Code of Medical Ethics © 2008–2009.

CODES OF ETHICS FOR OTHER MEDICAL PROFESSIONALS

Other professional organizations have developed codes of ethics that assist in guiding members' behavior. These organizations promote practicing their profession with honesty, integrity, and accountability. They are committed to respecting all laws, and avoiding involvement in any false, fraudulent, or deceptive activity. Two such groups of professionals include nurses and medical assistants.

Nurses' Code of Ethics

The American Nurses Association (ANA) has developed a code for nurses that discusses their obligation to protect patients' privacy, respect patients' dignity, maintain competence in nursing, and assume responsibility and accountability for individual nursing judgments. This code is found in Appendix A.

Code of Ethics of the American Association of Medical Assistants (AAMA)

Medical assistants may not be faced with the life-and-death ethical decisions that face the physician, but they will encounter many dilemmas regarding right and wrong on an almost daily basis. For example, how does the medical assistant handle a situation in which another employee violates confidentiality or uses foul language in front of a patient? How is a homeless patient treated whose body smells of urine and alcohol? What do we do if we make an error? What do we do if we observe a coworker making an error? These are issues involving ethics and doing the right thing at the right time. To provide guidance for this category of allied health professional, the AAMA has developed a Code of Ethics for Medical Assistants. This code is found in Appendix A.

Other professional organizations, including the American Dietetic Association, the American Health Information Management Association, the American Society for Medical Technology, and the American Society of Radiologic Technologists, have developed codes of ethics.

MED TIP

Know the code of ethics that relates to your professional practice. Many healthcare professionals keep a framed copy near their place of work to remind them of this responsibility.

BIOETHICAL ISSUES

Bioethical issues, resulting from advances in medical technology, are reported in newspapers and journals almost daily. Debates about cloning, harvesting embryos, and in-vitro fertilization were unknown two or three decades ago.

As we read in the Tuskegee case, there was very little protection for the men involved in the study. Unfortunately, there are examples of poor protection for the individual today. As recently as 2001, two students at two major universities died in government-sponsored clinical trials. Another concern is that ill or dying patients will rush into any treatment or research trial to try and save their life.

There is a real concern that expensive biotech treatments will be used for chronic illness when a more reasonably priced product is available. Patients may not be able to afford the co-pay or their out-of-pocket share. An ethical dilemma arises when the patient is no longer able to afford the treatment and the insurance company refuses to pay. The patient with a chronic disease may decide that "enough is enough" and decide not to take medication.

The privacy issue is a major concern when dealing with technological advancements. For example, scientists are now able to decode our genetic composition through the human genome project. But this also means that information about a person's future health, such as a 5-year-old child's future tendency for serious heart disease, may become available to others, including insurance companies. The question arises about to whom our health information should be made available.

Stem cell research has become an important topic among religious and even political groups. Some states are taking initiatives to promote the development of stem cell research to fight diseases such as Parkinson's disease. In California voters examined the potential economic value of stem cell research, and, based on that criterion, passed Proposition 71, which guarantees the spending of $3 billion in state funding over the next decade.

And finally, many scientists and politicians have examined the potential loss of lives in the case of a terrorist attack. The federal government is promoting Project Bioshield to promote the development of vaccines and preventive medications in quantities that can protect a large number of people. Economists and ethicists are concerned that the amount of money spent on these items will leave less for diseases that are becoming more prevalent. On the other hand, there is an optimistic approach that the research and development of this project could lead to finding medicines to treat diseases. And, in addition, this research may lead to fighting infections such as those caused by HIV and hepatitis.

Table 11.2 ■ illustrates a wide variety of medical issues relating to bioethics.

MED TIP

Adherence to bioethical principles involves the entire healthcare team, not just the physician.

TABLE 11.2 Medical Issues Relating to Bioethics		
Abortion	In-vitro fertilization	
Allocation of scarce health resources	Organ donation and transplantation	
Cloning	Quality-of-life issues	
Determination of death	Random clinical trials	
Euthanasia: active and passive	Stem cell research	
Fetal tissue research	Sterilization	
Genetic counseling	Surrogate parenthood	
Harvesting of embryos	Withdrawing treatment	
HIV, AIDS, and ARC	Withholding lifesaving treatment	

Organ and Tissue Donation

In the United States, people may voluntarily donate their organs and tissues to others. They can indicate their desire to do this in their advance directives or, in some states, on their driver's license. The most commonly donated organs and tissues are eyes (usually the cornea), heart, kidneys, skin, bone marrow, blood, liver, and lungs. In addition, the long bones of the body (tibia, fibula, femur, humerus, radius, and ulna) can also be transplanted. There are some organs and tissues, such as blood, bone marrow, and kidneys that can be donated by living persons. There is a law in the United States that prohibits the sale of organs. The only payment allowed is to cover the medical costs for the donor of the transplant.

Many more people need donor organs than in the past because dialysis and other medical advances are able to keep them alive longer as they wait for transplants. The **United Network for Organ Sharing (UNOS)** system, established in 1999, contains a database relating to every organ donation and transplant event occurring in the U.S. since 1986. UNOS is the legal entity in the U.S. responsible for allocating organs for transplant. They use a formula that gives half the weight to considerations of medical utility or need, and the other half to considerations of justice. Current estimates of people waiting for a transplant in the United States are estimated as high as 400,000. There are more than 106,000 people listed on the UNOS waiting list, and many of these people will die before they can receive a donor organ. Most of the needed organs are for kidneys.

Due to a severe shortage of donor organs, patients have resorted to going onto the Internet to search for a donor, and have even used ads, public broadcasts, and even billboards to advertise their need. Unfortunately, in some cases transplant departments have exaggerated the severity of their patient's condition in order to have him or her jump ahead on the UNOS list. UNOS has recently made changes in its allocation system to prevent this type of abuse. From an ethical perspective, the transplant surgeon still may have to make the life-or-death decision about who receives the first available organ (Figure 11.2 ■).

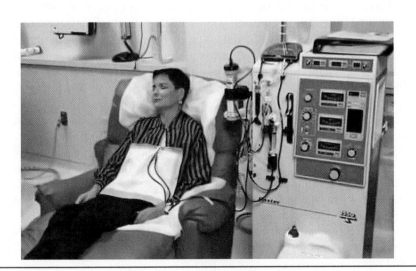

FIGURE 11.2
Patient Undergoing Hemodialysis while Waiting for a Kidney Transplant

The Ethics of Transplant Rationing

One of the most discussed bioethical issues today is who shall receive an organ transplant. The issue of organ transplantation adds a strong ethics component to medical ethics. These procedures are some of the most expensive of all medical procedures. Liver transplants cost about $250,000. In addition, the follow-up care to aid the transplant by suppressing the immune system can be more than $30,000 a year.

The criteria for rationing of transplants are controversial. The problem began back in the 1960s when kidney dialysis machines and centers were scarce. The centers had to establish screening committees to determine who should be allowed to have kidney dialysis. At a Seattle, Washington, dialysis center, a screening committee was composed of a lawyer, a physician, a housewife, a businessman, a minister, a labor leader, and a state government official that became known as the "God squad." One of the lay members of this committee recalled voting against a woman who was a known prostitute and a playboy ne'er-do-well. An observer to this process claimed that committee members were measuring patients according to their own middle-class, suburban standards.

Many believe that there is an element of "playing God" with the moral issues of removing human body parts from one person and placing them into another person's body. In many, if not most, cases, the donors are still alive when the discussions are held concerning the harvesting of their organs, adding another dilemma. Usually both a healthy donor and ill recipient do well after surgery. However, there are some exceptions. A 57-year-old man in New York donated a part of his liver to his 54-year-old brother. In this case, the recipient did well after surgery, but the donor unexpectedly died from surgical complications.

In some countries, it is legal to remove organs from a deceased person unless the person has made an objection. For example, in one small village in Pakistan there are many poor people who have long purple scars on their side resulting from surgery to sell a kidney, often for less than $1,700. However, the United States and Great Britain are among the countries still committed to the donation model for organs. Under the donation model, organs may be taken (**harvested**) only with the consent of the donor (or the donor's surrogate representative). The Uniform Anatomical Gift Act, which has been adopted in all states, permits competent adults to either allow or forbid the **posthumous** (after death) use of their organs through some type of written document, including a donor card. See Figure 11.3 ■. for a sample donor card.

Problems still arise over the allocation of scarce organs. Many ethicists and others believe that because there is a fixed supply of transplant organs, especially livers and hearts, clearly defined standards should be used by all transplant committees. One basis for determining the allocation of organs is to give them to patients who will benefit the most. This is the **social utility method of allocation.** It is based on careful screening and matching of the donor with the recipient to determine if there is a strong chance of the recipient's survival. Another favored approach is one of justice, which gives everyone an equal chance at the available organs. A controversial proposal would put younger patients higher on the waiting list.

Other methods used to allocate scarce transplant organs include a seniority (first-come, first-served) basis and a lottery method. Both of these methods cause concern because they may result in providing a scarce resource, such as a heart, to a patient whose need is not as great as a patient further down the seniority list. The lottery method may result in a patient with little chance for recovery, such as someone suffering from terminal cancer, receiving a scarce organ. When other criteria for selection are added, such as age, social status, or ability to give back something to the community, there is the suspicion that this is not a just system for all persons.

Organ Donor Card

I, _____, hereby make the following anatomical gift, if medically acceptable, to take effect upon my death.

_____Any organs or parts   _____Entire body

Only the following specific organs or parts:

_____

Limitations or special wishes if any:

_____

(Signatures of donor and witnesses appear on reverse side.)

Front of card

Organ Donor Card (side two)

Signed by the donor and the following two witnesses in the presence of each other.

Donor Signature: _____

Date of Birth: _____ Date signed: _____

City and State: _____

Witness Signature: _____

Witness Signature: _____

This is a legal document under the Uniform Anatomical Gift Act or similar laws.

Back of card

FIGURE 11.3
Organ Donor Card

A combination approach using basic "medical suitability," which measures the medical need and medical benefit to the individual patient, may be used first. After a decision is reached, then a seniority (first-come, first-served) basis is the most often used method.

Most people agree that selling organs is morally objectionable. The **National Organ Transplant Law of 1984** forbids the sale of organs in interstate commerce. This law seeks to protect the poor from being exploited, as they may be tempted to earn money by selling what they believe to be an unneeded organ, such as a kidney. There is also a concern addressed by this legislation that the donor organs should be located as close to the patient's locale as possible in order for a fast response when an organ becomes available.

There have even been suggestions that there should be a financial incentive for cadaver (a dead body used for dissection and study) organs. However, ethicists and members of the general public are against this proposal. They are very concerned that a "slippery slope" could develop by hastening the death of a person to harvest the organs.

Medicare has been expanded to fully fund kidney transplants, and most insurance plans will now fund heart transplants. A number of courts have questioned or even reversed decisions by Medicaid to not fund liver transplants. In a Michigan case, the court required the state to fund a liver transplant for an alcoholic patient. The court found in favor of the patient in spite of documentation that the patient's alcoholism most likely resulted in the need for the transplant (*Allen v. Mansour*, 681 F. Supp. 1232, E.D. Mich. 1986). See the case study, "Mantle's New Liver" at the end of this chapter.

A dramatic example of the painful decisions surrounding the issue of organ transplants is the situation that the state of Oregon faced in the 1980s. The state could either fund Medicaid coverage for 1,500 additional patients or continue to fund its organ transplant program for an anticipated thirty-four patients. Between 1985 and 1987, the state funded nineteen transplants at a cost of $1 million, only nine of these patients survived the transplant. Cost estimates for transplants in Oregon for the years 1987 to 1989 were $2.2 million. Because the amount was expected to double during the next two years, voters in Oregon believed that it was more cost effective to fund Medicaid, which provides basic healthcare for many, rather than fund transplants for the few patients who would require them. The public response to this new plan was slow. However, there was a nationwide response when a 7-year-old boy died without receiving a needed bone marrow transplant to treat leukemia. The new law resulted in several lawsuits as well as fundraising for transplants in Oregon. The lessons learned from Oregon's plight are many:

1. Medical resources are limited in all states.

2. The need for acute care, such as for transplants, is more visible than preventive care, such as prenatal care.

3. New medical discoveries and treatments, with their enormous costs, are likely targets for cost containment rather than older, more basic, medical treatments.

4. For new treatments to be funded, they must replace older, ineffective treatments.

These difficult issues mean that policymakers will have to examine all treatments on a cost/benefits basis and be ready to eliminate outdated and ineffective medical treatments. Information about organ transplants is found in Table 11.3 ∎.

ETHICAL ISSUES AND PERSONAL CHOICE

In some cases, the healthcare professional may have a personal, religious, or ethical reason for not wishing to be involved in a particular procedure. Ideally, this preference should be stated before one is hired. If a situation arises after an employee is hired, it should be discussed openly with the employer. The employee can request permission to refrain from participating in a procedure, such as a therapeutic abortion, if that procedure would violate the employee's values or religious beliefs. However, in some situations, the

TABLE 11.3	
Information about Organ Transplants	▷ The largest group of Americans awaiting organ transplants are those ages 50 to 64.
	▷ More than 28,000 transplants were performed in 2009.
	▷ People of all ages can be tissue and organ donors.
	▷ The heart is the only organ that cannot come from a live donor.
	▷ Organ donation does not conflict with the tenants of any major religion.
	▷ A person can register to be an organ donor at most state motor vehicle bureaus.
	▷ Even if a person is a registered donor, family members ultimately decide whether their relative's organs may be donated after death.
	▷ It is essential that everyone who wishes to donate their organs clarifies their wishes to family and friends.

inability of an employee to assist the physician may jeopardize the health and safety of the patient. In these cases, it may even be necessary for the employee to resign.

There are still many areas of medical ethics for which there are no conclusive answers. When should life support be withdrawn? Is **euthanasia** (intentionally killing the terminally ill) ever permissible? Should a baby's life be sacrificed to save the life of the mother? Should a baby be conceived in order to donate a needed organ to an ill or dying sibling? Scientific discoveries continue to present new medical possibilities and choices—but with these possibilities come more complicated ethical issues that must be addressed before choices can be made.

MED TIP

The ethical implications of these issues and dilemmas must be carefully examined by the healthcare professional. The ethics of the employer must be in agreement with the ethics of the healthcare professional.

THE ETHICS OF BIOMEDICAL RESEARCH

Ethics of the Biomedical Researcher

The relief of pain and suffering, the restoration of body functions and health, and the prevention of disability and death are all aims of healthcare. Human experimentation is considered necessary for medical progress to occur. Both animal testing and human testing have been used successfully to further medical knowledge and conquer disease.

Medical research almost always carries with it some degree of risk. Human beings cannot be used for testing purposes unless they consent to participate. Obtaining informed consent is particularly important in **nontherapeutic research,** or research that will not directly benefit the research subjects. The justification for all medical research is that the benefits must outweigh the risks. Many consider that this utilitarian, or benefit/cost, approach to decision making is a good model to use when examining medical research. Merely increasing knowledge is not considered an adequate justification for taking a risk with a human life. Medical researchers must abide by the standards for testing that have been established by their medical associations, such as the AMA and the ANA.

The Department of Health and Human Services (HHS) implements government standards for research. The government requires that all institutions that receive federal research funds, such as hospitals and universities, establish an **Institutional Review Board (IRB)** that oversees any human research in that facility.

Consent

Informed consent (as discussed in Chapter 5) is necessary when a patient is involved in therapeutic research. **Therapeutic research** is that form of medical research that may directly benefit the research subject. The research subject must be made aware of all the risks involved with the research. In addition, the subject must be informed about the type of research design that is used. These consist of:

- **Control group** who receive no treatment;
- Randomized study in which the subject is assigned at random to either the control or experimental treatment group (who receive treatment);
- Or a **placebo group** in which an inactive substance or an alternative type of treatment is given.

The physician conducting the research must explain all the facts relating to the research, even if this means that the patient may decide not to participate.

An African-American woman, Henrietta Lacks, unknowingly gave an incredible gift to research when a strain of cancer cells were saved from a tumor that was removed from her in 1951. Mrs. Lacks died a few months later from a virulent strain of cervical cancer. The tumor was sent to a researcher at Johns Hopkins where he was trying to find cells that would live indefinitely so that researchers could experiment on them. Mrs. Lacks' cancer cells were perfect as they multiplied rapidly and did not die in the lab. A cell line from them, called HeLa (named after Henrietta Lacks), have become immortal and are still used by researchers. They were used to develop the first polio vaccine, and helped produce drugs for numerous diseases including Parkinson's, leukemia, and the flu. Millions and millions of these cells have been produced and are now sold to researchers, and have generated millions of dollars in profit. However, the Lacks family has never benefitted from them, and Henrietta Lacks died in poverty. Even though rules about informed consent have changed in the last 60 years, nevertheless, patients still do not have much control over tissues and organs that are removed during surgery.

When Research Can Resolve Debate over the Best Treatment

Medical research does not always give the answers that the medical profession is looking for. Ethics becomes a concern when the results prove that the type of treatment subjects have been receiving has actually harmed patients. And in some cases, there is no definitive answer on the best treatment. For example, in the case of prostate cancer, men have been faced with the decision of having their cancerous prostate removed with the inherent danger of suffering from impotence and incontinence or leaving this slow-growing cancer alone. The latest research indicates that after six years there is little difference in the death rate between the men who had the cancer removed and the men who did not. However, the overall death rate from cancer by the end of their life is 50 percent lower in the men who had their prostate removed. A urologist at Johns Hopkins, Dr. Patrick Walsh, believes that death from this type of cancer should be prevented since the cancer moves into the bones and can be extremely painful. But the experts are still divided on the best treatment to use.

A research study with a happy ending is the case of premature baby, Jake Hoyt. The infant was born four months ahead of schedule weighing 1 pound, 10 ounces and was hospitalized for 102 days. On his eleventh day after birth he experienced one of the most frequent causes of death in premature infants when his intestines tore and failed. (This happens in as many as 10,000 of the 500,000 premature infants born every year.) There were two options for treating Jake. One choice was to insert a drain into the ruptured or torn part of the intestine. The other option was to perform surgery and remove the damaged portion of the intestine. Because Jake's condition was frail, he was given the drainage tube to pull out the waste products from his intestine rather than to put him through a surgical procedure requiring a general anesthetic.

His doctor made that decision, in part, based on the results of a pediatric research study at the Yale-New Haven Children's Hospital, in which it was determined that the outcome was the same whether the patient was treated with the surgery or the drainage tube. Until the research study took place, doctors were determining which treatment to use based on their own preference. During a four-year research period, when a baby was rushed into the operating room at a hospital participating in the study, the doctor was handed a randomly selected sealed envelope. Half of these envelopes gave instructions to insert the drain. The other half had instructions to perform the surgical procedure to remove the dead length of tissue. Because the results of the study showed no significant difference in the outcome of the two procedures, many doctors are performing the tubal insertion such as Jake received, rather than the surgical option. The surgical treatment often placed an additional burden on an ill infant. In this type of research study, all the infants received beneficial treatment.

Jake's mother stated that she is grateful that he received only the tubal procedure because his feeding and aftercare were much easier. He went home, with a functioning intestine, nine days before his due date weighing 5 pounds, 7 ounces. Doctors state that they no longer have to consider the tubal procedure as a "second-class" treatment (Figure 11.4 ■).

MED TIP

The physician is responsible for explaining to the patient all the risks involved in a research project. However, other healthcare professionals, such as nurses, pharmacists, and medical assistants, may become aware of information relating to a research project that needs to be conveyed to the attending physician. An example would be a patient who tells the nurse that he is taking a medication prescribed by another attending physician at the same time that he is taking an experimental drug from a medical researcher.

Conflicts of Interest

A conflict of interest can arise in medical research if the researcher's interests are placed above the interests of the patient. For example, medical researchers fearful of losing financial backing for research projects may state incorrect data or test results in order to have the research appear more successful than it is. In addition, it is a conflict of interest if physicians engaged in drug-testing research for pharmaceutical companies own stock in those companies. In both examples, the physicians may be improperly placing their own interests before the patient's interests.

Dr. Ezekiel Emanuel, who heads the Department of Clinical Bioethics at the National Institute of Health Clinical Center, believes that evidence shows that researchers who have

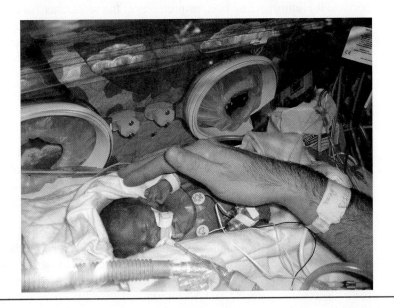

FIGURE 11.4
Premature Infant Does Well after Life-Saving Procedure
(Photo courtesy of Roselle-Hoyt family)

a financial tie to manufacturers will tend to interpret their data in a more favorable light when they are studying those companies' products. He recommends that the key to running important medical studies is to have people who can make independent judgments.

An unusual example of a conflict of interest occurred when a manufacturer of medical devices decided not to send a "Dear Doctor" letter of warning about defective equipment because it did not want to expose patients to "unnecessary device replacement." The Guidant Corporation, which manufactures implantable heart defibrillators, determined that two of their models had an electrical flaw. In fact, at least seven patients are known to have died when their defibrillators failed to work. These defibrillators are life-saving devices that are surgically implanted into the patient and control potentially fatal heart rhythms. A "Dear Doctor" letter was drafted as an internal memorandum alerting medical doctors to these defects, but the letter was never sent. The company finally alerted doctors to the defect when it became aware that the *New York Times* was going to publish an article about the problem.

Ethics of Randomized Test Trials

Many ethicists believe that it is unethical to use a control group when conducting medical experiments, as this group has no hope of benefiting from the experimental drug. A race-based control group may produce an additional ethical dilemma. For example, in the Tuskegee syphilis case at the beginning of the chapter, the Public Health Service used members of the black population who had untreated syphilis as a research group. These patients were not given an effective treatment for syphilis that was available at the time. A race-based selection of research patients is unethical unless there is evidence that they will benefit by the therapy. There are some diseases that affect only a particular portion of the population, such as Tay-Sachs disease that affects the Jewish population. In this instance, research participants in a study to eradicate Tay-Sachs disease would be drawn only from the Jewish population.

Problems with the Double-Blind Test

In a **double-blind test,** neither the experimenter nor the patient knows who is getting the research treatment. This is considered to be an objective means of gathering test data because it eliminates any bias, or preference, the researcher may have toward a specific research method or treatment. An ethical question arises with double-blind tests about the *process* of informed consent. Are the patients fully aware that they may not be receiving any treatment whatsoever? In some research situations, where the physicians discover an immediate positive effect of an experimental drug on the test group, the project will be adjusted so that the control group can also receive the treatment.

HUMAN GENOME PROJECT

The **Human Genome Project** was begun in the early 1990s as a research program by the federal government. The purpose was to determine or "map" the sequence of the total number of genes, estimated at 100,000, each of us has within the 23 pairs of human chromosomes. This complete set of genes is known as the **human genome.** It resembles a set of blueprints for the human being that is stored in the nucleus of each cell.

The goal of the Human Genome Project, which is supported by scientists in several countries, is to provide a map of where each gene is located on the 23 pairs, or 46 chromosomes. The U.S. portion of the genome project was divided between scientists in nine centers at both national laboratories and universities. This important project was estimated to cost between $3 and $5 billion and take fifteen to twenty years to complete.

However, the project was completed ahead of time in the year 2003 and has provided important information for both biological and medical researchers.

The Human Genome Project provides a better understanding of the process of human evolution. The most important information for medical researchers relates to an improved understanding of the relationship between certain genes and particular diseases. The hope is that this genome information will result in the eventual elimination or control of genetic diseases such as cystic fibrosis and sickle-cell anemia. Ultimately, a test for a gene could actually diagnose a medical condition before any symptoms even appear. The "maps" that have been created by this project make it ten times quicker to locate a particular gene on a linkage map.

MED TIP

A genome linkage map is similar to a roadmap in that it provides the location of where a particular gene (genetic material) is located on the chromosomes. **Chromosomes** are thread-like structures within the nucleus (center) of a cell that transmit genetic information.

There is currently an astonishing list of genes identified as **gene markers** that are responsible for disease. Some of these gene markers for disease are for colon cancer, amyotrophic lateral sclerosis (ALS), Type II (adult onset) diabetes, Alzheimer's disease, Huntington's disease, and achondroplastic dwarfism.

GENETIC ENGINEERING

The ability to alter the basic structure of life to correct a malfunction is the goal of genetic engineering. It has increased the prospect of curing genetic diseases and enhancing the genetic code of children. The new trait, as developed through genetic engineering, would then be passed along to succeeding generations. For example, it may be possible for scientists to develop a trait that would prevent the development of colon or breast cancer. This trait, if passed along to succeeding generations, could mean a more pain-free and longer life.

Cloning

Moral and ethical concerns are raised by critics who say that manipulating the human genetic code is "playing God." One of the most controversial examples of genetic engineering is in the area of human cloning. A **clone** is a group of genetically identical cells that come from a single common cell. Thus, cloning makes an exact replication of a parent or a cell. In 1997, a sheep named Dolly was cloned by a Scottish scientist who found a new way to reproduce sheep by fusing the nucleus of a cell taken from the udder of a 6-year-old sheep with the ovum from another sheep after the nucleus was removed. This resulted in the lamb's receiving the chromosomes from only one parent (the female), not two. Dolly was then a clone, or twin, of her 6-year-old mother. The birth of Dolly caught the public's attention. There was widespread speculation about the ability for human cloning. Shortly after Dolly was cloned in February 1997, President Clinton banned the use of federal funds for research on cloning human beings.

Researchers claim that one major reason for developing cloning in animals is to permit the study of genetic development and genetic diseases. It has been claimed that studying cloning in humans might eventually enable infertile couples to have children that are genetically related to them. Further claims state that cloning also reduces the risk of passing along some diseases that are caused by defective genes, as only nondefective chromosomes would be used in the cloning process. There has been speculation that cloning could be used to create "spare parts" by growing stem cells for particular areas of the body. It is not yet clear if there would be major advantages to human cloning.

One of the strongest arguments against human cloning is the effect it might have on human dignity. There is a concern that if we are able to control the creation of human beings, then we might also have the ability to limit the creation of defective human beings. The definition of "defective" could have very different meanings depending upon who supplies the definition. For example, a child born with crossed eyes or a clubfoot might be considered to be "defective" even though these are relatively easy-to-repair disorders. There are three reasons that are most frequently given to oppose cloning:

1. Health risks from the mutation of genes
2. Emotional risks
3. The risk of abusing the technology

Several early attempts at cloning produced disfigured animals with many abnormalities. Additionally, there is a concern about the emotional pressure of knowing that a person is perhaps the twin of a long dead brother, or even the notion that a person's sister is actually his or her mother. Finally, the abuse of this technology causes some people to equate cloning with a Hitler-like attempt to create only "perfect" human beings—in the case of Hitler, these would be members of the Aryan race.

The anti-abortion lobby promotes a ban on therapeutic cloning used for medical purposes, because 4-day-old embryos are destroyed in the process. This group believes that this practice is the same as taking a life.

Gene Therapy

Gene therapy, in which a needed gene is spliced, or connected, onto the DNA of body cells to control the production of a particular substance, is still in its infancy. The opportunities are limitless. For example, diseases such as PKU, caused by the absence of a single enzyme that can cause cognitive impairment if untreated, might be corrected by altering a person's genes to manufacture that enzyme. Many diseases involve dozens, or even hundreds, of genes and are more difficult to correct.

However, scientists are investigating many unanswered questions about gene therapy. The biotechnology companies, in particular, are expecting to earn millions with the development of their new medical techniques and products for gene therapy. But they are also raising troubling ethical and moral problems. Should gene therapy be used to create healthier fetuses? Should these companies develop tests to predict mental illness?

Fertility clinics are interested in testing their embryos for the newly discovered cancer gene, which would then allow parents to pick a child without that risk. Religious leaders have criticized scientists for patenting genes they discover, saying that no one can "own" genes.

Many people are concerned that gene therapy, performed to save lives, will eventually become gene enhancement to augment a desirable feature in our appearance or body function. For example, a wish for tall, blond children is an example of a misplaced use of gene therapy. Other ethical issues include whether it is right to provide a therapy to fight dwarfism, but not to let other children take it to add a few inches to their height. What about engineering hormones to turn average-sized children into basketball players? What are the implications for a society of people seven feet tall? Biotechnology's societal implications are becoming more complex as scientific discoveries increase.

Human Stem Cell Research

Stem cells are considered the master cells in the body that can generate specialized cells. In 1998, Dr. James A. Thompson, a University of Wisconsin researcher, became the first person to isolate stem cells. These cells, which can grow into any cell or tissue in the body, are extracted from the inner mass of an embryo. They are composed of 100 to 300 cells that are small enough to fit on the head of a pin. Scientists regard these cells as the building blocks of a new era of regenerative medicine in which the body can eventually heal itself. According to scientists, the stem cells can be used to treat a variety of diseases, including Parkinson's disease, Alzheimer's disease, stroke, and diabetes. For example, in the case of diabetes in which the pancreatic cells are ineffective, researchers can produce healthy pancreatic cells from embryonic stem cell lines that are then transplanted into a diabetic patient.

The controversy surrounding human stem cell research is not about the ability to end disease, as most people agree that this should be the purpose of medical research, but rather the use of frozen embryos to conduct the research. Cells are removed from frozen embryos, which are obtained in a variety of ways, including those that would be discarded by in-vitro fertilization clinics. Some of the embryos are grown in the laboratory especially for the purpose of stem cell research, some are obtained from terminated pregnancies, and a few are donated by couples who have excess embryos as a result of in-vitro fertilization.

This research has resulted in intense criticism from several fronts, including religious groups and abortion opponents, because the embryos used in the research are destroyed. These groups believe that the embryo is a living human being, and destroying them is therefore the same as killing a person. The issue is so controversial that Congress has banned all federal financing for stem cell research. However, this ban does not affect private stem cell research. In addition, the Food and Drug Administration (FDA), which oversees research therapy tested on people, presently has little jurisdiction over embryonic research.

Many states have widely opposing views on the research. For instance, a Massachusetts law enacted in 1974 prohibits using any live human fetus in experiments. On the other hand, Pennsylvania has introduced legislation to allow government-financed scientists to derive stem cells from embryos. A representative from South Dakota, Jay Duenwald, who introduced legislation to ban stem cell research, likened it to Nazi experiments. His legislation passed, and embryonic stem cell research is now a crime in South Dakota, punishable by as much as a year in jail and a $1,000 fine.

Many state spokespersons are not opposed to studies using frozen embryos to treat diseases like diabetes, but they fear what they consider negative uses, such as for cloning. President George W. Bush restricted federally funded research to stem cells that already had been obtained before August 9, 2001, but no new embryonic cells could be harvested after that date. While the ability to use stem cells that had been obtained before the August 2001 date still remains true, the ban on research has been lifted by President Obama's administration in 2009. While federal funding is now available for stem cell research, it is unclear about the amount that will actually be provided as research funding is limited.

One answer to the moral dilemma created by stem cell research is a new procedure that would not destroy embryos. In this method only one cell is removed from the embryo without destroying the embryo. This cell would be allowed to divide into two cells. One of these cells would then be tested for genetic defects and the other cell would be cultured to propagate new stem cells. If genetic defects were found in the first tested cell, then the cells would be discarded. Some ethicists have voiced a concern that removing even one cell might damage the embryo.

A more noncontroversial approach to stem cell research is offered by the researchers who use sources other than embryos. For example, blood stem cells can regenerate specialized cells to treat blood disorders such as leukemia. These blood stem cells are found in adult bone marrow, in umbilical cord blood, and in small amounts in the circulating blood stream. The hope is that these stem cells can be used in new ways to produce other types of cells such as neural and liver cells. This is far less controversial than embryonic stem cell use.

A "slippery slope" is often mentioned during a discussion of stem cell research. The use of the term "slippery slope" is meant to warn people that there are dangers associated with starting a practice that is ethically questionable. We can easily slip backwards down that slope and find that the uses for stem cells may be outweighed by the ethical dangers of harvesting them.

Whistleblowing

Whistleblowing occurs when employees publicly report a potentially dangerous situation in their organization to authorities who can take corrective action. The employee must

1. Exhaust all other channels for correcting the situation within the organization.
2. Have documented evidence that would convince an impartial and reasonable observer.
3. Have good reason to believe that by "blowing the whistle" and going public the necessary changes will be made to prevent harm and injury.

The ethical justification for whistleblowing is evident as it is a service to protect others. This is often done at great personal risk to the whistleblower. Often whistleblowers are subject to harsh treatment by others within their organization, even coworkers. Once a decision is made to "go public" with information, it is wise to consider all the alternatives. An anonymous complaint can be made to a regulatory agency such as the Environmental Protection Agency (EPA). The Occupational Safety and Health Act (OSHA) of 1970 prohibits any retaliation against an employee who files a complaint with OSHA. The Solid Waste Disposal Act and the Food and Drug Administration also protect employees against retaliation for "blowing the whistle." Whistleblowers who work for the federal government are protected by law from losing their jobs. As a last resort some people have leaked information to the press such as in the Guidant case mentioned previously.

Even though the lives of many whistleblowers have been negatively affected, most say that they could not have lived with themselves if they had remained silent.

MED TIP

Whistleblowing is always used as a last resort when all other methods for warning about a dangerous situation have failed.

HEALTHCARE REFORM

It is estimated that more than 50 million Americans are without adequate healthcare coverage and, thus, forgo preventive care. When they become sick, they are often very ill and receive inadequate, ineffective, and often costly care. There is a movement underway to ensure that every American has health insurance. But a continuing problem relates to economic and racial disparities. Some research indicates that African-Americans, Latinos, and American Indians are often lacking in treatment for conditions such as diabetes and high-tech heart surgery. Politicians are addressing the issues of the uninsured and the underinsured, but there is no one perfect solution. The governor of Massachusetts signed a bill in 2006 that made this the first state to require all its citizens to carry health insurance. In that state a person who can afford insurance and refuses to buy it faces a fine of $1,000. Businesses that do not provide medical insurance for employees would also face a fine. The poor in the state would have access to coverage with no premiums or deductibles, and low-income residents would receive subsidies.

Illness has been linked to as many as 50 percent of all personal bankruptcies in the United States. In many cases, according to a Harvard University study, the bankrupt individuals were middle-class, owned their own homes, and had health insurance at the onset of their illness. When people are too sick to work, they may lose their jobs as well as their medical insurance coverage. In many cases the co-payments, deductibles, and out-of-pocket expenses were so great that the bills could not be paid. The only escape is through filing for bankruptcy. When people are fortunate enough to recover and find another job, they are often denied insurance because of the pre-existing conditions of their health problems.

In addition to the high costs of medical care, the proportion of physicians who provide free care to the poor has declined dramatically during the past decade. In 2004–2005, 68 percent of physicians said they provided either free or discounted care to their low-income patients. This decreased from 78 percent who provided this service a decade earlier. This decrease has resulted in more patients either going without care, or using their local emergency room in lieu of a primary care physician. Pressures such as reduced reimbursement rates, high malpractice rates, medical school debt, and busy schedules have impacted on the physicians' ability to provide free care. However, almost 70 percent of physicians still offer some free care.

MED TIP

Medical office personnel must treat all patients with the same consideration for the patient's dignity no matter what their ability to pay.

Another problem that has driven up the cost of medical care is that physicians have encountered the need to practice a form of defensive medicine to avoid potential lawsuits. The estimate is that at least $100 billion of the United States $1.7 trillion annual healthcare bill is the cost of defensive medicine including cesarean deliveries, unneeded antibiotic therapy, and advanced imaging tests such as PET, MRI, and CT scans. In some cases, patients request these imaging procedures for aches, sprains, and cardiac assessment. As a result, some insurance companies have issued policy statements declaring that full body scans are medically unnecessary.

It is understandable that when unexpected situations occur, such as flu pandemics, it is necessary to ration healthcare services due to limited medications and vaccines, service providers, and treatments. For example, during a recent H1N1 flu outbreak there was a question about "who gets the vaccine in a flu outbreak?" Physicians argued that young people, rather than the elderly, should have limited vaccines first. Most people agreed with this decision.

However, many Americans are concerned that they are not receiving necessary healthcare on a daily basis due to rationing. There are arguments about whether women under 50 years of age should receive mammograms. There is ongoing debate about elderly patients having expensive procedures such as MRIs and CT scans. Many believe that a renewed interest in correcting inequalities in the healthcare system will solve some of these questions and problems.

On March 21, 2010 the House passed H.R.3590, the Patient Protection and Affordable Care Act (the Patient Protection Act) that had been approved by the Senate on December 24, 2009. This massive healthcare reform package, along with $400 billion in new revenue and taxes, was then signed into law by President Obama.

Major components of this law include:

▶ A "grandfather provision" so that individuals who already have healthcare coverage may retain that coverage if they desire.

▶ A similar "grandfather" provision applies to employers who currently offer coverage.

▶ Patients who are not eligible under Medicare and Medicaid will be required to maintain minimum coverage beginning after 2013. There is a penalty for failing to maintain this coverage.

▶ A tax credit and reduced cost sharing, on a sliding scale, for qualified individuals.

▶ an expansion of Medicaid.

▶ The act does not require employers to provide healthcare coverage. However, if they do not, they may be liable for an additional tax.

▶ Hospitals would be required to conduct periodic community health needs assessments.

The full impact of this law will be determined in the future.

POINTS TO PONDER

1. Why do students still learn about codes of ethics such as the Nuremberg Code?

2. Do all physicians follow the guidelines relating to euthanasia as discussed in the Opinions of the Council on Ethical and Judicial Affairs of the AMA? If not, why not?

3. What would you do if you knew that a patient suffering from cancer was part of a control group of research patients who were not receiving a drug that could benefit them?

4. What do you do when you observe unethical behavior by a coworker?

5. What do you do when you make a mistake?

6. In your opinion, what criteria should be used for selecting the recipient of a scarce organ such as a heart or liver? Would you include such factors as the patient's medical need, chance for success of the procedure, and the patient's responsibility for causing the illness? Why or why not?

DISCUSSION QUESTIONS

1. Explain what the AMA Principles of Medical Ethics statement on "improved community" means.

2. Discuss the freedom of choice that a physician has about accepting patients, as stated in the AMA's Principles of Medical Ethics.

3. What should healthcare professionals do if their ethical values differ from those of their employer? Discuss several options.

4. Describe several bioethical issues that modern-day healthcare professionals have to face.

5. Why are bioethical issues discussed in codes of ethics?

6. Do you think that a national health plan, which would provide medical coverage for all citizens, is a good idea in the United States? Why or why not?

7. Describe a situation in which the "slippery slope" of ethics may be a concern.

8. Should whistleblowers be protected by law from losing their jobs if they "blow the whistle" about an illegal or unethical action in their organization?

REVIEW CHALLENGE

Short Answer Questions

1. Describe the *social utility method* for the allocation of scarce organs.

   _____

   _____

2. Describe the *justice method* for the allocation of scarce organs.

   _____

   _____

3. Describe the *"medical suitability"* method for the allocation of scarce organs.

   _____

   _____

4. In your opinion, what criteria should be used to determine who will receive a flu shot when there is a only a limited supply.

   _____

   _____

5. What is whistleblowing? What federal laws might protect a whistleblower?

   _____

   _____

6. Define "slippery slope."

   _____

   _____

7. What do you say to a family member who says, "I don't want to be an organ donor because I'm afraid that if I'm unconscious they won't take good care of me?"

   _____

   _____

8. Explain what a double-blind test is and why it is used.

   _____

   _____

9. What is UNOS and what does it do?

   _____

   _____

10. What are your thoughts on the following guidelines on who should be excluded during a pandemic: people older than 85; those with severe trauma; severely burned older than 65; those with severe mental impairment such as Alzheimer's disease; and those with chronic disease such as heart failure, lung disease, or poorly controlled diabetes?

    _____

    _____

Matching

Match the responses in column B with the correct term in column A.

Column A

_____ 1. revocation
_____ 2. expulsion
_____ 3. censure
_____ 4. allege
_____ 5. posthumous
_____ 6. clone
_____ 7. euthanasia
_____ 8. ghost surgery
_____ 9. double-blind test
_____ 10. gene therapy

Column B

a. condemn
b. splicing onto the DNA of body cells
c. after death
d. research design
e. take away; recall
f. one physician substituting for another
g. force out
h. group of genetically identical cells
i. to assert
j. aiding in the death of another person

Multiple Choice

Select the one best answer to the following statements.

1. Nontherapeutic research

   a. will always benefit the research subject.
   b. does not directly benefit the research subject.
   c. is unethical.
   d. should be justified with the benefits outweighing the risks.
   e. b and d only.

2. A double-blind test means that

   a. neither the patient nor the researcher knows who is getting the treatment.
   b. the participants are visually impaired.
   c. the results will not be gained from an objective method for testing.
   d. the control group will eventually benefit from being in the experiment.
   e. there is an unethical practice taking place.

3. Many professional codes of ethics are based on

   a. current laws.
   b. mandates from the government.
   c. early writings of Hippocrates.
   d. outdated value systems.
   e. none of the above.

4. Stem cells are

   a. genetically identical cells from a single common cell used to create an identical organism.
   b. master cells in the body that can generate specialized cells.
   c. the same as chromosomes.
   d. the same as gene markers.
   e. none of the above.

5. What topics are included under the topic of bioethics?

   a. Stem cell research
   b. Fetal tissue research
   c. Random clinical trials
   d. a and b only
   e. a, b, and c

6. The Summary of Opinions of the Council on Ethical and Judicial Affairs of the AMA

   a. describes fee splitting as an acceptable practice.
   b. admonishes the surgeon against "ghost surgery."
   c. admonishes the physician to be sensitive to the need to assist patients in suicide.
   d. describes gene therapy as acceptable as long as it is for the purpose of altering human traits.
   e. all of the above.

7. Taking away a license to practice medicine is called

   a. revocation.
   b. censure.
   c. expulsion.
   d. a and c only.
   e. a, b, and c.

8. Medical issues relating to bioethics include

   a. harvesting embryos.
   b. DRGs.
   c. withdrawing treatment.
   d. HMOs.
   e. a and c only.

9. Conflicts of interest occur

   a. when there are financial interests present.
   b. if stock is owned by the physician in the company that sponsors the research.
   c. if the researcher can control the results of the research.
   d. if the patient's needs are not considered.
   e. all of the above.

10. A model for making ethical decisions requires that

    a. the potential consequences are not revealed in order to provide objectivity.
    b. the alternative of "not doing anything" is not an appropriate consideration.
    c. the ethical issues are defined in vague terms in order to look at all the dimensions of the problem.
    d. the facts be determined by asking who, what, where, when, and how.
    e. all of the above.

DISCUSSION CASES

1. *Mickey Mantle, Baseball Hall of Fame center fielder for the New York Yankees, received a liver transplant in 1995 after a six-hour operation. It took only two days for the Baylor Medical Center's transplant team to find an organ donor for the 63-year-old former baseball hero when his own liver was failing due to cirrhosis and hepatitis. Mantle was a recovering alcoholic who also had a small cancerous growth that was not believed to be spreading or life-threatening.*

There is usually a waiting period of about 130 days for a liver transplant in the United States. A spokesperson for the United Network for Organ Sharing (UNOS) located in Richmond, Virginia, stated that there had been no favoritism in this case. She based her statement on the results of an audit conducted after the transplant took place. However, veteran transplant professionals were surprised at how quickly the transplant liver became available.

Doctors estimated that due to Mantle's medical problems, he had only a 60 percent chance for a three-year survival. Ordinarily, liver transplant patients have about a 78 percent three-year-survival rate. There are only about 4,000 livers available each year, with 40,000 people waiting for a transplant of this organ. According to the director of the Southwest Organ Bank, Mantle was moved ahead of others on the list due to a deteriorating medical condition. The surgery was uneventful, and Mantle's liver and kidneys began functioning almost immediately. His recovery from the surgery was fast.

There were mixed feelings about speeding up the process for an organ transplant for a famous person. However, Kenneth Mimetic, an ethicist at Loyola University in Chicago, stated, "People should not be punished just because they are celebrities." The ethics of giving a scarce liver to a recovering alcoholic was debated in many circles. University of Chicago ethicist Mark Siegler said, "First, he had three potential causes for his liver failure. But he also represents one of the true American heroes. Many people remember how he overcame medical and physical obstacles to achieve what he did. The system should make allowances for real heroes."

Mickey Mantle died a few years later from cancer.

    a. As in the case of the liver transplant for Mickey Mantle, should the system make allowances for "real heroes"? Why or why not?

    _____

    _____

    b. Some ethicists argue that patients with alcohol-related end-stage liver disease (ARESLD) should not be considered for a liver transplant due to the poor results and limited long-term survival. Others argue that because alcoholism is a disease, these patients should be considered for a transplant. What is your opinion, and why?

    _____

    _____

    c. Analyze this case using the Blanchard-Peale Three–Step model in Chapter 1.

    _____

    _____

    _____

2. *Using the Tuskegee Syphilis Research Study at the beginning of this chapter, answer the following questions:*

a. Could this type of research study be conducted today? Why or why not?

_____

_____

b. Taking into account an average annual inflation rate of 5 percent over a period of thirty-seven years, the settlement of $37,500 would now be approximately $230,000, the $16,000 settlement would be $97,000, the $15,000 settlement would be $91,000, and the $5,000 settlement would be $30,000. In your opinion, was this a fair settlement? Why or why not?

_____

_____

c. The public knew about the study, so what should they have done?

_____

_____

d. Many scientists believe that using data from this type of experiment indirectly condones the experiments. Others believe that the suffering should not be in vain and, thus, be used for the good of others? In your opinion, how should the data be used that is obtained from an unethical experiment and how can we prevent this from happening again?

_____

_____

PUT IT INTO PRACTICE

Select a newspaper article relating to a medical ethics or bioethical issue. Explain the ethical issue and summarize the article. Discuss the people who could be adversely affected by this issue.

WEB HUNT

Using the website of the Department of Health and Human Services (www.hhs.gov), examine the statement on "National Organ and Tissue Donation Initiative." Click on the site for organ donation and discuss the steps that you would need to take in order to become an organ and tissue donor.

CRITICAL THINKING EXERCISE

What would you do to correct the imbalance in health care for low-income people?

BIBLIOGRAPHY

American Medical Association. 2008–2009. *Code of medical ethics Current opinions on ethical and judicial affairs.* Chicago: American Medical Association.

Barker, K. 2007. "Desperation Spurs Poor Pakistanis to Sell Kidneys." *Chicago Tribune* (Aug. 26), 1, 24.

Becker, A. 2010. "Cancer Treatment: Who Pays?" *Hartford Courant* (March 11), 1, A4.

Becker, A. 2009. "Stem Cell Funding a Victim of Deficit." *Hartford Courant* (Dec. 14), 1, 10.

Becker, G. 2006. "Should the Purchase and Sale of Organs for Transplant Be Permitted?" *Capital Ideas: The University of Chicago Graduate School of Business.*

Brody, J. 2007. "The Solvable Problem of Organ Shortages." *New York Times* (Aug. 28), 8D.

Brooks, D. 2009. "The Values Question." *New York Times* (Nov. 24) A33.

CCH Tax Briefing. 2010. "*Health care reform act.*" Washington, D.C.

"Cures for an Ailing System." 2007. *Newsweek* (Dec. 10), 78–84.

Espejo, R. 2003. *Biomedical ethics.* New York: Greenhaven Press.

Grady, D. 2010. "A Lasting Gift to Medicine that Wasn't Really a Gift." *New York Times* (Feb. 2), D5, D6.

Grady, D. 2002. "New Yorker Dies after Surgery to Give Liver Part to Brother." *New York Times* (Jan. 1), A17.

Graham, J. 2006. "Plan B Cap Lifted." *Chicago Tribune* (Aug. 25), 1, 23.

Graham, J. 2007. "Should Age Determine Who Gets a Kidney Transplant?" *Chicago Tribune* (Feb. 9), 1, 20.

Gorner, P., and P. Baniak. 1995. "Mantle's New Liver: A Question of Ethics." *Chicago Tribune* (June 9), Sec.1, 3.

Hall, M., and M. Bobinski. 2007. *Health care law and ethics: A nutshell.* St. Paul, MN: West Publishing.

Interlandi, J. 2009. "Not Just Urban Legend: Organ Trafficking Was Long Considered a Myth. But Now Evidence Suggests It Is a Real and Growing Problem, Even in America." *Newsweek* (Jan.19), 41–42, 45.

Klotzko, J., ed. 2001. *The cloning sourcebook.* New York: Oxford University Press.

Kotulak, R. 2003. "Gene May Be the Trigger to Arouse Stem-Cell Renewal." *Chicago Tribune* (October 23), 14.

Levine, C. 2004. *Taking sides.* New York: McGraw Hill.

Lock, M. 2001. *Twice dead: Organ transplants and the reinvention of death.* Los Angeles: University of California Press.

Manier, J. 2006. "Stem Cell Find May Not End All Concerns." *Chicago Tribune* (Aug. 24), 1, 22.

McNeil, D. 2009. "Shifting Vaccine for Flu to Elderly." *New York Times* (Nov. 24), D1.

Meier, B. 2006. "Papers Show Guidant Considered Warning Doctors of Hazards." *New York Times* (June 7), C1, C2.

Munson, R. 2007. *Intervention and reflection: Basic issues in medical ethics.* Belmont, CA: Wadsworth.

President's Council on Bioethics. 2003. *Stem cells: The administration's funding policy: Moral and political foundations.* Retrieved March 29, 2004 from the World Wide Web: http://bioethics/transcripts/sep03/session2.html.

Rabin, R. 2010. "Doctor-Patient Divide on Mammograms." *New York Times* (Feb. 16), D7.

Rackl, L. 2005. "Half of Bankruptcies Blamed on Illness, Medical Bills." *Chicago Sun Times* (Feb. 2), 1, 3.

Rubin, B. 2005. "Medical Bills Pave Way to Poorhouse, Study Says." *Chicago Tribune* (Feb. 2). 1, 26.

Shaw, B., and V. Barry 2006. *Moral issues in business.* Boston: Wadsworth Publishing Company.

"States Take on Healthcare." 2006. *USA Today* (April 10), 13A.

Tanner, L. 2008. "Report Suggests Who to Let Die." *Akron Beacon Journal* (May 5), A3.

Veatch, R. 2002. *The basics of bioethics.* Upper Saddle River, NJ: Prentice Hall.

Waldman, H. 2006. "Study Resolves Preemie Debate." *Hartford Courant* (May 25), 1, A6.

"When Doctors Hide Medical Errors." 2006. *New York Times* (Sept. 9), 14.

Wolffe, R. 2007. "As a Stem Cell Bill Passes, New Research Alters the Debate." *Newsweek* (Jan. 22), 46.

Ethical Issues Relating to Life

Learning Objectives

1. Define the glossary terms.
2. Discuss the ethical considerations relating to artificial insemination.
3. Describe the Baby M case.
4. Discuss the ethical considerations relating to surrogate motherhood and contraception.
5. List several ethical issues surrounding sterilization and contraception.
6. Explain the importance of *Roe v. Wade*.

Key Terms

Amniocentesis
Anencephalic
Artificial insemination
Artificial insemination donor (AID)
Artificial insemination husband (AIH)
Child Abuse Prevention and Treatment Act
Contraception
Embryo

Eugenic (involuntary) sterilization
Eugenics
Fetus
Gestational period
Harvested
Induced abortion
In-vitro fertilization (IVF)
Preimplantation genetic diagnosis (PGD)

Safe Haven Laws
Spontaneous abortion
Sterilization
Surrogate mother
Therapeutic sterilization
Unborn Victims of Violence Act
Viable

THE WILLOWBROOK STATE HOSPITAL CASE

Historical Case

Willowbrook State Hospital, an institution for the cognitively impaired (formerly called mentally retarded) children on Staten Island, experienced a large number of infectious diseases among its patients. Conditions at the hospital were not good, and most children suffered from hepatitis, measles, parasitic and respiratory infections. Hepatitis, in particular, was a problem, as many of the children were not toilet-trained and the disease was spread through an oral-intestinal route. Researchers determined that nearly all susceptible children became infected with hepatitis during their first year at the hospital.

Between the years 1956 and 1970, 10,000 children were admitted to Willowbrook Hospital. Of those children, almost 800 were entered into a research project to gain information about hepatitis with the hopes of eventually developing an immunization against the disease. All the parents of the children in the research project granted written consent. The children were injected with the same strain of hepatitis that was already prevalent in the hospital.

The physician-researchers in charge of the project received intense criticism for subjecting the children to the research. The researchers defended their actions by stating that:

a. The children that were used as subjects were unharmed or, at least, not made any more ill than they already were.

b. The children may have even benefitted, because they were placed on an isolated unit and thus were not exposed to the other infectious diseases.

c. The children in the study may have had a subclinical infection, which would render them immune to the hepatitis virus.

d. The children may have been better off as a result of the research, because the study added to the growth of information about the disease.

e. All the parents had given their informed consent.

The medical community was outraged about the experiment and raised the following objections:

a. Cognitively impaired persons, especially children, should not be used for research experimentation.

b. The children are unable to defend or speak for themselves.

c. There is a greater possibility of abuse with children than with adults.

d. The parents may have been coerced to grant consent, as the hospital was full and there was only space to admit children into the hepatitis unit.

e. The experiment did not appear to be therapeutic.

f. The benefits to the hospital and the community at large were minimal.

g. The experiments were designed to confirm *existing* studies about the effects of gamma globulin immunization for hepatitis.

h. Researchers withheld from the nonresearch children (control group) an inoculation that may have been effective against hepatitis.

Because the 800 children were isolated from other children, they did not acquire infectious diseases prevalent at the time. Ultimately, the claim that the children in the research study benefited from the project was upheld in court.

(Summarized from G. Pence. *Classic Cases in Medical Ethics.* McGraw Hill Publishing Company, 1990).

Issues relating to birth and life are especially difficult because they carry the extra burden of one's own personal values. There is widespread disagreement on when life begins and ends. However, all healthcare professionals must be willing to understand the topics and issues discussed by patients, physicians, and the federal court system.

Introduction

FETAL DEVELOPMENT
When Does Life Begin?

An issue that causes great controversy is the question of when life begins. Many people and various religions believe that life takes place at the moment of conception; therefore, any interference with this process, such as abortion or a morning-after pill, is the wrongful taking of another's life. The jurist, John T. Noonan is convinced that the most positive argument in favor of life beginning at the time of conception is due to the new being's receiving the genetic code at this time. He contends that a being with the genetic code is human.

Others believe that life does not begin until fourteen days after the egg and sperm unite to form an embryo. The **embryo** stage is the stage of development between the second and eighth week. During this time, the embryo is attached to the uterine wall. Some claim that life begins when the embryo becomes a **fetus** at about the third month of development, or around the ninth week of pregnancy. At this time the fetus starts to develop organs and has a pronounced heartbeat and a functioning brain. Still others claim that life does not begin for the fetus until birth occurs. There are perhaps as many claims about when life begins as there are weeks in the time before birth occurs, or the **gestational period,** which is usually around 40 weeks. See Figure 12.1 ■.

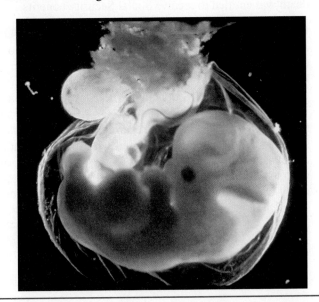

FIGURE 12.1
Embryo at 5–6 Weeks in Utero
(Petit Format/Nestle/Photo Researchers, Inc.)

This controversy has created an ethical dimension for many medical professionals. Physicians and other healthcare workers whose religious or personal beliefs lead them to oppose abortion cannot counsel women on ending a pregnancy, assist at abortions, or in any way terminate a pregnancy. Their religious beliefs must be respected by coworkers.

ASSISTED OR ARTIFICIAL CONCEPTION

Some couples desire children and have viable reproductive organs, but are unable to achieve pregnancy. These couples often seek medical assistance through their own physician or a fertility expert. Single women have also successfully used artificial insemination. Three of the most recent methods for assisted conception are artificial insemination, in-vitro fertilization (IVF), and surrogate motherhood.

Artificial Insemination

Artificial insemination (AI) is the injection into the female's vagina of seminal fluid that contains male sperm from her husband or partner (**artificial insemination husband, AIH**), or donor (AID) by some means other than sexual intercourse. Single women have also successfully used artificial insemination.

MED TIP

Do not confuse the abbreviation for artificial insemination donor (AID) with the abbreviation for the disease Acquired Immune Deficiency Syndrome (AIDS).

Artificial insemination has become a very common practice, resulting in thousands of babies being conceived. There are few legal problems if the husband's semen is used. However, in some cases, women have used their deceased husband's semen, which has caused problems concerning the child's rights in relation to the father. For instance, should the child be entitled to receive Social Security benefits from the deceased father's Social Security account? In a 1995 case, a federal administration law judge ruled that a child conceived from frozen sperm and born more than eleven months after her father's death was entitled to receive Social Security benefits.

Consent for Artificial Insemination Donor (AID)

An **artificial insemination donor (AID)** is a man who donates his semen for insemination of a woman who is not his wife. If the woman is married, problems may arise because the donor is unrelated to the woman. In response, many states have passed laws to address such issues, but none of these laws have prohibited the use of a donor's sperm.

Oklahoma was the first state to pass AID legislation that provides guidelines for both the physician and the hospital regarding the issue of consent. The 1967 Oklahoma statute specifies that both the husband and wife must consent in writing to the procedure. The reasons for this strict mandate are twofold. First of all, if the physician touches the woman without her consent, it could result in a charge of battery. Second, the husband might claim that the wife had committed adultery because the semen was not his.

MED TIP

Even if your state does not have a statute regulating AID, it is always wise to require consent in writing from both the husband and wife.

Legal Status of Offspring

The most common legal and ethical concern relates to the legitimacy of the child and the determination of who is responsible for the child's support. Several state statutes suggest that a child is legitimate if the husband consents to the AID. These statutes also state that the donor is not responsible for the child's support.

The Oklahoma statute also clarifies that a child conceived through artificial insemination is legitimate and entitled to all the rights of a naturally conceived child. Thus, a child born as a result of AID must receive support from the nondonor husband. Similarly, California holds the husband responsible for child support, as if he were the natural father, if he consented in writing to the AID procedure.

Ethical Considerations in Artificial Conception

Many moral and ethical problems surround the issue of AID. AID records, which contain the identity of the sperm donor, are considered confidential and handled in the same manner as adoption papers: Thus they are not made a part of a public record.

While most states require that only a licensed physician should perform artificial insemination, this does not guarantee that it will be done in an ethical manner. In one famous case, a fertility physician was convicted for using his own sperm (*James v. Jacobson,* 6 F.3d 233, 4th Cir. 1993).

In the case of a married couple using AID, assisted conception can cause future problems for both the couple and the child. The husband may resent his wife and the child if his sperm was not used. The child may question his or her parentage. Even though the husband signs the consent before the AID procedure, there is no guarantee that he will treat the child as his own once it is born.

Record keeping surrounding donor-assisted conceptions is often incorrect or nonexistent. Although there is usually an effort by fertility clinics to keep records relating to the donors of eggs and sperm, not all people notify the clinics when they become pregnant. In some cases, the parents believe that the baby looks like both of them, even if a donor egg or sperm was used. There is a belief among some members of the medical community that this may be a healthier approach for the family. Many couples prefer to keep the details of the baby's conception between themselves and their doctor.

MED TIP

If the information is available, it is important to note on a child's health record if the child is the result of artificial insemination. In some cases, the medical history of the donor is known and can be added to the child's record. However, the topic should never be discussed in front of the child. It is up to the parents to determine if they wish to talk to the child about his or her heritage.

In-Vitro Fertilization

Some couples have viable reproductive cells (ovum and sperm), but conception does not occur for them using the natural means of sexual intercourse. In this situation **in-vitro fertilization (IVF)** has been helpful. In this process, ovum and sperm cells are combined outside of the woman's body. These cells are grown in a laboratory and later implanted into the woman's uterus. Until the early 1990s, this procedure was considered experimental, but this attitude has changed, and several insurers now pay for the procedure.

The physician needs to carefully explain the entire procedure to the couple, including what happens to the unused cells. In most cases, the unused cells, even when they are fertilized embryos, are destroyed. There are moral and ethical issues involved in destroying, or what some people believe to be "killing," these embryos.

In some cases, the fertilized cells are not destroyed but frozen for possible future implantation. While several babies have been born using frozen embryos, this procedure has created legal and ethical problems. Custody battles have challenged the "ownership" of the frozen embryos. In a 1989 divorce case, a Tennessee couple contested the ownership of frozen embryos in their divorce proceedings. The trial judge ruled that the embryos were children, and he awarded custody to the mother. However, the appellate court granted joint custody. The case then went to the Supreme Court in Tennessee, which ruled that if the parties did not agree, the embryos should be destroyed. In this case, the couple did not agree, and the embryos were destroyed *(Davis v. Davis,* 842 S.W.2d 588, Tenn. 1992).

Some attorneys suggest that a married couple should place their wishes in writing about what should happen to their embryos in the case of a death or divorce. But there is still no guarantee that a court would accept the couple's decision, or that one partner could enforce an agreement, even if written, against the wishes of the other partner. Thus, the legal status of embryos remains unclear.

Surrogate Motherhood

An infertile couple, either married or gay, who do not wish to adopt a child may use a surrogate or gestational mother who agrees to bear the child for them. Conception usually takes place by means of artificial insemination using the husband's viable sperm. In-vitro fertilization can also be accomplished without using the surrogate mother's genes; instead, the ovum of the wife, if she is fertile, or another woman is combined with the husband's sperm and then implanted into the **surrogate mother.** A contract is established between the couple wanting the child and the surrogate mother, who must give up the child at birth. The couple may pay as much as $20,000–$25,000 for the medical expenses of the surrogate mother; however, because of the U.S. Constitution's prohibition on slavery, the baby cannot be bought. Currently, few, if any, laws regulate surrogate motherhood, and it is legal in most states.

Many surrogate cases end up in court because either the surrogate mother or the contractual parents changed their mind. This often occurs when the baby is born with a health problem or defect. In a Washington, D.C. surrogate case, both the surrogate mother and the contracting couple refused to claim an HIV-positive baby.

A problem arises, too, if the surrogate mother changes her mind when the baby is born, as occurred in the famous Baby M case. Most surrogacy agreements now stipulate that the woman who carries the baby cannot also donate the egg.

The Baby M Case

The Baby M case resulted from a surrogate parenting contract between Mary Beth Whitehead and Mr. and Mrs. Stern. Initially, Mrs. Whitehead had agreed to a surrogate motherhood arrangement—in which she would give up the child at birth—with the Sterns in return for $10,000. A Michigan attorney and a New York infertility clinic handled this agreement. Mrs. Whitehead was then inseminated with Mr. Stern's sperm in 1985. On March 7, 1986, Baby M was born. She was named Sarah Elizabeth by the Whiteheads and Melissa Elizabeth by the Sterns. The baby was turned over to the Sterns on March 30. The next day, the Sterns temporarily returned the baby when Mrs. Whitehead threatened suicide. On May 5, Mr. Stern went to the Whitehead residence with a court order to return the baby to his custody. However, Richard Whitehead had escaped to Florida with the child. Three months later, both the Whiteheads and the child were located by a private detective and Baby M was returned to the Sterns on July 31. Mrs. Whitehead was allowed visitation rights pending the outcome of the trial.

The New Jersey Supreme Court eventually granted parental rights to the natural mother, who had since remarried. However, the court granted the Sterns continuing custody of the baby, saying it was in the best interests of the child. The decision allowed overnight stays and vacations with the natural mother. The Sterns did not appeal this decision (*In re Baby M,* 537 A.2d 1227, N.J. 1988).

Ethical Considerations with Surrogate Motherhood

Many ethical and legal problems surround surrogate motherhood. Is it right to ask a surrogate mother to give up all rights to a baby she has carried for nine months? Does, or should, the child have an emotional or physical link to the surrogate mother? Will the relationship between the husband and wife be altered if the husband's sperm is implanted into another woman? What is the sibling relationship toward the surrogate baby? Can the contract between the surrogate mother and the couple be enforced?

There have also been "compassionate" cases such as the situation in which a 48-year-old grandmother carried triplets for her daughter who was unable to bear children. However, some religions oppose this procedure as immoral.

Other ethical dilemmas relating to surrogate motherhood include the following:

▶ Potential court battles over custody of a child conceived outside of marriage.

▶ Potential embarrassment for the gestational (surrogate) mother, whose actions some people have likened to prostitution.

▶ Potential harm to the surrogate mother's own children when they learn she has given one child away and received money in return.

▶ Future emotional distress when the child learns that he or she was deliberately taken away from the natural mother.

▶ Reducing birth to a legal arrangement and the exchange of money.

There are two very strong and opposite opinions regarding surrogacy. On the one hand, opponents of the practice state that they have a moral objection to commercial surrogacy. They believe it to be the equivalent of baby selling, because the mother is often paid a fee over and above the costs of the delivery. On the other hand, there are many people who believe that surrogacy, as a viable alternative for infertile people, is both a pro-life and pro-family option. For some couples, age restrictions and a limited number of adoptable children has limited their ability to have a family. In addition, infertility treatments can take both an emotional and a financial toll on couples (Figure 12.2 ■).

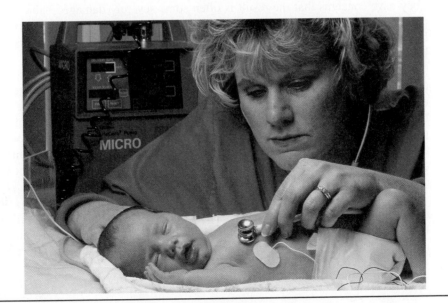

FIGURE 12.2
A Physician Examining a Newborn

Fertility Drugs

One of the more recent advances in the treatment of fertility problems, or the inability of the female to conceive, is the use of fertility drugs. These drugs increase female hormones and the production of ova, thus enhancing the ability to conceive a pregnancy.

However, the use of fertility drugs increases the woman's chance of having a multiple birth. While the birth of twins to a woman who has taken fertility drugs is not unusual, there is also a chance that she may conceive as many as eight embryos at a time. These babies are all underweight and usually are born prematurely. The "baby boom" resulting from aggressive fertility treatments has resulted in thousands of miscarriages, stillbirths, infant deaths, and disabled children. While there have been many advances in premature care allowing tinier babies to survive, the statistics relating to the survival of babies in multiple births is ominous. Even if all the babies live, they often suffer severe life-long medical problems.

The multiple birth trend began in the 1970s with the advent of fertility drugs. It is estimated that there are many more sets of twins and triplets born every year as a result of these drugs. In 1998, the first set of octuplets to *all* survive even one day were born in Houston, Texas. They weighed from 10.3 ounces to one pound, 10 ounces and only one of the babies was breathing without a respirator. One of the babies died a week after birth. Ten years later, in 2008, the second set of octuplets to survive were born to a California mother, who already had six other children. These babies are all premature and, thus, require an immense effort in order to survive. They are also at risk for long-term complications such as cerebral palsy. Neither of these mothers wished to have 'selective reduction' in order to increase the chances for the remaining fetuses to survive.

Selective Reduction or Harvesting Embryos

Because there is little chance that all seven or eight babies of a multiple pregnancy will survive, physicians may recommend that some of the embryos be "**harvested**" or removed. This procedure, also called selective reduction, is performed by entering the uterus and removing some of the embryos, leaving only two or three. The embryos removed are usually destroyed, although there have been some attempts to freeze discarded embryos for later use in stem cell research.

Many ethicists speak out against the widespread practice of using fertility drugs. They have concerns that the result is often some severely damaged babies. While most physicians believe that it is up to the couples to decide if they wish to have a multiple birth, many physicians believe that the indiscriminate use of fertility drugs is in danger of becoming reckless.

On the other hand, one couple had physicians use an embryonic 'harvesting' approach to make sure that they would have a child who did *not* inherit a gene for colon cancer. Their combined family had a high incidence of death from this type of cancer: it had killed his mother, her father, and her two brothers. This couple had used **preimplantation genetic diagnosis (PGD)** to screen for this disease. Doctors eventually examined several of the couples eight-cell embryos in a petri dish to determine which one did not carry a gene for colon cancer. That one embryo was implanted in the mother and developed into a little girl who was free of the deadly gene.

There are a growing number of parents who are selecting to use PGD to test for genes that cause diseases that are either untreatable or severe. Diseases that can be detected with PGD include cystic fibrosis, sickle cell anemia, and Huntington's disease. This type of testing can also be used for less severe problems such as a predisposition for arthritis or obesity.

CONTRACEPTION

Contraception stems from two words—*contra,* or against, and *conception,* meaning the union of the male sperm and the female ovum. Therefore, contraception is any action taken to prevent pregnancy from occurring. Birth control drugs, condoms, a tubal ligation of the female, and a vasectomy of the male are all forms of contraceptive techniques. Abstinence from sexual intercourse and noncoital sex are also means of avoiding pregnancy.

It is important to bear in mind that the Catholic Church has, as a tradition, condemned contraception. In addition, several states still have laws that prohibit selling contraceptives to minors.

However, many people do not consider contraception and sterilization to be moral issues. In fact, many ethicists and moral philosophers only address these issues when discussing the subject of a coerced sterilization, such as the sterilization of criminals, the cognitively impaired, or irresponsible mothers.

MED TIP

Note that the term 'mentally retarded' is no longer an acceptable term. The correct terminology includes 'cognitively challenged,' 'cognitively impaired,' and 'developmentally delayed' depending on the particular circumstances. It is wise to determine the correct use of these terms in your field of practice. In addition, there will most likely be further terminology changes in order to protect people from discrimination.

In 1965, Connecticut's law banning contraceptives was challenged in a case known as *Griswold v. Connecticut.* Prior to 1965, Connecticut imposed a criminal penalty on any physician who prescribed contraceptives for a married woman who the physician believed would be harmed by a pregnancy. The U.S. Supreme Court struck down the Connecticut law, declaring that it was the woman's constitutional right to privacy to use contraceptives if she wished (*Griswold v. Connecticut.* 381 U.S. 479, 1965). Justice William O. Douglas, who wrote the majority opinion, asked the question, "Would we allow the police to search the sacred precincts of marital bedrooms for telltale signs of the use of contraceptives? The very idea is repulsive to the notions of privacy surrounding the marriage relationship." Eight years later, this ruling had a major effect on the *Roe v. Wade* decision, which concluded that a woman's right to privacy included the right to abortion (*Roe v. Wade,* 410 U.S.113, 1973).

STERILIZATION

Sterilization is the process of medically altering reproductive organs so as to terminate the ability to produce offspring. It may be the result of surgical intervention such as a vasectomy (surgical removal or tying of the vas deferens to prevent the passage of sperm) in the male or a tubal ligation (tying the fallopian tubes) in the female. While sterilization is usually considered an elective or voluntary procedure, it can also be therapeutic, incidental, or an involuntary action. Sterilization can be incidental if the procedure is performed for another purpose, such as in the case of a hysterectomy for uterine carcinoma. It can also be a side effect of treatments such as chemotherapy.

Voluntary Sterilization

Voluntary or elective sterilization of competent persons presents few legal problems—although there are religions that oppose sterilization. Sterilization is becoming the most popular method of contraception, or birth control, in the United States. However, the failure of sterilization procedures to prevent births is the most common reason for "wrongful conception" or "wrongful pregnancy" cases.

Sterilization is sought for a variety of reasons: economic, personal, therapeutic, and genetic. Some couples, for economic reasons, do not want to assume the additional expense of raising a child. Other couples just do not want any more children. **Therapeutic sterilization** is sought if the mother's health is in danger. Genetic reasons include the fear of having a child with a genetic defect.

Currently, no state prohibits the voluntary sterilization of a mentally competent adult. The sterilization patient receiving Medicaid payments must sign a special consent thirty days prior to having the procedure. Written consent should always be given before a sterilization procedure is performed. Implied consent is not sufficient.

Voluntary Sterilization of Unmarried Minors

The voluntary sterilization of unmarried minors poses special problems. Some state statutes authorize such sterilization if a parent or guardian will also consent. However, many state statutes forbid sterilization of an unmarried minor. Therefore, most physicians are very reluctant to sterilize a minor without a court order. In addition, most physicians do not want to perform this procedure on a young person unless there is a medical reason.

Consent for Sterilization

In an early case relating to sterilization, *Skinner v. Oklahoma,* the court held that a law permitting sterilization of habitual criminals violates the equal protection clause of the Fourteenth Amendment. The court stated that the right to bear children is one of the basic

civil rights of man and is fundamental to the very existence of the human race (*Skinner v. Oklahoma,* 316 U.S. 535, 1942). As a result of the case, a patient, even though a criminal, must grant consent for the surgical procedure of sterilization.

For most surgical operations, the patient's written consent is all that is necessary. Without consent, this procedure, or operation, could be considered battery. In cases of sterilization, many hospitals and physicians also require the consent of the spouse. Spousal consent should always be encouraged. However, in most cases, performing sterilization without spousal consent has presented very little legal risk. In a case in Oklahoma, a husband sued his wife's physician for performing sterilization without his consent. The court dismissed the suit and stated that he had not been legally harmed,

because his marital rights do not include a childbearing wife (*Murray v. Vandevander,* 522 P.2d 302, Okla. Ct. App. 1974).

Currently, no federal law requires consent from one spouse for another spouse's sterilization. Because sterilization procedures are permanent, consenting individuals must be at least 21 years of age.

Therapeutic Sterilization

Therapeutic sterilization may be necessary if the mother's life or mental health is threatened. In some cases, it is necessary to remove a diseased organ, such as in cancer of the uterus or ovaries, in order to preserve the patient's life. This operation would result in sterilization, but it would be incidental and thus would not be classified as a sterilization procedure.

Eugenic Sterilization

Eugenic (involuntary) sterilization, considered to be unethical by most people, is the sterilization of certain categories of persons, such as those who are insane, cognitively impaired, or epileptic, in order to assure that they won't pass on the defective gene to their children. Some states still authorize the involuntary sterilization of wards of the state who are genetically impaired. The procedure must be proven to the courts to be in the best interests of the mentally disabled person. However, this practice is no longer as common as it once was. Recent research demonstrates that most forms of cognitive impairment are not hereditary.

Between 1929 and 1975 about 65,000 people in the United States underwent involuntary sterilization. Many of these people were believed to be unfit to have children based on criteria that were dictated by state boards. The politicians and scientists who supported eugenics during those years believed that by sterilizing the cognitively disabled or impaired, the insane, and persons with epilepsy, they would ensure that undesirable traits would not be passed along to future generations. As a result of flawed thinking, the plan was agreed to by state legislatures. Eugenics boards, established in many states, resulted in many poor white and African American women either tricked or forced to undergo sterilization. Larry Womble, a state Representative from North Carolina, made this statement about the sterilization of 7,500 people (mostly women) in North Carolina alone, "This was really genocide. It cut off their bloodline and took away all their dignity." There is a movement underway to provide financial reparations for the eugenics victims who are still alive.

Some state statutes still allow sterilization without the consent of the patient or the patient's agent. However, this practice has lost favor. Several states have included categories of persons, such as sexual deviates and habitual criminals, who may also be sterilized for the purpose of preventing procreation. Those procedures include providing a notice to the person or the person's representative, guardian, or nearest relative; a hearing by a board designated by statute to perform a review; and an opportunity to appeal to a court. For instance, in a civil lawsuit brought by a single, deaf mother of two who was unable to speak, the mother alleged that several social workers and physicians conspired to sterilize her against her will. The court decided in her favor (*Downs v. Sawtelle,* 574 F.2d 1, Cir. 1978).

MED TIP

It is important to remember that anyone who castrates or sterilizes another person without following the procedures required by law is personally liable (civilly or criminally) for assault and battery.

Negligence Suits Related to Sterilization

Many negligence claims involve cases where a woman has become pregnant after a sterilization procedure. In an Oklahoma case, a physician assured his patient that she was sterile after he performed such a procedure in August 1980. She subsequently became pregnant and delivered a baby in October 1981. She successfully argued that because of the physician's negligence in performing the operation, she incurred $2,000 in medical expenses and would require $200,000 to raise the child. This case went to an appeals court, which ruled that parents could not recover the expenses for raising a healthy child, but they were entitled to the expenses resulting from the unplanned pregnancy (*Goforth v. Porter Med. Assoc., Inc.,* 755 P.2d 678, Okla. 1988).

In some cases, the negligence occurs during the sterilization procedure. For example, in *McLaughlin v. Cooke,* a physician was found negligent for mistakenly cutting an artery while performing a vasectomy. This error resulted in excessive bleeding and tissue necrosis, and the testicle eventually had to be removed. The physician was found to be negligent because he did not intervene soon enough to prevent the necrosis from happening (*McLaughlin v. Cooke,* 774 P.2d 1171, Wash. 1989).

Ethical Issues Surrounding Sterilization and Birth Control

Regardless of one's religious beliefs, healthcare professionals must realize that sterilization and birth control present ethical issues because of the risks surrounding these procedures. The ethical issues surrounding contraception and sterilization include the following:

▶ Eugenic sterilization is particularly abhorrent to most people. It carries a stigma of attempting to determine who shall live and who shall die. **Eugenics** is the science that studies methods for controlling certain characteristics in offspring.

▶ Is it morally acceptable for public schools, receiving federal and state funding, to dispense contraceptive devices, such as condoms, birth control pills, and information?

▶ Some courts suggest that habitual and violent sex offenders should be ordered to undergo sterilization. Is this morally and ethically acceptable?

▶ Some people believe that women who receive public funds such as Medicaid should not continue to have children by unknown fathers and thus increase the welfare rolls. Is it ethical and morally acceptable to require these women to seek sterilization before they are allowed welfare money?

▶ Many hospitals refuse to allow sterilization procedures on their premises. What is the ethical implication of this restriction if this is the only hospital in the area?

▶ Some people believe that mentally incompetent women should be sterilized to prevent a pregnancy from occurring if men take advantage of them. Many believe that this is a violation of a woman's rights.

▶ Are children being treated as property?

▶ Is human life being destroyed (for example, by harvesting of embryos) to achieve live birth of some healthy children?

▶ Some people believe that issues of contraception can interfere with the relationship between husband and wife.

These are some of the questions and issues that patients, physicians, other healthcare professionals, and policymakers are considering. There are no easy answers. Some people refuse the use of any contraceptive device for any reason, based on their religious beliefs. However, not all people hold identical beliefs regarding the ethics of using contraceptives.

ABORTION

Abortion has become a major issue in the United States. Even though the number of abortions declined somewhat during the 1990s, about 1.2 million legal induced abortions are performed every year.

Abortion is the termination of a pregnancy before the fetus is **viable,** or able to survive outside the uterus. (There have been some cases of viable aborted fetuses with birth defects who were allowed to die.) An abortion may be spontaneous or induced.

A **spontaneous abortion** is one that occurs naturally without any interference. It is also referred to by the layperson as a miscarriage. A spontaneous abortion can result from an illness or injury of the mother, her physical inability to bear a child, or other causes. An **induced abortion,** or one that is caused by artificial means such as medications or surgical procedures, is used to save the life of the mother and/or to destroy the fetus. An induced abortion is also used to destroy life. The laws have focused only on induced abortions performed for the purposes of destroying the fetus.

Under common law in the nineteenth century, abortions performed prior to the first fetal movements, which occur at or about six weeks, were not illegal. However, legal and illegal abortions were being performed that were painful and often resulted in the mother's death. The AMA adopted an anti-abortion position in 1959, which was quite influential and resulted in political action to control abortions. States began passing statutes that made induced abortions a crime, whether they occurred before or after fetal movements, unless they were performed to save the mother's life.

In the 1960s and 1970s, states amended these laws to permit induced abortion only if the physical or mental health of the mother was threatened, if the child was at serious risk of congenital defects, or when the pregnancy was the result of a rape or incest. More laws continued to be passed, and in 1973, the major case affecting abortion, *Roe v. Wade,* was tried.

Roe v. Wade

In *Roe v. Wade,* the United States Supreme Court declared a Texas criminal abortion law, which prohibited all abortions not necessary to save the life of the mother, to be a violation of the woman's right to privacy under the Fourteenth Amendment of the Constitution (*Roe v. Wade,* 410 U.S. 113, 1973). Jane Roe (a pseudonym), a single pregnant woman, challenged the District Attorney of Dallas County, Henry Wade, when she believed that her "right to privacy' under the Fourteenth Amendment was violated by a Texas antiabortion statute. This 1973 case gave strength to the argument that a woman should be allowed the right to have privacy over matters that relate to her own body, including pregnancy. While the Supreme Court refused to determine when life begins, it did recognize that states would have an interest in protecting the potential lives of their citizens. Therefore, the Court tried to clarify the extent to which states can regulate and even prohibit abortion. To set up guidelines, the Supreme Court adopted a three-step process relating to the three trimesters of pregnancy.

1. First trimester—During the first three months of pregnancy, the decision to have an abortion is between the woman and her physician. The state may, however, require that this physician be licensed in that state. During the first trimester, the fetus is generally not viable, or able to live outside of the uterus.

2. Second trimester—During the second three months of pregnancy, the court determined, "the State, promoting its interest in the health of the mother, may, if it chooses, regulate the abortion procedure in ways that are reasonably related to maternal health." If the fetus is viable, which occurs at around six months, the Supreme Court believes the states have a compelling interest in the life of the unborn child, and so abortions could be prohibited at this stage except when necessary to preserve the life or health of the mother.

3. Third trimester—The Supreme Court determined that by the time the final stage of pregnancy (seventh through the ninth month) has been reached, the state has a compelling interest in the unborn child. This interest would override the woman's right to privacy and therefore justify stringent regulation of and even prohibit *all* abortions except to save the life of the mother or to protect maternal health.

Historical Progression of Cases Affecting Abortion

Since *Roe v. Wade,* a steady progression of abortion cases have reached the Supreme Court to challenge that ruling. The following briefly summarizes some of the cases that resulted in major changes to the *Roe v. Wade* decision.

In a 1976 case, the Supreme Court ruled it unconstitutional to require a pregnant woman to obtain her husband's consent, or if she was a single minor under the age of 18 to obtain parental consent in writing before she could obtain an abortion. However, the Court failed to determine any guidelines for obtaining parental consent if the minor is too immature to understand the nature of the procedure (*Planned Parenthood of Central Missouri v. Danforth,* 428 U.S. 52, 1976).

The following year, the Supreme Court examined a Connecticut statute that denied Medicaid payment for first-trimester, medically necessary abortions. In this case, the Court considered the argument that because Medicaid covered pregnancy and childbirth expenses, states were obligated to subsidize nontherapeutic abortions. However, the Supreme Court voted six to three that states may refuse to spend their public funds to provide nontherapeutic abortions (*Maher v. Roe,* 432 U.S. 464, 1977).

In 1980, the Supreme Court upheld the Hyde Amendment, which prohibits the use of federal funds to pay for Medicaid abortions. The Court ruled that the states are not compelled to pay for Medicaid recipients' medically necessary (therapeutic) abortions. However, the Court allowed states to fund these abortions if they wished to do so (*Harris v. McRae,* 448 U.S. 297, 1980).

The next year, the Supreme Court upheld a Utah statute requiring the physician to notify, if possible, the parents or guardian before an abortion is performed on a minor. In *H. L. v. Matheson,* a physician had advised the minor patient that an abortion would be in her best interests, but that he would not perform the procedure without her parents' consent. The Court ruled that a state statute could require a parental notice, when possible, and that this did not violate the constitutional rights of the immature minor. However, the Court also declared in this case that a state may not legislate a blanket power for parents to veto their daughter's abortion (*H. L. v. Matheson,* 450 U.S. 398, 1981).

In 1990, the Supreme Court upheld the federal statute that prohibited federally funded family planning clinics from giving abortion advice (*Rust v. Sullivan,* 500 U.S. 173, 1991).

The most significant case was the 1992 *Planned Parenthood of Southeastern Pennsylvania v. Casey,* in which the Supreme Court examined Pennsylvania's law that restricted a woman's right to abortion. This case was important because it rejected the trimester approach used in *Roe v. Wade,* which limited the regulations states could issue on abortion based on the stage of the fetus's development. Instead of the trimester approach, the Court looked at the abortion rules in terms of whether they placed "an undue burden on the mother." In this case, undue burden meant placing a substantial obstacle in the path of a woman's seeking an abortion before viability of the fetus. The Court ruled that it is an undue burden to require spousal consent (*Planned Parenthood of Southeastern Pennsylvania v. Casey,* 50 U.S. 833, 1992). This ruling has been upheld in several subsequent cases in which the husband could not prevent the mother from aborting the child.

MED TIP

It is always wise to remember that it is not the duty of anyone, except the physician, to advise the patient concerning such topics as sterilization and abortion.

Partial Birth Abortion

Currently, as a result of *Roe v. Wade,* the law states that a woman may terminate a pregnancy for any reason until the fetus is viable (able to survive outside the womb). After that point, which is about 24 weeks, or toward the end of the second trimester, an abortion is permitted by law only if the mother's health or life is at risk. An exception to the 24 week time limit is the state of Nebraska which recently passed a law prohibiting any abortion after 20 weeks. Many people are uncomfortable allowing late-term abortions, as there is a very narrow margin at this stage between a fetus and a baby. Due to advanced treatment of premature infants, many survive when the delivery takes place at a very early stage during the pregnancy. In a few cases, a late-term abortion has resulted in the delivery of a live baby.

A partial birth abortion is performed in one of several ways. One method is a two-day process in which absorbent fibers are inserted into the mother's cervix to gradually dilate it overnight. If she is 20 or more weeks pregnant, she also receives an injection of digoxin, a heart medication, into her amniotic fluid, which stops the fetus's heart. The next day, the fetus is removed by using forceps and suction. This procedure, known as dilation and evacuation (D&E), is used for second-trimester pregnancies. Another procedure involves allowing the fetus to enter the birth canal while still alive, and then removing the brain contents with suction. Many state legislatures oppose procedures that allow the fetus to enter the birth canal while still alive (partial birth abortion).

Many women wait until the second trimester to have an abortion because they do not have the money to pay for one any earlier. They cannot use Medicaid, which would ordinarily pay for medical care for the poor. Rep. Henry Hyde (R-Ill.) sponsored the Hyde Amendment, a law stating that federal funds cannot be used for an abortion except to save the life of the mother or in the case of incest or rape. As expected, there is a great deal of controversy about late-term abortions.

Incompetent Persons and Abortion

Difficult ethical issues surround situations in which incompetent persons may be subjected to unplanned or unwanted pregnancies. Many believe that if the incompetent person were able to speak for herself, she would not wish to be pregnant as a result of incest or rape. In some of these cases, abortions have been performed using a welfare agency as the *guardian ad litem* (a guardian appointed by the court to speak on behalf of the incapacitated party). In a 1987 case, a profoundly cognitively impaired woman became pregnant as a result of a sexual attack while she was a resident in a group home. The attacker was unknown. In this case, the *guardian ad litem,* rather than the girl's mother, spoke on behalf of the patient, since the mother and daughter had little contact. The family court authorized an abortion in this case (*In re Doe,* 533 A.2d 523 R.I., 1987).

Plan "B" Contraceptive Pill

The "morning after" or "Plan B" pill for use as a contraceptive, particularly in the case of rape, has raised many ethical questions. This pill contains a high dose of a contraceptive that can prevent a pregnancy if taken within 72 hours following intercourse. It works by releasing hormones that prevent ovulation and the implantation of a fertilized egg. There is divided opinion about the use of this pill by religious organizations, such as the Catholic Church, and rape crisis counselors. Catholic hospitals are opposed to administering this pill to rape victims in their emergency rooms if the woman is carrying a fertilized egg. Many will only allow the drug to be administered to nonovulating women. In some states, such as Illinois, there is a requirement that all pharmacies carry this drug. In some more conservative states, such as Arkansas, lawmakers passed a law that protects pharmacists from having to fill the prescription for the "morning after" pill based on moral reasons. Rape crisis counselors believe that it is morally indefensible to deny this pill to rape victims.

Opposition to Abortion

People have very strong, and often differing, viewpoints about abortion. Many people, because of their religious and moral beliefs, believe that *Roe v. Wade* protects the "personhood" of the mother and neglects the "personhood" of the fetus. According to this viewpoint, abortion is killing a human being and thus constitutes murder. The opponents of abortion believe that while *Roe v. Wade* protected a woman's right to choose an abortion under the fourteenth Amendment, the fetus was not covered under this amendment. *Roe v. Wade* does not declare when human life begins. An initiative is underway in some state legislatures to include a definition of a person as human life from the time of conception.

In 2004, the U.S. Congress passed a law called the **Unborn Victims of Violence Act.** This law is designed to provide legal penalties for any harm that is done to an unborn child at federal facilities such as military bases or in crimes that cross state lines. The law treats all unborn life as a person.

Almost forty states have statutes that grant varying degrees of legal standing to a fetus. These are statutes that relate to criminal matters, murder and homicide, and permit civil wrongful-death suits.

Employee's Right to Refuse to Participate in Abortions

Hospital employees have the right to refuse to participate in performing an abortion, and a hospital cannot dismiss the employee for insubordination. An employee can abstain from assisting in an abortion procedure as a matter of conscience or religious conviction. (See conscience clause in Chapter 4.)

MED TIP

Healthcare professionals must keep in mind that people have very strong, and often differing, viewpoints about abortion. Their viewpoints must be respected even when they differ from the employee's viewpoint. However, no one should be required to participate in an action, such as abortion, if it is against his or her beliefs.

Funding for Abortion

Funding for abortion procedures has been another area of great controversy. Under the Hyde Amendment, the U.S. Congress limited the types of medically necessary abortions for which Medicaid monies may be spent.

There are many arguments both for and against abortion. Pro-choice advocates argue that women have the right to choose what to do with their bodies. They argue that legalized abortions are safer for the woman. They cite statistics showing that deaths from illegal abortions—and there were thousands of deaths before *Roe v. Wade*—have diminished to just a few deaths when they are performed correctly in a hospital or clinic. They further argue that a woman has the right to an abortion when she is the victim of rape or incest.

The right-to-life advocates argue that no one has the right to deny a life. They believe that the embryo, no matter how young, is a human life; that it is morally wrong to take a human life; and that the right of the unborn child should take precedence over the right of the mother not to be pregnant. They also argue that those who carry out an abortion diminish humanity for everyone involved, including the mother, the physician, and the healthcare professionals.

Whenever healthcare reform is discussed in Congress the question of funding abortion is always a contentious issue. Some members of Congress will not approve any legislation that includes using federal funds for abortions.

Ethical Issues Surrounding Abortion

Abortion raises a multitude of ethical issues, even for those who believe abortion, in general, should be legal. See Table 12.1 ■ for ethical issues and questions surrounding abortion.

Baby Doe Regulations

In the 1980s, a tiny baby in Bloomington, Indiana, was born with Down syndrome and other disabilities. This baby, known as Baby Doe, was born with a hole between the trachea and the esophagus, which made normal feeding impossible. The parents refused to grant consent for surgery that would correct the blockage. The hospital went to court to get permission to perform the life-saving surgery on the baby's esophagus. The court refused to grant the request, stating that it was the parents' right to make medical decisions for their baby. However, the court did appoint a public guardian who could appeal the ruling on behalf of the baby. Baby Doe died before the public guardian was able to take the case to the Supreme Court.

This was considered to be a case of withholding treatment rather than of mercy killing or euthanasia, since food, water, and repair of the medical condition were withheld. The belief is that the treatment would not have been withheld if the baby had been less disabled.

The Baby Doe case became national news. The public protested about withholding treatment from a disabled (Down syndrome) infant. As a result Congress enacted legislation, the **Child Abuse Prevention and Treatment Act** of 1987, that prohibited the withholding of medical treatment solely because the infant was disabled. The government entered the picture with legislation preventing any healthcare providers, such as hospitals, from receiving federal financial aid if they discriminated against handicapped infants. In other words, the same medical treatment that is given to non-handicapped infants must also be given to handicapped infants. Because most, if not all, hospitals receive some government aid, this law went into effect in virtually all hospitals. Notices about the Baby Doe regulation must now be posted in all maternity and pediatric wards as well as in neonatal intensive care units. In addition a hotline telephone number is also posted so that anyone can call with information about life-saving measures being withheld from a baby.

1. Many private citizens do not wish their tax money to be spent on funding abortions for women on Medicaid. They cite both moral and economic reasons for their opposition.	**TABLE 12.1** **Ethical Issues and Questions Surrounding Abortion**
2. One of the most vocal opponents of induced abortion is the Catholic Church, which believes that abortion, performed at any time from conception of the fetus to a full-term baby, is immoral. The Catholic Church and others condemn this action as the deliberate taking of a life, or "killing" the unborn child. It is considered morally wrong for anyone of the Catholic faith to have an abortion or to assist in the procedure.	
3. Many people believe that abortion is thought to be a moral decision as it results in the loss of a human life.	
4. Is it a violation of the rights of an incompetent person to have to submit to an abortion for eugenic reasons?	
5. Is it appropriate for the government to deny the need for spousal consent for abortion?	
6. Should abortion be used as a means for gender selection of children?	

This law has been changed slightly to allow parents to have some say in their handicapped infant's medical treatment. An unexpected side effect of the Baby Doe regulation is that some mothers are opting for a late-term pregnancy abortion out of fear that they would have to turn over the decisions regarding their handicapped infant to the courts.

There are many ethical questions that arise out of Baby Doe regulations. For example,

- Should strangers become the advocates for handicapped infants' medical treatments if they are in disagreement with the parents' decisions?
- Would it be better to spare the handicapped infant a life that may include suffering and future surgical procedures?
- Should all modern technology that is available to save life be used no matter what the consequences for the child?

On a more positive outlook, it should be noted that there are thousands of children born with Down syndrome who are able to live a full and meaningful life.

In the Matter of Baby K

Baby K was an **anencephalic** (missing a brain and spinal cord) infant whose mother requested that her baby daughter receive a mechanical ventilator to assist with the baby's breathing. The doctors had recommended that life-saving measures not be used since the infant could not see, hear, or interact with her environment. They further recommended that Baby K only be given nutrition, fluids, and kept warm. Baby K survived longer than other anencephalic children, and even though unconscious, was kept alive in a nursing home. She had several episodes of difficulty breathing and was transferred to a hospital for treatment. Both the hospital and Baby K's father joined in a lawsuit against the mother to request that aggressive life-saving measures be discontinued for the child.

Baby K's mother disagreed with the hospital's wishes to withhold life-saving measures such as respiratory assistance. She requested that the hospital follow the guidelines of the federal law, Emergency Medical Treatment and Active Labor Act (EMTALA), which prohibited hospitals from "dumping" patients who are unable to pay for their care. The court upheld the mother's request. It stated that while they understood the physicians' dilemma when faced with having to provide medical care that they consider to be morally and ethically incorrect, nevertheless, the statute (EMTALA) had to be upheld (*Matter of Baby K,* 16 F.3d 590, 4th Cir. 1994).

Conscience Clause in Contraception and Abortion

Some healthcare professionals have embraced a conscience clause by refusing to provide medication or care when their religious beliefs are challenged. In Texas a pharmacist refused to sell the morning-after pill to a rape victim. In Chicago an ambulance driver refused to drive a patient for an abortion. And in California, a gay woman seeking artificial insemination, was turned away by fertility specialists. These cases have caused legal and even political battles. The patients filed lawsuits and complaints, and the workers cited religious discrimination after being fired or disciplined. And patient advocates, and some members of the general public, point out that medicine has a long tradition of healers putting the needs of their patient first. There is no simple answer to this dilemma.

Some anesthesiologists are refusing to assist in sterilization procedures. And occasionally a respiratory therapist has refused to remove ventilators from terminally ill patients. Some gynecologists refuse to prescribe contraceptives. In every case, there is some other healthcare professional who can provide the patient service. But hospital administrators, physicians, lawyers, ethicists, and patient advocates are all trying to balance each person's conflicting rights as well as defuse this contentious situation. There are many observers who say that a patient's needs must come first. But, on the other hand, the rights of employees to practice their religious beliefs is also a paramount freedom. At present, there is no easy or clear answer to this dilemma.

> **MED TIP**
>
> Always clarify your own values and beliefs with your employer when you are hired. Everyone has the right to religious freedom. Most employers want to know ahead of time if they need to make adjustments to assignments.

GENETIC COUNSELING AND TESTING

Genetic Counseling and Testing

The science of genetics, discovered by Austrian botanist and priest Gregor Mendel, is the study of heredity and its variations. It describes the biological influence that parents have on their offspring.

> **MED TIP**
>
> The study of genetics should not be confused with eugenics. Eugenics, the science that studies methods for controlling certain characteristics in offspring, is also called selective breeding. Hitler practiced eugenics when he tried to eliminate the Jewish population in favor of an Aryan one.

Genetic counseling is usually performed by geneticists who have a master's or higher degree, or by physician geneticists who are medical doctors with special training in genetics. Genetic counselors meet with a couple, usually one-on-one, before pregnancy occurs to discuss the potential for passing on a defective gene (Figure 12.3 ■).

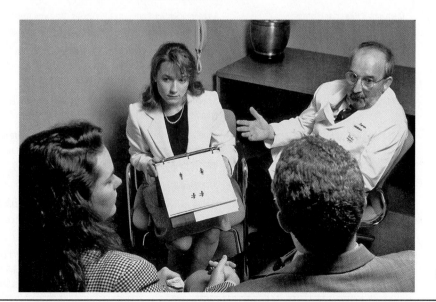

FIGURE 12.3
Genetic Counseling with Prospective Parents

Genetic counseling has emerged as a legitimate means to identify couples who are at risk of passing on a genetic disease to their offspring. Over 2,000 human diseases have been identified as having a genetic factor, including Tay-Sachs disease, sickle-cell anemia, and cystic fibrosis. In these recessive gene diseases, each parent must pass on a copy of the defective gene in order for the disease to be produced in the child. Therefore, persons who carry the recessive gene for these disorders can be tested before marriage, with the option of making a decision to remain childless. Other conditions for which genetic testing is available include Huntington's chorea, retinoblastoma, Down syndrome, and phenylketonuria (PKU). These and other hereditary disorders are explained in Table 12.2 ■.

Prenatal Testing

Patients believe they have a right to be informed of their medical conditions. A better-educated public with greater access to medical information via the Internet is now demanding to know the results of testing.

The most common means of genetic testing during a pregnancy is through **amniocentesis.** In this test, the physician uses a needle to withdraw from the uterus a small amount of amniotic fluid that surrounds the fetus. This fluid is tested for the presence of genetic defects such as Tay-Sachs disease and Down syndrome. The physician carefully introduces the needle into a portion of the uterus in which there is the least likelihood of

TABLE 12.2 Hereditary Disorders	Disorder	Characteristics
	Cooley's anemia	Rare form of anemia or reduction of red blood cells. More common in people of Mediterranean origin.
	Cystic fibrosis	Disorder of exocrine glands causing an excessive production of thick mucus. Affects organs such as the pancreas and respiratory system.
	Down syndrome	Moderate to cognitive impairment. Child may have a sloping forehead, flat nose, lowset eyes, and general dwarfed physical growth. More commonly seen when the mother is over 40. However, not all forms of Down syndrome are hereditary.
	Duchenne's muscular dystrophy	A progressive wasting away of muscles. May also have heart and respiratory problems. Caused by a recessive gene and more common in boys.
	Hemophilia	Bleeding disorder in which there is a deficiency in one factor necessary for blood to clot. The mother carries the recessive gene and passes it on to the males. Found almost exclusively in boys.
	Huntington's chorea	A condition in which there are bizarre involuntary movements. May have progressive mental and physical disturbances.
	Phenylketonuria (PKU)	A metabolic disorder in infants that, if untreated, can result in cognitive impairment. Is treated with a special diet. Most states require a screening test for PKU. Affects mainly Caucasians.
	Retinoblastoma	A cancerous tumor of the eye that is fatal if untreated.
	Sickle-cell anemia	Severe, chronic, incurable disorder that results in anemia and causes joint pain, chronic weakness, and infections. Occurs more commonly in people of Mediterranean and African heritage.
	Tay-Sachs disease	A deficiency of an enzyme leading to cognitive impairment and blindness. Transferred by a recessive gene and more commonly found in families of Eastern European Jewish descent. Death generally occurs before the age of 4.

touching the fetus. Prior to the procedure, physicians must discuss all the risks with the patient, such as the risk of damage to the fetus and of causing early labor. A consent form must be signed, as the procedure is invasive.

> ## MED TIP
>
> Genetic testing is not always performed for the purpose of termination of a pregnancy. In many cases, parents are better able to plan for the care of the child if they have advance information about a potential for genetic defects.

Conceiving Donor Siblings

The U.S. Constitution protects a fundamental right to procreate, and any limitation on the right must, of necessity, be very narrow. Ethicists have looked for a solution to the problem of women conceiving a donor sibling whose organs and tissues can be used to save the sibling's life, and then aborting the fetus if it is not a match. One viable solution is to protect the right of the donor sibling to live by withholding the results of tissue tests until after the baby is born.

This is a difficult ethical dilemma for many people who believe that an embryo is a live human being and harvesting them is a means of destroying their life. This gray area of ethics does not seem to have a clear answer at present.

The Uniform Anatomical Gift Act has implemented legal safeguards to prevent women from becoming pregnant with the specific purpose of aborting the fetus to sell the fetal tissues or organs, or donate them to a relative. (See Chapter 5 for more information on the Uniform Anatomical Gift Act.)

Genetic Testing of Newborns

It is estimated that between 3 and 5 percent of all newborns have a hereditary or congenital disorder, and one-fourth of all hospitalizations and deaths among babies are due to these disorders. Routine genetic screening on newborns has become standard in many hospitals.

Almost all states have passed laws requiring phenylketonuria (PKU) testing on infants immediately after birth so that treatment, such as dietary restrictions, can begin right away. PKU is a relatively rare (5.4 per 100,000 infants) metabolic disease that accounts for only 0.8 percent of all cognitively challenged institutionalized people. Without this treatment, PKU babies face cognitive impairment, and even death.

In addition, federally funded voluntary screening centers exist to screen for sickle-cell anemia. Due to the growing use of artificial insemination, donors of semen are routinely screened to rule out genetic diseases.

Ethical Questions Regarding Genetic Testing

Genetic testing and counseling has provided assistance for parents who wish to make rational decisions regarding their family planning. Some parents want to avoid the birth of children with crippling impairments such as with Duchenne Muscular Dystrophy, which is caused by a recessive gene, and more commonly found in boys.

Medical researchers believe that if all people who are carriers of diseases caused by a dominant gene, such as Huntington's disease, produced no children with the disease, then the disease would become eradicated. Many ethical and moral questions arise when examining these issues:

1. Do parents have the right to be informed of all the results of a genetic test? The duty of the physician *is* to inform the patient of all the results of testing. This is especially difficult for some physicians who oppose abortion, because they know that there is a likelihood the parents may seek an abortion if the testing indicates a defective baby.

2. It is now almost routine to tell patients that genetic testing might uncover unexpected unpleasantness, such as the discovery that they might be at risk for Alzheimer's disease, but that they will be given all the information if they ask. Occasionally, a case of "misidentified paternity" (incorrect identity of the father) is discovered in this type of testing. Researchers at the University Hospital of Cleveland estimate that 1 to 10 percent of all people may have misidentified paternity.

3. Does a person have a right to have children who are likely to be impaired? For example, after having a series of tests, including an amniocentesis, a woman may be informed that the baby she is carrying will be born with a neural tube defect such as spina bifida. Because this child will have a difficult life, including painful surgeries, the mother may be advised to abort. But many people who are opposed to abortion would elect to deliver the baby and spend the time during pregnancy preparing to care for a handicapped child. There is no legal sanction either for or against abortion in this case. Each decision must be based on the free choice of the parents.

4. Is society ever justified in requiring people to submit to genetic screening and counseling?

5. Do a small number of people with the potential for a disease or genetic condition, such as PKU, justify the expense of testing all babies?

6. Should public funds be used to pay for genetic testing when the parents are unable to pay? Many people believe that indigent patients should have the same access to genetic testing that the rest of the population has. However, if genetic problems are discovered, according to the Hyde Amendment, public funds cannot be used to pay for an abortion.

7. Should we limit the types of diseases or disorders that can be tested for using a test such as PGD? For example, is using the test to determine a predisposition for cancer of the same importance as testing for mild skin conditions and obesity?

These and other difficult questions face the parents and physicians every time genetic testing is performed.

WRONGFUL-LIFE SUITS

Wrongful Life

In some cases, a baby is born with severe defects that greatly affect the quality of life for the child. A wrongful-birth claim or lawsuit is often brought against a physician or laboratory by the parents of a child born with these genetic defects. The parents may claim that they were not informed in a timely fashion that their child might have defects. They believe that this lack of information meant that they did not have the option of deciding whether to abort the child.

Some lawsuits are also brought when sterilization has failed. Parents have brought lawsuits against a physician or laboratory for breach of duty when it negligently failed to inform the parents of an unfavorable genetic test result or a failed sterilization. In general, the courts have rejected wrongful-life lawsuits brought against hospitals or physicians by children with genetic defects who claim they were injured by the action of being born. The courts reason that it is impossible to assess a dollar amount of damages for being alive as opposed to being dead.

Smith v. Cote is an example of such a case. The court awarded damages for wrongful birth but not for wrongful life. The court ruled that the physician was negligent by failing to test for the mother's exposure to rubella and to inform her of the potential for birth defects. Rubella in pregnant women during the first trimester can cause defects, such as deafness, in the fetus. In this case, the mother claimed that she might have sought an abortion if she had known all the facts surrounding her pregnancy. However, the court refused to award the child damages for the "wrong" of being born (Smith v. Cote, 513 A.2d 341 N.H., 1986).

MED TIP

It is important for all healthcare workers to take the issue of their own health seriously. They need to alert their employer if they contract a contagious disease such as rubella, which could cause serious complications if a pregnant patient or coworker were to become infected.

Wrongful Conception/Wrongful Pregnancy

A 1991 case in New Mexico presented many ethical concerns. In this case, the parents of a healthy baby were awarded the cost of raising the child to adulthood when they conceived a child after an unsuccessful tubal ligation (sterilization). The physician ligated (tied) only one of the mother's tubes and failed to inform her of this negligence (Lovelace Medical Ctr. v. Mendez, 805 P.2d 603, N.M. 1991).

In another case a geriatric mother (a medical term for a pregnant woman over 35) who was not advised by her doctor that her age put her unborn child at a greater risk for birth defects, sued when she gave birth to a child with Down syndrome. The court found in favor of the family to seek financial damages for the added cost of raising a child with a disability. Wrongful-birth lawsuits are increasingly awarding financial damages to parents. But wrongful-life lawsuits, in which the disabled children sue the physicians, have generally been rejected by the courts.

MED TIP

The best method to avoid wrongful conception/wrongful pregnancy lawsuit is for the physician to advise the parents, in writing, that there are always a small number of failures in these procedures.

Safe Haven Laws

The **Safe Haven Laws** create a safe alternative to leaving unwanted babies in unsafe places such as on doorsteps and in dumpsters. These laws allow a parent to voluntarily give up custody of an infant thirty-one days or younger to a hospital Emergency Room (ER), or a police or fire station. For example, in Connecticut an ER nurse will talk to the parent about the child's medical history. The ER will also give the parent information on how to contact the Department of Children and Families (DCF) services. The infant is then turned over to DCF who are required by law to contact both parents of its intent to keep custody of the child and seek termination of parental rights. If the parents' names or addresses are unknown then DCF will place a newspaper notice. The parent(s) can change their mind and try to regain custody, but they must act quickly and make a request to the court for an attorney to represent them. The court will schedule a hearing within 30 days of DCF's application and the termination of parental rights can be granted at the first hearing. DCF will attempt to place the child for adoption within thirty days.

These laws are meant to protect babies whose parent(s) are unable to care for them. The laws do not provide protection to parents if abuse or neglect has already occurred. It also does not allow for the abandonment of older children. States vary on administration of these laws.

MED TIP

It's important to know the Safe Haven Law in your state. They vary somewhat from state to state.

POINTS TO PONDER

1. What do you say to a patient who asks for family planning advice?

2. How would you react to a coworker who tells you she has recently had an abortion?

3. Can you relate to the dilemma faced by a surrogate mother who is giving up her baby to the contractual parents? Why or why not?

4. What would you say to a person who does not share your religious or moral views concerning abortion?

5. What are some of the daily issues faced by parents who have children born with hereditary disorders?

6. In your opinion, should cells or tissue from aborted fetuses be used in the treatment of diseased or disabled persons? Why or why not?

DISCUSSION QUESTIONS

1. Discuss the ethics of minors having the same access to contraceptives as adults.

2. Should there be mandatory testing for genetically transmitted diseases? Why or why not?

3. Discuss the history of U.S. Supreme Court decisions relating to abortion since *Roe v. Wade*.

4. What are the ethical implications relating to abortion?

5. Discuss some of the ethical implications relating to sterilization.

6. What are some of the ethical implications relating to fertility drugs?

7. Discuss the ethical implications relating to an artificial insemination donor (AID).

8. How is the traditional notion of family challenged by the new reproductive technologies?

9. Should genetic counseling include recommendations by the medical personnel?

REVIEW CHALLENGE

Short Answer Questions

1. Why are the terms 'cognitive impairment' or 'cognitively challenged' preferred over the term 'mental retardation' for children with autism or Down syndrome?

   _____

   _____

2. What are some of the ethical issues surrounding sterilization?

   _____

   _____

3. What consent is required for sterilization?

   _____

   _____

4. Why is selective reduction or the "harvesting" of embryos used?

   _____

   _____

5. What are some of the considerations when using a surrogate mother?

   _____

   _____

6. What is in-vitro fertilization (IVF)?

   _____

   _____

7. What is the difference between an embryo and a fetus?

   _____

   _____

8. Who should make the life and death decisions of severely disabled babies? Discuss your answer.

   _____

   _____

9. In your opinion, is it ever proper to hasten the death of a severely disabled baby? Explain your answer.

   _____

   _____

10. Discuss the Child Abuse and Prevention Treatment Act.

   _____

   _____

Matching

Match the responses in column B with the correct term in column A.

Column A

_____ 1. fetus
_____ 2. embryo
_____ 3. in-vitro fertilization
_____ 4. anencephalic
_____ 5. genetics
_____ 6. AID
_____ 7. AIH
_____ 8. surrogate
_____ 9. gestation period
_____ 10. viable

Column B

a. time before birth during the development of the fetus
b. artificial insemination by husband
c. born without a brain and spinal cord
d. able to survive
e. biological influence of parents on their offspring
f. second to twelfth week of development
g. artificial insemination by donor
h. ovum and sperm combined outside of the mother's body
i. substitute
j. third month of development until birth

Multiple Choice

Select the one best answer to the following statements.

1. The current laws relating to artificial insemination
   a. do not forbid artificial insemination.
   b. state that the donor father must provide a portion of the child's support.
   c. provide for the records that relate to the donor to remain open.
   d. clarify the child's legitimacy.
   e. all of the above.

2. The Baby M case is an example of
   a. problems encountered with fertility drugs.
   b. problems relating to the practice of eugenics.
   c. problems encountered as a result of the use of a surrogate.
   d. problems encountered due to involuntary sterilization.
   e. problems encountered as a result of genetics.

3. Ethical issue(s) relating to contraception is/are
   a. dispensing contraceptives in schools receiving federal funds.
   b. requiring sex offenders to undergo sterilization.
   c. providing contraceptives for women on Medicaid.
   d. sterilization of mentally incompetent women.
   e. all of the above.

4. A miscarriage is the same thing as a/an
   a. induced abortion.
   b. spontaneous abortion.
   c. drug-induced abortion.
   d. conscience clause.
   e. eugenics.

5. A genetic disorder that causes severe joint pain, chronic weakness, and infections and is more prevalent in people of African heritage is
   a. Tay-Sachs disease.
   b. hemophilia.
   c. cystic fibrosis.
   d. sickle-cell anemia.
   e. Cooley's anemia.

6. Genetic testing of the newborn is required by law for
   a. Tay-Sachs disease.
   b. phenylketonuria.
   c. retinoblastoma.
   d. Down syndrome.
   e. Cooley's anemia.

7. A disease that could cause serious birth defects for an unborn child if the pregnant mother is exposed to it during her pregnancy is
   a. Down syndrome.
   b. Huntington's disease.
   c. cystic fibrosis.
   d. rubella.
   e. retinoblastoma.

8. Withdrawing a small amount of amniotic fluid from the uterus for genetic testing is called
   a. induced abortion.
   b. eugenics.
   c. amniocentesis.
   d. spontaneous abortion.
   e. drug-induced abortion.

9. A person that is appointed by the court to defend a lawsuit on behalf of an incapacitated person is a/an
   a. donor.
   b. surrogate.
   c. AID.
   d. AIH.
   e. *guardian ad litem.*

10. Tay-Sachs disease
    a. results from an enzyme deficiency.
    b. is more common among people of Eastern European descent.
    c. is curable if diagnosed early.
    d. a, b, and c.
    e. a and b only.

DISCUSSION CASES

1. *Using the Willowbrook State Hospital Case discussed at the beginning of the chapter, respond to the following questions.*

   a. What are the pros (positives) of this study?

   _____

   b. What are the cons (negatives) of this study?

   _____

   _____

   c. Is society ever justified in permitting this type of research when the outcome benefits only some members of society? Why or why not?

   _____

   _____

   d. Should public funds be used to pay for this type of research on children? Why or why not?

   _____

   _____

   e. Some say that the final outcome of the Willowbrook case falls into a "gray area" of ethics in which there is no one clear answer. If this is the case, then, in your opinion, where do we draw the line on testing children?

   _____

   _____

2. *Your sister and her husband are having difficulty becoming pregnant. She comes to you as a healthcare professional and asks your thoughts on what they might do to conceive a child.*

   a. What are some topics that you might discuss with your sister and her husband?

   _____

   _____

   b. Who would you recommend that they speak with about this problem?

   _____

   _____

   c. Is there an ethical problem in giving medical advice to a family member? Why or why not?

   _____

   _____

3. *Your neighbor's 18-year-old unmarried daughter has just given birth to a baby boy. The neighbor is concerned that neither she, nor her daughter, can take care of this baby. She asks you what you suggest that she should do?*

   a. What can you tell her about the Safe Harbor Law in your state?

   _____

   _____

b. In your opinion, is giving her advice about this law within the code of ethics of your chosen health-care profession?

_____

_____

c. Is this a legal and /or ethical problem?

_____

_____

PUT IT INTO PRACTICE

Contact your local chapter of Planned Parenthood and a Right-to-Life organization and request information on their organization and services. Compare the philosophies and missions of the two organizations as stated in their printed materials. What do they have in common? What are the differences?

WEB HUNT

Using the website of the National Institute of Health (www.nih.gov), click on the Office of Rare Diseases heading. Using the list provided by the office, determine which of the hereditary disorders in Table 12.1 is considered a rare disease.

CRITICAL THINKING EXERCISE

What would you do if your best friend's daughter comes into the office where you work seeking birth control pills? You know that her mother does not know that she is sexually active.

BIBLIOGRAPHY

Ali, L. and R. Kelley. 2008. "The Curious Lives of Surrogates." *Newsweek*, (April 7), 45, 51.

Archibold, R. 2009. "Octuplets, 6 Siblings and Many Questions." *New York Times*, (Feb. 4), A14.

Devettere, R. 2000. *Practical decision making in healthcare ethics: Cases and concepts.* Washington, DC: Georgetown University Press.

Glanton, D. 2006. "Sterile Victims Stand Up, Decry Legacy of Eugenics." *Chicago Tribune* (Sept. 6), 4.

Harmon, A. 2006. "Couples Cull Embryos to Halt Heritage of Cancer." *New York Times* (Sept. 3), 1, 20.

Hathaway, W., and H. Hathaway. 2006. "Pill Sharpens Abortion Division." *Hartford Courant* (March 13), 1, A4.

"Huge Settlement in Baby-Birth Suit." 2007. *Chicago Tribune.* (April 24), Sec. 2, 3.

Lachman, V. 2004. "Frontiers of Biomedicine." *Advance for Nurses.* King of Prussia, PA: Merion.

Levine, C. 2005. *Taking sides.* New York: McGraw Hill.

Munson, R. 2007. *Intervention and reflection: Basic issues in medical ethics.* Belmont, CA: Wadsworth.

Noonan, J. 2003. "An Almost Absolute Value in History." In R. Munson, *Interventions and reflection* (pp. 83–86). Belmont, CA: Wadsworth Publishing.

Rabin, R. 2007. "As Demand for Donor Eggs Soars, High Prices Stir Ethical Concerns." *New York Times,* (May 15), F6.

Stein, R. 2006. "A Medical Crisis of Conscience." *Hartford Courant*, (Aug. 8), D3, D4.

Zuckman, J. 2001. "House OKs Bill on Fetus as a Victim." *Chicago Tribune*, (April 27), 1, 28.

Weil, E. 2006. "A Wrongful Birth?" *New York Times Magazine*, (March 12), 48–53.

Waldman, H. 2006. "When Doctors Deliver Anguish." *Hartford Courant*, (Nov. 19), 1, A6.

Death and Dying

Learning Objectives

1. Define the glossary terms.
2. Discuss the difference between cardiac and brain-oriented death.
3. Describe the Harvard Criteria for a Definition of Irreversible Coma.
4. Discuss the pros and cons of euthanasia.
5. Provide examples of ordinary versus extraordinary means used in the treatment of the terminally ill.
6. List and discuss the five stages of dying as described by Dr. Kübler-Ross.

Key Terms

Active euthanasia
Brain death
Cardiac death
Cardiopulmonary
Comatose
Curative care
Electroencephalogram (EEG)
Expired
Hospice

Hypothermia
Life support systems
Mercy killing
Palliative care
Passive euthanasia
Persistent vegetative state (PVS)
Principle of double-effect
Quality of life

Respite care
Rigor mortis
Substitute judgment rule
Terminally ill
Viatical settlements
Withdrawing life-sustaining treatment
Withholding life-sustaining treatment

CASE OF MARGUERITE M. AND THE ANGIOGRAM

Marguerite M., an 89-year-old widow, is admitted into the cardiac intensive care unit in Chicago's Memorial Hospital at 3:00 A.M. on a Sunday morning with a massive heart attack (myocardial infarction). Her internist, Dr. K., who is also a close family friend, has ordered an angiogram to determine the status of Marguerite's infarction (heart attack). Dr. K. knows that the angiogram and resulting treatment need to be done within the first six hours after an infarction in order to be effective. Therefore, the procedure is going to be done as soon as the on-call surgical team can set up the angiography room. The radiologist, who lives thirty minutes from the hospital, must also be in the hospital before the procedure can begin. At 4:30 A.M. the team is ready to have Marguerite, who is barely conscious, transferred from the intensive care unit (ICU) to the surgical suite.

Coincidentally, at 4:30 A.M. Sarah W., an unconscious 45-year-old woman, is brought in by ambulance with a massive heart attack. The emergency room (ER) physicians, after conferring with her physician by phone, conclude that she will need a balloon angiography (dilating an obstructed blood vessel by threading a balloon-tipped catheter into the vessel) to save her life. When they call the surgical department to have the on-call angiography team brought in, they are told that the room is already set up for Dr. K.'s patient. They do not have another team or surgical room for Sarah. A decision is made that because Sarah needs the balloon angiography in order to survive, they will use the angiography team for her.

Dr. K. is called at home and told that his patient, Marguerite, will not be able to have the angiogram. The hospital is going to use the angiography team for Sarah, because she is younger than Marguerite and has a greater chance for recovery. Unfortunately, it took longer than expected to stabilize Sarah before and after the procedure and the six-hour "window" when the procedure could be performed on Marguerite passed. Marguerite expired (died) the following morning.

1. Do you believe that this case presents a legal or an ethical problem, or both?

2. What do you believe should be the criteria for a physician to use when having to choose a solution that will benefit one patient at the expense of another?

3. How can Dr. K. justify this decision when speaking to the family of Marguerite M.?

4. What options does a member of the angiography team or a caregiver for Marguerite have if he or she disagrees with this decision?

I ssues relating to death and dying are especially sensitive, as they are topics that are ultimately faced by everyone. The questions are difficult to contemplate, even though they are critical. For example, should a feeding tube be inserted when a patient can no longer be fed by mouth? Should a ventilator be attached when the patient can no longer breathe independently? Should CPR be attempted when the heart stops beating? There are no definitive agreements within the medical profession on many of the issues relating to death and dying. The one point of agreement is that the dying patient must be treated with dignity.

THE DYING PROCESS

Death is inevitable for everyone. Modern medicine has enabled people to live longer and survive diseases such as pneumonia that once caused the elderly to die quickly. Infections can be treated and eliminated. The elderly, who may welcome death at the end of a long life or illness, can now be kept alive by medical technology. This has caused ethical and moral dilemmas for the healthcare profession. It is important to remember that professional codes of ethics usually include a statement about the healthcare professional's duty to preserve the dignity and life of the patient.

LEGAL DEFINITION OF DEATH

Determining when a person has died is important for a variety of reasons. Obviously, the most important reason is that no one wants to make the mistake of treating living patients as though they were dead. A person who has died, or is said to have **expired,** is no longer treated the same way as a living human. This in no way means that the body of a deceased person, also known as a corpse, can be handled in a disrespectful way.

The actual determination of death has also become critical in the past few decades due to advances in medicine such as organ transplantation and life-support systems. **Life-support systems,** such as ventilators/respirators and feeding tubes, allow medical practitioners to sustain for additional weeks, months, or even years a person who, according to all traditional standards, has died. The classic case is that of Karen Ann Quinlan.

Karen Ann Quinlan Case

On April 15, 1975, 21-year-old Karen Ann Quinlan was admitted to a New Jersey hospital after becoming unconscious from a combination of a prescription drug and alcohol. She suffered **cardiopulmonary** (heart and breathing) arrest and was placed on a respirator after her pulse was restored. She received a tracheotomy (a surgical incision into the trachea to assist in ventilation), had a nasogastric (NG) feeding tube inserted through her nose and into her stomach to receive nourishment, and was considered to be in a **comatose,** or permanently vegetative, condition. Her **electroencephalogram (EEG),** which measured brain activity, was abnormal, but a brain scan showed her brain activity to still be within normal limits. Months passed with no change in Quinlan's comatose condition, but her physical condition continued to deteriorate. She lost weight, dropping from 115 pounds to 70 pounds by September, and her body became rigid.

Karen's father appealed to the court to appoint him guardian, which it ultimately did. He requested that the extraordinary procedures, such as the respirator, be discontinued. The Superior Court denied this request. Many other legal battles took place, and eventually the respirator was discontinued. However, Quinlan continued to breathe on her own even after the respirator was discontinued. The hospital continued to feed Karen by artificial means, and she lived in a coma for ten years before she died on July 11, 1985. The Quinlan case was groundbreaking because it represented the first time a family had requested a court to approve the removal of a respirator from a permanently comatose patient and won the case (*In re Quinlan,* 355 A.2d 647, N.J. 1976).

The insertion of a nasogastric (NG) tube is a serious decision when the patient is comatose. An NG tube used as a feeding tube is a life-extending treatment as it will continue to provide nutrition and hydration long after a patient is able to take nourishment on his or her own. (A feeding tube can also be surgically inserted directly into the stomach through the abdomen.) An incompetent person, unable to make decisions on his or her own behalf, raises one of the most difficult ethical problems for those persons who must decide whether to withdraw nutrition and hydration. The reason for this is that there is no one clear definition of incompetence.

A physician may recognize that the patient may have an inability to make decisions regarding his or her own care. But mental incompetence is often not enough when determining to withdraw life support measures. Physicians must make a determination based on mental competence, physical condition, and the possibility of recovery. If the patient has periods of incompetence as well as lucid moments, then the courts will want decisions followed that are made during the patient's lucid moments. The family will also have to be consulted. Thus, there is not a simple answer to when to remove an NG tube or withhold nutritional or other life support measures.

> **MED TIP**
>
> The right to accept or reject medical treatment is each person's fundamental right.

Criteria for Death

Certain criteria or standards assist in the determination that death has occurred. Some indications, in addition to the loss of a heartbeat, include a significant drop in body temperature, no pupil response to light, loss of body color, no response to pain, **rigor mortis** (stiffness that occurs in a dead body), and biological disintegration. However, these symptoms may not appear until several hours after death, or not at all if life-support equipment is used.

While the criteria for death vary, this becomes problematic when a general consensus for the definition of *death* is needed. For instance, because a deceased person's organs can be removed for transplantation into a living body, if permission has been granted by the deceased prior to death or by the deceased's relatives, it is important to determine if and when death has occurred.

In one unusual case, an emergency room doctor pronounced a 20-month-old little girl, Mackayala Jespersen, dead after drowning in her backyard swimming pool. The doctor made this pronouncement based on the flat-line heart and brain tracings taken after she had been given an hour of CPR. As a police detective was photographing her dead body for record-keeping purposes, she took a deep breath. This occurred thirty-nine minutes after being pronounced dead. Other children have survived **hypothermia** (the state in which body temperature is below normal range) when they fell into ice-cold water. But this little girl's case is unusual because all of the proper procedures to determine death were followed, and the criteria used to define death were met. However, she was still alive.

Dr. Susan Tolle, director of the Center for Ethics in Healthcare at the Oregon Health and Science University in Portland stated, "Clearly, medicine needs to get it right 100 percent of the time. . . . There can be no errors, ever." But there is a real concern that errors may still occur as there is no one reliable test to determine exactly when a person has died. There is a continuing controversy over whether to use a cardiac definition of death or a brain-oriented definition of death. Even then, in some cases it is difficult to determine if someone is alive or dead.

Cardiac Death

Traditionally, death was defined as **cardiac death,** or death in which the heart has stopped functioning. A person who suffered an irreversible cessation of respiratory and circulatory function was considered dead. Medically trained personnel can make this determination based on lack of pulse or breathing. A cardiac death is considered a legal death.

In most situations, the cardiac determination of death is effective. However, using only the cardiac definition of death creates some problems. In fact, there is documentation of cases in which people lived even when their hearts stopped functioning. Several years ago, at the University of Utah, a heart patient named Barney Clark lived for four months with an artificial heart while he waited for a heart transplant. He was able to be partially active while connected to the artificial heart, although his own heart was no longer beating.

The definition for a cardiac death means that there is an irreversible loss of all cardiac function. In some cases, the cessation of breathing and pulse are reversible, such as in a drug overdose or hypothermia. This prolonged absence of oxygen can result in neurological damage. A patient who has suffered a cardiac arrest and is "clinically dead" may successfully be resuscitated with CPR. This person cannot be considered dead because the cessation of breath and pulse is not irreversible.

MED TIP

The terms *cardiac* and *cardiopulmonary,* referring to the heart and the lung function, are interchangeable as a legal definition of death.

Another serious problem with using only the cardiac-oriented definition of death involves organ transplantation. In many cases, if the surgeon waits until all cardiac function has ceased, many of the potential donor's organs are useless as transplants. Obviously, it is not ethical or moral to change the definition of death in order to increase the number of organs available for transplant. However, many people believe that a cardiac-oriented definition of death is inadequate.

Brain-Oriented Death

The whole-brain-oriented definition of death has gained favor in many countries, including the United States. Under this definition, death occurs when there is irreversible cessation of all brain function. It is based on the premise that the brain is responsible for all bodily functions, and once the brain stops functioning, all other bodily functions will stop. Most states accept this definition of death. One exception is New Jersey, which uses the traditional cardiac criteria to determine death.

MED TIP

Modern technology has made it possible to maintain heart and lung function for hours, and even days, after all brain function has stopped.

In most states, if the whole brain is dead, then the person is considered deceased. A **persistent vegetative state (PVS)** is an irreversible brain condition in which the patient is in a state of deep unconsciousness. If it persists for a few months it is almost always irreversible. The diagnosis for PVS is usually made by a neurologist and confirmed by two consulting neurologists after a brain-injured patient has been in a coma for at least six months. A dilemma occurs in the case of a patient whose heart and respiratory functions are maintained by mechanical means, such as a ventilator, but who has no brain activity. The patient's brain is dead, but because technology is sustaining cardiopulmonary functioning, the body is still alive. Discontinuing the ventilation support for a patient would result in the cardiac death of the patient. A moral dilemma confronts physicians when they have to definitely determine whether such a person has died.

The issue of death becomes extremely complex when a patient is comatose. In 1968, the Harvard Medical School published a report that outlined criteria for determining when a patient was in an irreversible coma or loss of consciousness, which, according to the study, meant the patient was brain-dead. This was regarded as the first and most important sign of impending death. This irreversible coma or loss of consciousness was then followed by a cessation of heartbeat and blood circulation. The Harvard Criteria for a Definition of Irreversible Coma includes consideration of whether the patient

1. Is unreceptive and unresponsive, with a total unawareness of externally applied, and even painful, stimuli.

2. Has no spontaneous movements or breathing, as well as an absence of response to stimuli such as pain, touch, sound, or light.

3. Has no reflexes, has fixed dilated pupils, lack of eye movement, and lack of deep tendon reflexes.

The Harvard Criteria also specified the required tests, including an electroencephalogram (EEG), to determine the absence of brain activity. Harvard recommended that these tests should be repeated again after 24 hours.

In the years since setting the criteria, there have been no known patients who have recovered after being declared in an irreversible coma using the Harvard Criteria. This irreversible coma is known as **brain death.** Because the Harvard Criteria use the diagnosis of brain death as the necessary condition for withdrawing life-support, such as mechanical ventilators or respirators, it emphasizes that the patient must be declared dead before any effort is made to take him or her off a respirator. Otherwise, according to the Harvard Committee, the physicians would be turning off a respirator on a person who, in a strict sense, is still alive.

However, the Harvard Criteria is now coming under careful scrutiny and criticism because they are the main criteria used to determine a person's eligibility to become an organ donor. There are patients who are in a persistently vegetative state but may show some evidence of consciousness. Some ethicists believe that if there is some level of consciousness, then the patient is not dead. This is a real concern for those who are involved in determining when a person's organs can be used for donation.

Furthermore, recent studies indicate that some vegetative patients, while unresponsive, may actually have brain activity indicating awareness, and even a wish to communicate.

It is estimated there are currently as many as 37,000 people in the United States who are in a persistently vegetative or minimally conscious state.

To protect the patient, and also protect a physician against malpractice suits, an outside medical opinion should be sought before terminating a life-support system. This issue has actually had a bearing in a criminal case. In Arizona, a murder defendant argued that it was not his criminal action that caused the death of the victim, but rather the actions of the physician who discontinued the life-support system. In this case, the court rejected the defendant's argument, holding that brain death was the valid test for death in Arizona. The court found that the victim's brain function had ceased as a result of the defendant's criminal action before the life-support was discontinued (*State v. Fierro,* 603 P.2d 74, Ariz. 1979).

Uniform Determination of Death Act

In the 1980s, the American Bar Association, the American Medical Association, the Uniform Law Commissioners, the American Academy of Neurology, and others approved a Uniform Determination of Death Act (UDDA). This law was adopted by a number of states. It says

> An individual, who has sustained either (1) irreversible cessation of circulatory and respiratory functions, or (2) irreversible cessation of all functions of the entire brain, including the brain stem, is dead.

Many groups, such as Orthodox Jews, many Catholics, and right-to-life proponents, object to the brain-death criteria. These groups believe acceptance of the brain-death criteria in all circumstances would legitimize practices they consider immoral, such as euthanasia and abortion.

MED TIP

Many phrases are used to refer to a deceased person, such as *passed away, passed on, departed,* and *left this world.* It is important to know which one is used in a particular family so as to be as compassionate as possible when discussing the death of a family member or loved one.

In caring for the critically ill or those patients who are considered to be **terminally ill,** where death is inevitable, there are several ethical considerations: (1) withdrawing versus withholding treatment, (2) active euthanasia versus passive euthanasia, (3) direct versus indirect killing, and (4) ordinary versus extraordinary means.

Withdrawing versus Withholding Treatment

Withdrawing life-sustaining treatment, such as artificial ventilation, means to discontinue it after it has been started. **Withholding life-sustaining treatment** means never starting it. Healthcare practitioners often find it more difficult to withdraw treatment after it has been started than to withhold treatment. However, many people believe that both are ethically wrong.

Starting a life-sustaining treatment, even on a temporary basis, allows the physician more time to evaluate the patient's condition. The physician may believe that if the treatment is ineffective, it can be stopped. However, in some cases, it has been necessary to get a court order to discontinue a treatment, such as a respirator, that has already been started.

Patients have the legal right to refuse treatment as well as food, even if they are not terminally ill. In a 1986 California case, a young woman with cerebral palsy, who had no use of her voluntary muscles, was unable to take her own life as she wished to do. She hospitalized herself and then stated her intent to refuse any food and to have her nasogastric (feeding) tube removed so that she could eventually die of starvation. The California Court of Appeals held that she had the right to refuse nutrition and hydration in order to end her life. She won her lawsuit and had the nasogastric tube removed. As recently as 1997, she continued to live and be cared for at home without the use of a feeding tube (*Bouvia v. Superior Court,* 225 Cal. Rptr. 287, Cal. App. 1986).

Active Euthanasia versus Passive Euthanasia

The word *euthanasia* literally means "good death" from the Greek word *eu* meaning "good" and *thanatos* meaning "death." However, the word has become much more complicated than simply providing a "good death" for another person. Most people equate the term euthanasia with "actively doing something" to create that good death. Other terms that people use instead of the term euthanasia are assisted suicide, right to die, and aid-in-dying. And, in fact, suicide has also been equated with euthanasia. There are differing viewpoints on whether euthanasia is ethical or unethical. Many people believe that euthanasia is a humane treatment of terminally ill patients in order to put an end to their suffering and pain. At the present time it is illegal in all states except Oregon and Washington.

Most people believe that there is a distinction between actively killing a patient (active euthanasia or assisted suicide) and allowing a patient to die by forgoing treatment (passive euthanasia). This moral distinction is approved by the AMA, Roman Catholic moral theology, and the President's Commission for the Study of Ethical Problems in Medicine and Biomedical and Behavioral Research. It is not accepted by Orthodox Judaism.

Active euthanasia, the intentional killing of the terminally ill, involves a second party directly introducing a lethal dose of medication, such as by injection, into the dying person. It is illegal in all jurisdictions in the United States, with the possible exceptions of Oregon and the state of Washington. The voters in Oregon have twice voted to give terminally ill patients, under carefully limited circumstances, the right to ask for a doctor's prescription to end their lives. The Oregon law requires a second medical opinion and the determination that the patient is in fact terminally ill and not just depressed. There has not been a stampede demanding death by prescription in Oregon, however. From 1997 to 2001, only 70 people in Oregon used this law. This law in Oregon is still being challenged and allows physician-assisted suicide (PAS) but not homicide. The state of Washington voted to allow physician-assisted suicide (called Initiative 1000 or Washington's Die with Dignity Act) in November, 2008.

Rather than directly killing a patient, some physicians have sought to allow a patient-assisted suicide. In this type of assistance, also called voluntary euthanasia, a physician provides a patient with the medical know-how or the means (a prescription) to enable a patient to end his or her own life. Jack Kevorkian first gained notoriety in June 1990 when he assisted in the suicide of Janet Adkins, a Michigan woman who was in the early stages of Alzheimer's disease. Since that time, he has assisted in the suicides of many other patients. In response to Kevorkian's actions, the state of Michigan enacted a law making assisted suicide a felony punishable by up to four years in prison. Kevorkian, however, ignored this law and went on to assist several more people with their suicides. He was released after serving a sentence in a Michigan prison.

While active euthanasia is illegal, **passive euthanasia,** or allowing a patient to die naturally, is legal everywhere. Passive euthanasia involves withholding medical interventions that would only serve to sustain the life. This includes hydration (supply of fluids) and nutritional feeding. The patient is to be kept clean, warm, and protected from infection and pain as much as possible. The dying patient is medicated to be pain free, but no lethal doses are administered. The dying process is neither inhibited nor accelerated.

There is always the concern that chronically ill and dying patients may be pressured to choose euthanasia in order to spare their families further emotional or financial strain. Any pressure of this type can lead to serious ethical and moral questions.

MED TIP

The term *passive euthanasia* is falling out of favor by organizations such as the Roman Catholic Church. The phrase "allow to die" is used instead.

Arguments in Favor of Euthanasia

People who favor euthanasia offer the following justifications:

- Respect for patient self-determination. Individuals should have the right to determine the outcome of their lives.
- Euthanasia provides a means for harvesting viable organs.
- It provides relief for the family of a patient with an irreversible condition or terminal disease.
- It provides a means to end a terminally ill person's suffering.

Arguments in Opposition to Euthanasia

Many people oppose euthanasia in any form (active or passive) for several reasons, including the following:

- There is no certainty regarding death. Many terminally ill patients have been known to recover.
- Modern technology may find a cure for a terminal disease.
- Families who are undergoing stress due to the financial burden of a dying relative may be examining euthanasia just to relieve that burden.
- If euthanasia is allowed, then it might be used indiscriminately.
- It is not good for society to have physicians kill patients or for patients to kill themselves.
- There is value and dignity in every human life.
- When physicians and other healthcare professionals become involved in any form of euthanasia, it erodes the very ethical basis of the professions.
- The sick and dying may have a fear of involuntary euthanasia if euthanasia is legalized.
- Judeo-Christian religious beliefs declare that only God has dominion over life.

Slippery Slope Argument of Assisted Suicide

Some ethicists are concerned that if our society were to allow assisted suicide, it could lead to a form of legalized murder. This "slippery slope" argument against permitting assisted suicide is that it would eventually lead to a diminishing of our respect for life. Their warning is that once we set out upon the climb, or slope, toward helping a patient die, we can easily slip into allowing many other persons to die who are not terminally ill, such as the elderly, disabled, or unproductive.

Signing a living will document is meant to prevent a medical staff from using "extraordinary" measures, such as ventilators, to keep us alive. However, there is documentation that an elderly woman, who had signed a living will, was then denied treatment that she expected and needed. Even though the complications she suffered after surgery were treatable, the medical staff misinterpreted the intent of her living will. They stood by doing nothing for twenty minutes as they watched her die. Consumer activist and attorney Wesley Smith is fearful that assisted suicide would not be restricted for dying people as a "last resort" but, instead, death would be hastened for people who were not terminal.

There is the added danger that if assisted suicide were legal, it might lead to situations such as allowing defective infants to die. Smith cites the example of a baby boy born prematurely with kidney problems. Only a court order demanding that his doctors use life-saving methods (dialysis) saved his life. This boy eventually came off dialysis and today lives a full life. According to Smith, legalizing euthanasia and assisted suicide would be a disservice to the people who are the most powerless such as the disabled, critically ill, and indigent.

There are many people who believe that pain and depression can be treated and should not be a reason for assisted suicide to take place. Most people agree that this is not just a religious matter. Mercy killing, a form of assisted suicide, is against the law but it still occurs. Some physicians have prescribed very high doses of narcotics to patients with terminal cancer knowing that, while the high dose will relieve the pain, it might also cause their death. In most cases, however, this death would be unintended by the physician and the high dose of narcotic would only be meant as a comfort measure for a dying patient.

U.S. Supreme Court Justice Benjamin Cardoza once wrote the following words about an early movement to legalize euthanasia, "Just as life may not be shortened, so its value must be held as equal to that of any other, the mightiest or the lowliest."

A concern that many ethicists voice is the rise in the suicide rates, particularly in the elderly, since the rise in euthanasia advocacy and the media attention to Jack Kevorkian. Barbara Haight, who directs a program to prevent suicide among the elderly at the University of South Carolina College of Nursing, believes that the attention paid to euthanasia by the media has "made suicide more acceptable to people who once would not have considered it because of religious and family concerns."

Individual healthcare professionals must remember that active euthanasia violates the medical profession's ethics and is against the law. The Nancy Cruzan case is an example of a situation in which the removal of a feeding tube was a form of active euthanasia *within* the law.

The Nancy Cruzan Case

On January 11, 1983, 25-year-old Nancy Cruzan was involved in an automobile accident that left her in a vegetative state until her death eight years later. A feeding tube was implanted in her in a Missouri hospital. Three years after the accident, her parents, who had been granted guardianship, believed that she would never regain consciousness. The family sought legal assistance from the American Civil Liberties Union and requested that the feeding tube be removed. The judge ruled in favor of the Cruzans, but the case was appealed. The U.S. Supreme Court overturned the judge's decision and ruled against the Cruzans because under Missouri law, hydration or nutritional support could not be withdrawn from an incompetent patient unless clear evidence demonstrated that this is what the patient would have requested. Several years later, new evidence became known when two of Cruzan's former co-workers came forward. They both stated that she had said she would not wish to be maintained like Karen Quinlan. In December 1990, a judge complied with the Cruzans' wish to have their daughter's feeding tube removed. In reaction to this verdict, right-to-life protestors demonstrated outside the rehabilitation center where Cruzan was being kept alive. The feeding tube was removed on December 14, 1990, and she was pronounced dead twelve days later on December 26, 1990 (*Cruzan v.*

Director, Missouri Dep't. of Health, 497 U.S. 261, 1990). In 1996 the Cruzan family went through another tragedy when Nancy's father, Joe Cruzan, hanged himself in the family home. His family and friends believed that he was unable to emotionally recover from his daughter's long, drawn-out death.

Both the Karen Quinlan and the Nancy Cruzan cases are considered to be landmark cases in medical law and ethics because they established an individual's right to refuse to receive medical care. Because both these cases lasted over a period of several years, the cases also illustrated the need for people to let family members know both verbally and particularly in writing what their wishes are for life-sustaining medical care if they become incompetent.

MED TIP

Families often ask for advice from healthcare workers on what course of action they should take for a dying loved one. Remember that the physician is the only healthcare professional who can advise the patients or their families on a course of medical treatment.

Terri Schiavo: "The Face That Moved a Nation"

In October 2003, the face of Terri Schiavo smiling at her mother caught the interest of the U.S. public and the governor of Florida, Jeb Bush (Figure 13.1 ■). Terri had been in a persistent vegetative state since 1990. Her husband, Michael, and her parents were friendly until a jury awarded $1 million to Terri, under Michael's control, in a medical malpractice lawsuit. The parents contend that Michael stopped his wife's therapy and used the money to pay lawyer's fees in an attempt to have his wife's feeding tube removed. Terri's husband stated that he wanted to fulfill his wife's wishes that she not be kept living in a comatose or vegetative state. Her parents opposed having the tube removed, declaring that she is not comatose but rather appears to smile, blink, and is able to follow balloons and her parents as they move about her room.

Physicians who examined Terri over the years indicated that she could respond to pain, blink her eyes, and raise her leg when asked to do so. In 2003, a speech pathologist stated that Terri uttered "stop" in response to a medical procedure that was being done to

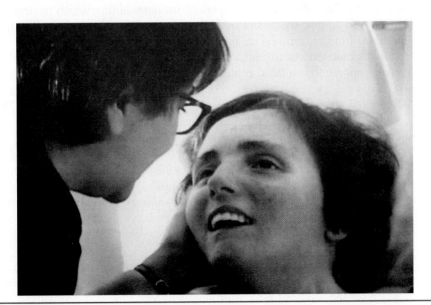

FIGURE 13.1
Terri Schiavo

her. One doctor stated that she was not in a "persistent vegetative state," based on the evidence he found when he examined her.

Terri's feeding tube was removed as ordered by the court. There was a great amount of media attention over her case, including a photo of Terri Schiavo smiling up at her mother on the front page of many national newspapers. One week after the feeding tube was removed, Governor Jeb Bush and the Florida legislature ordered that the feeding tube be reinserted. It was. In fact, Terri's feeding tube was removed and reinserted three times before the final removal. She died thirteen days after the feeding tube was removed, which was fifteen years after her collapse at the age of 26, and seven years after her court battle began.

Direct versus Indirect Killing

In some situations, an action can lead to two effects: one that is intended and even desirable, and another that is unintended and undesirable.

A person's death may result from another person's intended action or inaction. For instance, if a nurse intentionally ignores a patient who is choking because she or he wants the patient to die, the nurse has killed the patient.

However, death may be an unintentional result of another person's action. For example, if a high-risk patient dies from an anesthetic, the patient's death was not intended or desired. A surgeon who is morally opposed to abortion may have to remove a cancerous uterus in a pregnant woman; the death of the fetus is not intended or desired, but is the indirect result of treating the disease. The death, in this case, would be morally tolerable, even by members of religions opposed to abortion, because death of the fetus was not the intended purpose of the surgery.

These actions fit within the **principle of double-effect,** which recognizes that an action may have two consequences: one desired (and intended or morally good) and one undesired (and unintended). Groups such as the AMA and the Catholic Church oppose direct killing but accept undesired and unintended deaths. The courts generally make the same distinctions.

Ordinary versus Extraordinary Means

Another important distinction concerns the difference between ordinary and extraordinary means. This distinction is important for determining which treatments are morally required. To do this, we cannot simply separate common means, such as fluids and feeding tubes, from uncommon means, such as respirators, because in some situations even common procedures or treatments may be considered extraordinary. Many believe that it is inappropriate to use the complexity of the technology to determine what treatment to use or not use. For example, is it morally right to force a nasogastric feeding tube into a 90-year-old pneumonia patient who does not wish to have this treatment? In other situations, it may be considered an ordinary means of treatment to temporarily use a respirator on a 90-year-old woman who is recovering from a choking episode.

The term *ordinary* refers to a treatment or procedure that is morally required, such as fluids and comfort measures. *Extraordinary measures* refer to those procedures and treatments that are morally expendable. Some professionals use the terms *appropriate* and *inappropriate* instead of *ordinary* and *extraordinary*. A treatment is considered morally expendable, or inappropriate, if it does not serve any useful purpose. For example, a commonsense judgment would determine that chemotherapy would be useless in the final days of a cancer patient's life.

Even if a treatment may serve the useful purpose of prolonging life, it may not be morally justified if it involves a grave burden. This was discussed in the President's Commission for the Study of Ethical Problems in Medicine and Biomedical and Behavioral Research. In addition, Pope Pius XII issued the following statement on prolonging life:

> Normally one is held to use only ordinary means—according to circumstances of persons, places, times, and culture—that is to say, means that do not involve any grave burden for oneself or another.

These are difficult issues to encounter. The administration of fluids, nutrition, and routine nursing procedures such as turning a patient may result in what the patient believes is a grave burden. These treatments may cause further pain and discomfort. In addition, they may actually be useless to recovery, but as in the case of turning bedridden patients, are considered necessary nursing care or ordinary means of care.

Right to Die Legislation or Right to Refuse Treatment

Patients have the right to refuse treatment. In extreme cases in which the patients' refusal places their lives in danger, legal action sometimes results. The following is an example of such a case.

In January 1978, the Tennessee Department of Human Services filed a lawsuit seeking to have a *guardian ad litem* appointed to care for 72-year-old Mary Northern, who had no living relatives and suffered from gangrene of both feet. This condition required removing both her feet in order to save her life. During the court hearings, even though she was alert and lucid, Northern did not have the capacity to understand the severity or the consequences of her disease process, as demonstrated by her insistence that her feet were black because of dirt and that her physicians were incorrect about the seriousness of her infection. The court determined that she was in imminent danger of death without the amputation and authorized the state's commissioner of human services to act on her behalf in consenting for the surgery. However, on May 1, 1978, before Mary could be stabilized for surgery, she died of a blood clot from the gangrenous tissue (*State Dep't. of Human Services v. Northern*, 563 S.W.2d 197, Tenn. Ct. App.1978).

STAGES OF DYING

Dr. Elisabeth Kübler-Ross devoted much of her life to the study of the dying process. She divided the dying process into five stages that she believes the patient, family members, and caregivers all go through. The five stages are denial, anger, bargaining, depression, and acceptance. According to Kübler-Ross, these stages overlap and may not be experienced by everyone in the stated order, but all are present in the dying patient. The five stages of dying or grief are summarized in Table 13.1 ■.

		TABLE 13.1
Denial	A refusal to believe that dying is taking place. This may be a time when the patient (or family member) needs time to adjust to the reality of approaching death. This stage cannot be hurried.	**Five Stages of Dying (or Grief)**
Anger	The patient may be angry with everyone and may express an intense anger toward God, family, and even healthcare professionals. The patient may take this anger out on the closest person, usually a family member. In reality, the patient is angry about dying.	
Bargaining	This involves attempting to gain time by making promises in return. Bargaining may be done between the patient and God. The patient may indicate a need to talk at this stage.	
Depression	There is a deep sadness over the loss of health, independence, and eventually life. There is an additional sadness of leaving loved ones behind. The grieving patient may become withdrawn at this time.	
Acceptance	This stage is reached when there is a sense of peace and calm. The patient makes comments such as, "I have no regrets. I'm ready to die." It is better to let the patient talk and not to make denial statements such as, "Don't talk like that. You're not going to die."	

QUALITY-OF-LIFE ISSUES

Quality of life refers to more than just what a person experiences at one moment in time. It includes many dimensions such as physiological status, emotional well-being, functional status, and satisfaction with life in general. A medical procedure or intervention, such as aggressive treatment for a terminal illness, will have an impact on the physical, social, and emotional well-being of the patient. This impact can be measured to assess the intangible costs and consequences of the disease or illness. These quality-of-life measurements can assist with making healthcare decisions based not only on clinical factors and costs, but on issues that the patient believes are important. Measures used to assess quality of life include

- General health
- Physical functioning
- Role limitations, such as within the family structure
- Pain

- Social function
- Vitality
- Mental health

Questions are asked relating to each of these dimensions by the healthcare professional to create a patient's health profile. Two useful quality-of-life measurement instruments are the Functional Living Index: Cancer (FLIC) and the Arthritis Impact Measurement Scale (AIMS). The results of these measurement tests can aid the practitioner and the patient in making quality-of-life decisions, such as whether to extend life with the use of support systems (Figure 13.2 ■).

USE OF MEDICATIONS

A four-year study of over 8,000 dying patients was published in the *Journal of the American Medical Association* in November 1995. Families reported that half of the patients who were able to communicate in their last days spent most of the time in moderate or severe pain. Physicians often have a reluctance to overprescribe pain medications for

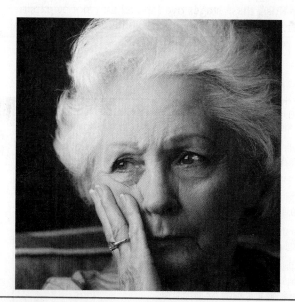

FIGURE 13.2
Anxiety on the Face of an Elderly Woman

patients out of a fear that the patient may become addicted to the drug. However, in the case of a dying patient who may not live long enough to become addicted, there is a belief among many physicians that the patient's pain and suffering should be controlled with the use of adequate medications. The Hippocratic tradition of medicine stated that it is a fundamental responsibility of physicians to relieve pain (Figure 13.3 ■).

Currently, 9 million Americans live with cancer, and the estimate is that about 60 percent of those patients will eventually die of the disease. Surveys indicate that one-third of patients receiving active therapy, such as chemotherapy, and two-thirds of patients with an advanced disease have significant pain. Yet only about half of the patients receive adequate pain control.

MED TIP

Even though a nurse may believe that a dying patient requires more pain medication, she or he cannot increase the dosage or administration times without a physician's order.

HOSPICE CARE

Hospice, a multidisciplinary, family-centered care, is a system that is designed to provide care and supportive services to terminally ill patients and their families. The hospice movement, which originated in France, has a commitment to keep patients with a terminal illness as pain-free as possible. Our modern-day hospice is modeled after Saint Christopher's Hospice in London, which was started by Dr. Cicely Saunders in 1966. She established a facility with a homelike atmosphere where terminally ill patients, both young and old, find comfort until death. Hospices, based on Dr. Saunders's model, are found throughout the world. The hospice service is available both in a facility such as Dr. Saunders's model and also in the patient's own home, where a hospice worker provides daily care if needed.

There is mounting evidence that hospice care can provide a better way to die. It is advertised as "death with dignity." Hospice care is focused on providing comfort measures, emotional support, and a final environment as pain-free as possible for the patient. There is now a much greater understanding of the use of narcotics for terminally ill cancer patients.

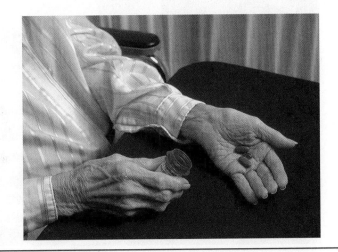

FIGURE 13.3
**Older Adults May Need
Special Assistance
with Medication**

Whenever possible, patients are kept awake and alert so that they can spend some of their last moments with their family members. Additional services, such as pastoral and respite care for the family, are part of the hospice philosophy. The staff consists of specially trained personnel who have experience and interest in caring for the dying patient. The patient is usually only hospitalized in a hospice unit during the final weeks of life. Hospice care is meant to liberate patients from their pain and suffering so that they can truly live until they die (Figure 13.4 ■).

PALLIATIVE CARE

Palliative care is the total care of patients whose disease is no longer responsive to curative therapy. This type of care, consisting of comfort measures, is meant to provide a relief of pain and suffering so the patient can die with dignity. Comfort measures include frequent turning and bathing, gentle massage, providing oral fluids, and listening to the patient. Palliative care emphasizes symptom control, such as for pain, shortness of breath,

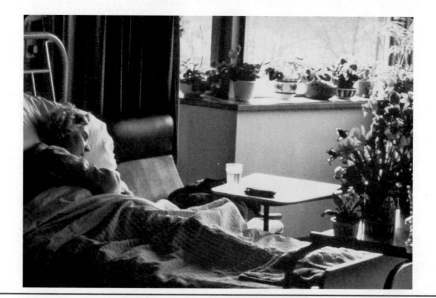

FIGURE 13.4
An Elderly Hospice Patient

and supportive therapy for depression. Palliative care is not euthanasia, nor do the health-care professionals giving this type of care passively allow people to die.

Palliative care, which is the opposite of **curative care** in which we attempt to cure the patient's disease, requires healthcare professionals who understand the need for compassion rather than surgical or medical interventions. What palliative care can do is to make the end-of-life period a meaningful experience for the patient rather than something of which to be frightened.

Some critics of modern-day healthcare believe that our culture has a built-in bias that "everything that can be done will be done" for the dying patient. Some physicians have stated that aggressive treatment for the elderly, such as chemotherapy, at acute care hospitals can be inhumane. And once they are started they cannot be withdrawn. Many dying patients do not wish to lose the opportunity to make decisions about their quality of life and give up control over their care. But this may not mean that they wish to have extraordinary measures taken to prolong their life. Dr. Dennis McCullough uses the term "slow medicine" meaning that a compassionate approach to caring for aging loved ones does not require aggressive and even painful procedures. He believes that because nine out of ten people who live into their 80s will be unable to care for themselves at a certain point, they must make their choices clear to their caregivers ahead of time. If they do not wish heroic measures, such as CPR, to be taken, then this must be stated in writing.

VIATICAL SETTLEMENTS

Viatical settlements allow people with terminal illnesses, such as AIDS, to obtain money from their life insurance policies by selling them. The term *viatical* comes from the Latin term *viaticum,* which were the money and supplies given to Roman officials before taking on a risky journey for the empire. (*Viaticum* is also the Roman Catholic sacrament given to the dying patient.) A viatical settlement means that in exchange for a 20 to 50 percent discount on the face value of the patient's insurance policy, he or she can have immediate access to the money. The patient names the settlement company as the recipient of the death benefit. In return, the viatical settlement company assumes complete responsibility for the insurance policy, including making all the premium payments. The owner then receives no further benefits from the insurance. At the time of the patient's (viator's) death, the viatical settlement company receives the death benefit from the policy.

Many terminally ill patients have used the money to provide for medical and nursing care during their final illness. However, others have used the money to enjoy a vacation with family members or to pay for experimental medical treatments that health insurance companies will not cover.

There are problems with viatical settlements, including tax liabilities and a potential loss of means-based entitlements such as Medicaid. Because the payment to the patient is less than the face value of the insurance policy, the patient could be "giving away" a significant amount of money to the settlement company. In addition, terminally ill patients often live much longer than they expected with their illness, and the small payment by the settlement company may not be enough to help them.

ADVANCE DIRECTIVES

The Federal Patient Self-Determination Act of 1991 mandates that adult patients admitted into any healthcare facility that receives funding from either Medicare or Medicaid must be asked if they have an advance directive or wish to have information about these self-determination directives. Ideally, people make decisions about advance directives before they are in a situation in which they are being admitted to a hospital or nursing home. If these documents—such as a living will, durable power of attorney for health-care, Uniform Anatomical Gift Act, or do not resuscitate (DNR) order—have to be drawn up after a patient has entered a facility, then it should be done in a nonstressful manner.

Advance directives are popularly known as living wills. These documents became popular about thirty years ago when medical technology made it possible for people to be kept alive in unpleasant and fragile conditions for long periods of time. Advance directives limit the type and amount of medical care and treatment that patients will receive if they should become incompetent and have a poor prognosis. It is important that directives are placed in writing; it is not sufficient for a person to just tell someone what his or her wishes for treatment are. The courts typically enforce written advance directives. For additional discussion about advance directives, see Chapter 5.

MED TIP

All healthcare professionals should be aware that it is also acceptable for a patient to write an advance directive asking to receive *maximum* care and treatment for as long as possible.

The **substitute judgment rule** is used when decisions must be made for people who cannot make their own decisions. Under this rule a person, committee, or institution will attempt to determine what the person would do if she or he were competent to make their own decisions. However, there is always speculation about what decision the patient would actually make if they were competent, even though they may have indicated their wishes to another person at an earlier time. Therefore, when there is a lack of an advance directive, most decision makers will rule in favor of using all interventions such as tube feedings. This is a case in which the principle of beneficence is followed because it operates in the interests of the patient. A subjective judgment of a committee or institution may or may not be what the patient would request if able to do so. Therefore, an advance directive is clearly the recommended document to advise the best course of treatment for the patient.

Without an advance directive from the individual patient, treatments that might be ordered for patients include CPR, mechanical breathing or respirator, tube feedings, kidney dialysis, chemotherapy, intravenous therapy, surgery, diagnostic tests, antibiotics, and transfusions.

MED TIP

It is recommended that all persons over the age of 18 place in writing their wishes about what type of treatment they should receive if they become incompetent. The advance directive should be specific about treatments such as CPR, tube feeding, and ventilators.

CHOICES IN LIFE AND DEATH

Suicide

Is it morally permissible to allow competent persons to consent to their own deaths? Voluntary euthanasia and suicide are considered to be morally different. Voluntary euthanasia, or **mercy killing,** is the action (or inaction) of a second person to help or hasten the death of the person who wishes to die. Suicide involves only the actions of the person seeking death. Suicide is considered to be morally wrong and is illegal in most states.

However, no state currently punishes people who attempt suicide, although they may be placed in psychiatric care if they present a danger to themselves. Many religions condemn suicide and euthanasia.

The Case of the Conjoined Twins

A marathon fifty-hour operation to separate 29-year-old Iranian twins joined at the head resulted in their deaths during the surgical procedure in July 2003. The twins, Ladan and Laleh Bijani, made a desperate plea to surgeons to give them a chance at living independent lives. The twins knew that the operation carried deadly risks, but knowingly accepted the risks, according to their physicians. Many of their physicians and relatives tried to talk the twins out of having the procedure. But the women gave instructions to their next-of-kin that they wished to be separated under all circumstances, no matter what the surgeons encountered during the surgery. Dr. Benjamin Carson, who was a part of the neurosurgical team to separate the twins, said that he was persuaded to proceed with the operation based on the medical evidence and the strong desire of the twins to be separated. He stated, "These were individuals who were absolutely determined to be separated. The reason I felt compelled to become involved is because I wanted to make sure they had their best chance."

However, during the operation, the surgeons found that contrary to their first impression, the twins' brains were fused together, and a vein graft failed, causing the twins to hemorrhage and die. After the death of the twins, Dr. Carson said that in hindsight he believes it was unwise for the medical team to tacitly agree to continue with the surgery to separate the twins no matter what they encountered during the surgery.

There have been many ethical debates about the separation of conjoined twins, such as Ladan and Laleh, who have little chance of both surviving such a surgery. Michael Grodin, director of medical ethics at the Boston University School of Medicine, stated, "The key issue is that they were adults and could understand the risks and benefits and make decisions on their own." He went on to say, "Obviously, if the chances were 100 percent that the twins were going to die, then the surgeons shouldn't have offered it. To do so would have been akin to participating in an assisted suicide." Grodin and other ethicists agree that no one knows exactly where the ethical cut-off point should be for an operation or procedure in which the odds for recovery are poor.

Some parents have opted not to have their conjoined twins separated because one would ultimately die during the separation if they share key organs. In the case of each twin receiving a kidney or a limb, the surgeons will often recommend separation. In the case of a shared heart, the decision becomes an ethical dilemma since both twins may die during the separation.

Mechanical Heart Recipient

The first implanted mechanical heart, a grapefruit-sized plastic and titanium four-pound heart called an AbioCor, was implanted into a 59-year-old man, Robert Tools, in July 2001. This patient did quite well with his mechanical heart until he suffered a severe stroke from a blood clot that was believed to be caused by the mechanical device. Mr. Tools was unable to take anticoagulant medications to reduce the risk of blood clots forming. He spent the final days of his life partly paralyzed and breathing through a ventilator. Before he had the mechanical heart transplant, Mr. Tools had been on the brink of death with end-stage heart failure and had been given little chance of surviving more than thirty days. Up until the time of his stroke, he expressed gratitude after the surgery and said that he had no regrets. Robert Tools lived for five months with his mechanical heart. The manufacturers of the mechanical heart said the success of the AbioCor is measured by how well it extends life and restores life's quality.

POINTS TO PONDER

1. What do you say to a dying patient who asks you, "Why me?"
2. What are some major concerns of family members of a dying patient?
3. Does an individual have the right to determine when he or she wishes to die? Why or why not?
4. What are the benefits of hospice care for the terminally ill?
5. What is your opinion regarding Jack Kevorkian's behavior?
6. Why is the ability to determine when death has occurred so critical in today's healthcare environment?
7. What is cardiac death?
8. Can a patient write an advance directive requesting maximum care?

DISCUSSION QUESTIONS

1. Explain the statement, "Healthcare practitioners often find it more difficult to withdraw treatment after it has started than to withhold treatment."
2. Describe a situation in which passive euthanasia might be acceptable.
3. Discuss reasons against the practice of euthanasia.
4. What are the pros and cons of a viatical settlement?

REVIEW CHALLENGE

Short Answer Questions

1. Explain the substitute judgment rule.

2. What does palliative care include?

3. Explain the "slippery slope" argument of assisted suicide.

4. What is the difference between withdrawing versus withholding life-sustaining treatment?

5. Do you think the courts acted properly in granting Michael Schiavo control over his wife's feeding tube?

6. How might the Schiavo case affect future court decisions of the same nature?

7. Describe the differences between ordinary and extraordinary means to keep a person alive.

8. What are some of the arguments opposing euthanasia?

Matching

Match the responses in column B with the correct term in column A.

Column A

_____ **1.** proxy
_____ **2.** expired
_____ **3.** mercy killing
_____ **4.** comatose
_____ **5.** rigor mortis
_____ **6.** hypothermia
_____ **7.** stages of dying
_____ **8.** cardiac death
_____ **9.** brain death
_____ **10.** active euthanasia

Column B

a. body temperature is below normal
b. person acting on behalf of another person
c. legal definition of death
d. euthanasia
e. stiffness that occurs in death
f. vegetative condition
g. legal term for killing a patient
h. died
i. irreversible coma
j. Kübler-Ross's reflection on the dying process

Multiple Choice

Select the one best answer to the following statements.

1. The practice of allowing a terminally ill patient to die by forgoing treatment is called

a. active euthanasia.
b. passive euthanasia.
c. mercy killing.
d. a and c.
e. b and c.

2. An electroencephalogram is used to

a. reverse a coma patient's condition.
b. measure cardiopulmonary function.
c. measure brain function.
d. reverse the condition of hypothermia.
e. reverse the condition of rigor mortis.

3. The Uniform Determination of Death Act

a. provides a definition of active euthanasia.
b. provides a definition of brain death.
c. is also called the doctrine of double effect.
d. mandates that everyone entering a nursing home must provide a written document stating the care he or she wishes to receive.
e. discusses the treatments that might be used for a comatose patient.

4. Criteria or standards for death include

a. rigor mortis.
b. hypothermia.
c. loss of body color.
d. biological disintegration.
e. all of the above.

5. What is the ethical term used to morally justify the removal of a cancerous uterus from a pregnant patient?

a. mercy killing
b. extraordinary means
c. ordinary means
d. doctrine of double effect
e. advance directive

6. Another term meaning death is

a. comatose.
b. expired.
c. proxy.
d. terminally ill.
e. hypothermia.

7. A hospice provides for

a. palliative care.
b. pain medications.
c. in-patient care.
d. home care.
e. all of the above.

8. Extraordinary care means that when caring for a comatose patient, one should include

a. CPR and mechanical breathing.
b. chemotherapy.
c. turning and hydration.
d. a and b only.
e. a, b, and c.

9. The Karen Ann Quinlan case involved

a. mercy killing.
b. removal of hydration from a comatose patient.
c. removal of a respirator from a comatose patient.
d. a heart transplant.
e. court order for a surgical procedure on an incompetent patient.

10. Terms referring to heart and pulmonary function include

a. cardiac.
b. comatose.
c. hypothermia.
d. cardiopulmonary.
e. none of the above.

DISCUSSION CASES

1. Analyze the Marguerite M. case at the beginning of this chapter using the Seven-Step Decision Model found in the first chapter.

    a. _____

    b. _____

    c. _____

    d. _____

    e. _____

    f. _____

    g. _____

2. Donald Hamilton, an alert 55-year-old man, was diagnosed with inoperable pancreatic cancer. His prognosis was poor; he was given about six months to live. He underwent several series of chemotherapy treatments, but they were of no benefit. He continued to lose weight, suffered from nausea, and became weaker. After three months of chemotherapy treatments, he stated that he wanted no further treatment. He became bedridden and was admitted into a nursing home for terminal care. Donald's son, who lived in another state, arrived at the nursing home and demanded that his father's physician be called immediately. The son wanted his father to be hospitalized and placed on chemotherapy immediately. When the physician explained that there was little hope for the father's recovery, the son threatened to sue the physician for withdrawal of care.

    a. Identify the ethical issues in the case.

    _____

    _____

    b. In your opinion, does the son have a legitimate reason to sue the physician? Why or why not?

    _____

    _____

    c. What are the possible solutions to this case?

    _____

    _____

    d. What might the physician have done to prevent the confrontation with Donald's son?

    _____

    _____

3. Lois, who is in the last stages of breast cancer, was recently admitted into a hospice program. Her husband, Henry, is relieved to have a hospice nurse come into their home and help with the care of his wife. After Lois had been receiving care for a week, Henry asked when he should take Lois into the hospital out-patient department for more chemotherapy. The hospice nurse said, "I thought that you understood that since treatments would no longer help Lois and she would ultimately die, that she would not receive any more treatments once she entered the hospice program." Henry said he did not understand this and insisted that he wanted everything done to save Lois.

a. How could this misunderstanding have been avoided?

_____

_____

b. What discussions should Lois and Henry have had with each other before Lois went into a hospice program?

_____

_____

c. What could hospice programs do to better inform the general public of their purpose?

_____

_____

PUT IT INTO PRACTICE

Find a recent obituary in your local newspaper. What information does it give about the deceased person? What would you like to read about yourself if you could write your own obituary?

WEB HUNT

Search the website of the National Hospice and Palliative Care Organization (www.nhpco.org), and look under "find a hospice program." Using this listing, find a hospice in your area.

CRITICAL THINKING EXERCISE

What would you say if you were asked for your opinion on who in our society has the right to determine who should and should not live?

BIBLIOGRAPHY

Abelson, R. 2007. "A Chance to Choose Hospice, and Hope for a Cure." *New York Times.* (Feb. 10), A1, C4.

Altman, L. 2001. "Artificial-Heart Patient is Bleeding in the Brain." *New York Times* (Nov. 21), 14.

American Medical Association. 2008–2009. *Code of medical ethics: Current opinions on ethical and judicial affair.* Chicago: American Medical Association.

Arras, J., and B. Steinbock, 2002. *Ethical issues in modern medicine.* Mountain View, CA: Mayfield.

Bauers, S. 2006. "Dueling Schiavo Memoirs to Duke it Out." *Hartford Courant* (Feb. 26), H5.

Bell, M. 2004. "Judge in Florida Voids Terri's Law." *Chicago Tribune.* (May 7), 4.

Black, H. 2009. *Black's law dictionary.* 8th ed. St. Paul, MN: West Publishing.

Bor, J., & E. Niedowski. 2003. "A Great Emptiness: The Deaths of Conjoined Twins." *Hartford Courant,* (July 9) 1, A4.

Brody, J. 2009. "One Piece of Health Reform: Avoiding 'Bad' Deaths. *New York Times* (August 18), D7.

Brown, D. 2001. "Surgeon in Doomed Operation on Twins Speaks Out." *Hartford Courant* (July 12), A5.

Bufill, J. 2003. "Ethical Dilemmas at the Beginning of Death." *Chicago Tribune* (Nov. 28), 21.

Caplan, L., J. McCartney, and D. Sisti. 2006. *The case of Terri Schiavo.* Amherst, NY: Prometheus Books.

Devettere, R. 2000. *Practical decision making in healthcare ethics: Cases and concepts.* Washington, DC: Georgetown University Press.

Espejo, R., ed. 2003. *Biomedical ethics: Opposing viewpoints.* San Diego, CA: Greenhaven Press.

Fernandes, C. 2009. "Coming to Know the Limits of Healing." *New York Times* (Sept. 8), D5.

Foley, K. 2001. "Pioneer in the Battle to Avert Needless Pain and Suffering." *New York Times* (Nov. 6), F5.

Hall, M., ed. 1947. *Selected writings of Benjamin Nathan Cardoza.* New York: Fallon Publications, 388.

Healy, M. 2010. "Vegetative Patients Shown to Be Aware." *Harford Courant* (Feb. 5), A7.

Hoffman, J. 2006. "The Last Word on the Last Breath." *New York Times* (Oct. 10), F1.

Kampert, P. 2003. "The Face That Moved a Nation." *Chicago Tribune* (Oct. 23), 1, 25.

Levine, C. 2005. *Taking sides: Clashing views on controversial bioethical issues.* Guilford, CT: McGraw-Hill.

McCullough, D. 2008. *My mother, your mother: Embracing slow medicine, the compassionate approach to caring for your aging loved one.* New York: HarperCollins Publisher.

Munson, R. 2004. *Raising the dead.* New York: Oxford University Press.

President's Commission for the Study of Ethical Problems in Medicine and Biomedical and Behavioral Research. 1983. *Deciding to forego life-sustaining treatment: Ethical, medical, and legal issues in treatment decisions.* Washington, DC: U.S. Government Printing Office.

Quill, T. 2005. "Terri Schiavo: A Tragedy Compounded." *The New England Journal of Medicine, 352,* 1630–33.

Smith, W. 2003. *The slippery slope from assisted suicide to legalized murder.* New York: Times Books.

Von Stamwitz, A. 2010. "An Ill Father, a Life-or-Death Decision." *New York Times* (Jan. 26), D5.

Codes of Ethics

A

HIPPOCRATIC OATH

I swear by Apollo Physician and Asclepius and Hygieia and Panaceia and all the goddesses, making them my witness, that I will fulfill according to my ability and judgment this oath and this covenant:

To hold him who has taught me this art as equal to my parents and to live my life in partnership with him, and if he is in need of money to give him a share of mine, and to regard his offspring as equal to my brothers in male lineage and to teach them this art—if they desire to learn—without fee and covenant; to give a share of precepts and oral instruction and all other learnings to my sons and to the sons of him who has instructed me and to pupils who have signed the covenant and have taken an oath according to medical law, but to no one else.

I will apply dietetic measures for the benefit of the sick according to my ability and judgment; I will keep them from harm and injustice.

I will neither give a deadly drug to anybody if asked for it, nor will I make a suggestion to that effect. Similarly I will not give to any woman an abortive remedy. In purity and holiness I will guard my life and my art.

I will not use the knife, not even on sufferers from stone, but will withdraw in favor of such men as are engaged in this work.

Whatever houses I may visit, I will come for the benefit of the sick, remaining free of all intentional injustice, of all mischief and in particular of sexual relations with both female and male persons, be they free or slaves.

What I may see or hear in the course of treatment or even outside of the treatment in regard to the life of men, which on no account one must spread abroad, I will keep to myself holding such things shameful to be spoken about.

If I fulfill this oath and do not violate it, may it be granted to me to enjoy life and art, being honored with fame among all men for all time to come; if I transgress and swear falsely, may the opposite of all this be my lot.

Reprinted from *Ancient Medicine: Selected Papers of Ludwig Edelstein,* O. Temkin, and C. Temkin, eds. (Boston, MA: Johns Hopkins University Press, 1967), p. 6.

THE NUREMBERG CODE

1. The voluntary consent of the human subject is absolutely essential. This means that the person involved should have legal capacity to give consent; should be so situated as to be able to exercise free power of choice, without the intervention of any element of force, fraud, deceit, duress, overreaching or other form of constraint or coercion; and should have sufficient knowledge and comprehension of the elements of the subject matter involved as to enable him to make an understanding and enlightened decision. This latter element requires that before the acceptance of an affirmative decision by the experimental subject there should be made known to him the nature, duration and purpose of the experiment; the method and means by which it is to be conducted; all conveniences and hazards reasonable to be expected; and the effects upon his health or person which may possibly come from his participation in the experiment.

   The duty and responsibility for ascertaining the quality of the consent rests upon each individual who initiates, directs, or engages in the experiment. It is a personal duty and responsibility which may not be delegated to another with impunity.

2. The experiment should be such as to yield fruitful results for the good of society, unprocurable by other methods or means of study, and not random and unnecessary in nature.

3. The experiment should be so designed and based on results of animal experimentation and knowledge of the natural history of the disease or other problem under study that the anticipated results will justify the performance of the experiment.

4. The experiment should be so conducted as to avoid all unnecessary physical and mental suffering and injury.

5. No experiment should be conducted where there is *a priori* reason to believe that death or disabling injury will occur; except, perhaps, in those experiments where the experimental physicians also serve as subjects.

6. The degree of risk to be taken should never exceed that determined by the humanitarian importance of the problem to be solved by the experiment.

7. Proper preparations should be made and adequate facilities provided to protect the experimental subject against even remote possibilities of injury, disabilities, or death.

8. The experiment should be conducted only by scientifically qualified persons. The highest degree of skill and care should be required through all stages of the experiment of those who conduct or engage in the experiment.

9. During the course of the experiment the human subject should be at liberty to bring the experiment to an end if he has reached the physical or mental state where continuation of the experiment seems to him to be impossible.

10. During the course of the experiment the scientist in charge must be prepared to terminate the experiment at any stage, if he has probable cause to believe, in the exercise of good faith, superior skill, and careful judgment required of him that a continuation of the experiment is likely to result in injury, disability, or death to the experimental subject.

Reprinted from *The Trials of War Criminals Before the Nuremberg Military Tribunals* (Washington, DC: U.S. Government Printing Office, 1948).

NURSES' CODE OF ETHICS (AMERICAN NURSES ASSOCIATION)

The American Nurses Association (ANA) has developed a code for nurses that discusses the nurses' obligation to protect the patient's privacy, respect the patient's dignity, maintain competence in nursing, and assume responsibility and accountability for individual nursing judgments. This code states the nurses' ethical responsibilities and is summarized here:

1. The nurse provides services with respect for human dignity and the uniqueness of the client, unrestricted by considerations of social or economic status, personal attributes, or the nature of the health problems.
2. The nurse safeguards the client's privacy by judiciously protecting information of a confidential nature.
3. The nurse acts to safeguard the client and the public when healthcare and safety are affected by the incompetent, unethical, or illegal practices of any person.
4. The nurse assumes responsibility and accountability for individual nursing judgments and actions.
5. The nurse maintains competence in nursing.
6. The nurse exercises informed judgment and uses individual competence and qualifications as criteria in seeking consultation, accepting responsibilities, and delegating nursing activities to others.
7. The nurse participates in activities that contribute to the ongoing development of the profession's body of knowledge.
8. The nurse participates in the profession's efforts to implement and improve standards of nursing.
9. The nurse participates in the profession's efforts to establish and maintain conditions of employment conducive to the high quality of nursing care.
10. The nurse participates in the profession's efforts to protect the public from misinformation and misrepresentation and to maintain the integrity of nursing.
11. The nurse collaborates with members of the healthcare profession and other citizens in promoting community and national efforts to meet the health needs of the public.

Reprinted with permission from *Code for Nurses with Interpretative Statements,* copyright 1985 (American Nurses Publishing: American Nurses Foundation/American Nurses Association, Washington, DC).

CODE OF ETHICS OF THE AMERICAN ASSOCIATION OF MEDICAL ASSISTANTS (AAMA)

The AAMA has developed a Code of Ethics for Medical Assistants. The introduction says, "The Code of Ethics of AAMA shall set forth principles of ethical and moral conduct as they relate to the medical profession and the particular practice of medical assisting."

The Code then states:

Members of the AAMA dedicated to the conscientious pursuit of their profession, thus desiring to merit the regard of the entire medical profession and the respect of the general public which they serve, do hereby pledge themselves to strive for:

Human Dignity

I.   Render service with full respect for the dignity of humanity;

Confidentiality

II.   Respect confidential information obtained through employment unless legally authorized or required by responsible performance of duty to divulge such information;

Honor

III.   Uphold the honor and high principles of the profession and accept its disciplines;

Continued Study

IV.   Seek continually to improve the knowledge and skills of medical assistants for the benefit of patients and professional colleagues;

Responsibility for Improved Community

V.   Participate in additional service activities aimed toward improving the health and well-being of the community.

In addition to the Code of Ethics of the AAMA, a creed, or statement of intent, has been developed by this organization. The creed states:

I believe in the principles and purposes of the profession of medical assisting.
I endeavor to be more effective.
I aspire to render greater service.
I protect the confidence entrusted to me.
I am dedicated to the care and well-being of all people.
I am loyal to my employer.
I am true to the ethics of my profession.
I am strengthened by compassion, courage, and faith.

Case Citations

Abernathy v. Sister of St. Mary's, 446 S.W. 2d 599 (Mo. 1969).

Agnew-Watson v. County of Almeda, 36 Cal. Rptr. 2d 196 Ct. App. (Cal. 1994).

Allen v. Mansour, 681 F. Supp. 1232, E.D. (Mich. 1986).

In re Axelrod, 560 N.Y.S.2d 573, App. Div. (1990).

In re Baby M, 537 A.2d 1227 (N.J. 1988).

Barnes Hospital v. Missouri Commission on Human Rights, 661 S.W.2d 534 (Mo.1983).

Benduburg v. Dempsey, 19 F.3d 557,11th Cir. (1994).

Big Town Nursing Home v. Newman, 461 S.W.2d 195 (Texas Civ. App.1970).

Blank v. Palo Alto-Stanford Hosp. Ctr., 44 Cal. Rptr. 572 (Cal. Ct. App. 1965).

Bondu v. Gurvich, 473 So. 2d 1307 (Fla. Dist. Ct. App. 1984).

Bouvia v. Superior Court, 225 Cal. Rptr. 287 (Cal. App. 1986).

Buchanan v. Kull, 35 N.W.2d 351 (Mich.1949).

Buckley v. Hospital Corp. of America, Inc., 758 F.2d 1525, 11th Cir. (1985).

Court v. Commonwealth of Massachusetts, 321 U.S. 158 (1944).

Child Protection Group v. Cline, 350 S.E.2d 541 (W. Va. 1986).

Cline v. Lund, 31 Cal. App. 3d 755 (1973).

Cruzan v. Director, Missouri Dep't of Health, 497 U.S. 261 (1990).

Darling v. Charleston Community Mem. Hosp., 211 N.E. 2d 253 (1965).

Davis v. Davis, 842 S.W.2d 588 (Tenn. 1992).

DeMay v. Roberts, 9 N.W.146 (Mich. 1881).

Doe v. Borough of Barrington, 729 F.Supp. 376 (N.J. 1990).

In re Doe, 533 A2d 523 (R.I. 1987).

Downs v. Sawtelle, 574 F.2d 1, Cir. (1978).

Estate of Berthiaume v. Pratt, 365 QA.2d 792, Me. (1976).

Fair v. St. Joseph's Hosp., 437 S.E.2d 875 (N.C. App. 1933).

Garcia v. Elf Atochem, N. Am., 28 F.3d 446, 5th Cir. (1994).

Goff v. Doctors General Hospital, 333 P.2d 29 (Cal. Ct. App. 1958).

Goforth v. Porter Med. Assoc., Inc., 755 P.2d 678 (Okla. 1988).

Grijalva v. Shalala, 946 F. Supp. 747 (Ariz. 1996).

Griswold v. Connecticut, 381 U.S. 479 (1965).

Grubbs v. Medical Facilities of America, Inc., 879 F. Supp. W.D. (Va. 1995).

Guilmet v. Campbell, 385 Mich. 57, 188 N.W.2d 601 (1971).

Harris v. McRae, U.S. 297 (1980).

Harvet v. Unity Med. Ctr., 428 N.W.2d 574 (Minn. Ct. App. 1988).

Hayes v. Shelby Memorial. Hosp., 726 F.2d 1543, 11th Cir. (1984).

Heller v. Ambach, 433 N.Y.S.2d 281 (1979).

Hickman v. Sexton Dental Clinic, P.A. 367 S.E.2d 453 (S.C. Ct. App. 1988).

H.L. v. Matheson, 450 U.S. 398 (1981).

Hurlock v. Park Lane Med. Ctr. Inc., 709 S.W.2d 872 (Mo. Ct. App. 1985).

James v. Jacobson, 6 F.3d 233, 4th Cir. (1993).

Jeczalik v. Valley Hosp., A.2d 90 (N.J. 1981).

Jenkins v. Bogalusa Comm. Med. Ctr., 340 So.2d 1065 (La. Ct. App.1976).

Kern v. Gulf Coast Nursing Home, Inc., 502 So.2d 1198 (Miss. 1987).

Lambert v. Bessey, 83 Eng. Rep. 220 (1681).

Landeros v. Flood, 551 P.2d 389 (Cal. 1976).

Landau v. Medical Board of California, 71 Cal. Rptr. (Cal. App. 1998).

Love v. Heritage House Convalescent Ctr., 463 N.E.2d 478 (Ind. Ct. App. 1983).

Lovelace Medical Ctr. v. Mendez, 805 P.2d 603 (N.M. 1991).

Maher v. Roe, 432 U.S. 464 (1977).

Mandel v. Doe, 888 F2d. 783 11th Cir. (1989).

McLaughlin v. Cooke, 774 P.2d 1171 (Wash. 1989).

Matter of Baby K; 16F.3d, 590 4th Cir. (1994).

Minn. Stat., §214.18(s), (4).

Mohr v. Williams, 104 N.W.12 (Minn. 1905).

Moon Lake Convalescent Center v. Margolis, 435 N.E.2d 956 (Ill. App. Ct. 1989).

Morena v. South Hills Health System, 462 A.2d 680 (Pa. 1983).

Morrison v. MacNamara, 407 A.2d 555 (D.C. 1979).

Murray v. Vandevander, 522 P.2d 302 (Okla. Ct. App. 1974).

Norton v. Argonaut Ins. Co., 144 So.2d 249 (La. App.1962).

O'Neill v. Montefiore Hosp., 202 N.Y.S2d, 436, App.Div. (1960).

Pardazi v. Cullman Med. Ctr., 838 F.2d 1155, 11th Cir. (1988).

Parrish v. Clark, 145 So. 848 (Fla. 1933).

People v. Gandotra, 14 Cal. Rptr. 2d 896 (11th Cal. App. 1992).

People v. Smithtown Gen. Hosp., 736, 402 N.Y.S.2d 318, Sup. Ct. (1978).

Planned Parenthood of Central Missouri v. Danforth, 428 U.S. 52 (1976).

Planned Parenthood of Southeastern Pennsylvania v. Casey, 50 U.S. 833 (1992).

Polonsky v. Union Hospital, 418 N.E.2d 620 (Mass. App. Ct. 1981).

Poor Sister of St. Francis v. Catron, 435 N.E.2d 305 (Ind. Ct. App. 1982).

Prince v. Commonwealth of Massachusetts, 321 U.S. 158 (1944).

Quinby v. Morrow, 340 F.2d 584, 2d Cir. (1965).

In re Quinlan, 355 A.2d 647 (N.J. 1976).

Rodgers v. St. Mary's Hospital, 556 N.E.2d 913 (Ill. App. Ct. 1990).

Roe v. Wade, 410 U.S.113 (1973).

Rowland v. Christian, 443 P2d. 561 (Cal. 1968).

Rust v. Sullivan, 500 U.S. 173 (1991).

St. John's Reg. Health Ctr. v. American Cas. Co., 980 F.2d 1222, 8th Cir. (1992).

Satler v. Larsen, 520 N.Y.S.2d 378, App. Div. (1987).

In re Schroeder, 415 N.W.2d 436 (Minn. Ct. App. 1987).

Skinner v. Oklahoma, 316 U.S. 535 (1942).

Smith v. Cote, 513 A.2d 341 (N.H. 1986).

Starks v. Director of Div. of Employment Section, 462 N.E.2d 1360 (Mass. 1984).

State v. Fierro, 603 P.2d 74 (Ariz. 1979).

State Dep't. of Human Services v. Northern, 563 S.W.2d 197 (Tenn. Ct. App. 1978).

Swanson v. St. John's Lutheran Hosp., 597 P.2d 702 (Mont. 1979).

Teeters v. Currey, 518 S.W.2d 512 (Tenn.1974).

Thompson v. Brent, 245 So.2d 751 (La. App.1971).

Thor v. Boska, 113 Cal. Rptr. 296, Ct. App. (1974).

Tugg v. Towney, 864 F. Supp. 1201, S.D. (Fla. 1994).

United States v. Busse, Dey, Lupulescu, and Failla, 833 F.2d 1014 (U.S. App. 1987).

United States v. NME Psychiatric Hosps., Inc., No. 94-0268.

Watson v. Idaho Falls Consol. Hosp., Inc., 720 P.2d 632 (Idaho 1986).

Weaver v. Ward, 80 Eng. Rep. 284 (1616).

Williams v. Summit Psychiatric Ctrs., 363 S.E.2d 794 (Ga. App. 1987).

Wis. Stat., §252.15(8).

Winkleman v. Beloit Memorial Hospital, 484 N.W. 2d, 211 (1992).

Woolfolk v. Duncan, 872 F. Supp. 1381, E.D. (Pa. 1995).

Zatarain v. WDSU-Television, Inc., WI 16777 E.D. (La. 1995).

Zucker v. Axelrod, 527 N.Y.S.2d 937 (1988).

Glossary

Note: number in parentheses indicates chapter where key term is found.

Abandonment   withdrawing medical care from a patient without providing sufficient notice to the patient. (5)

Accreditation   a voluntary process in which an agency is requested to officially review healthcare institutions, such as hospitals, nursing homes, and educational institutions, to determine compliance. (3)

Acquired immunodeficiency syndrome (AIDS)   a disease resulting in infections that occur as a result of exposure to the human immunodeficiency virus (HIV), which causes the immune system to break down. (5)

Active euthanasia   actively ending the life of or killing a patient who is terminally ill. (13)

Addiction   an acquired physical or psychological dependence on a drug. (7)

Administrative law   a branch of law that covers regulations set by government agencies. (2)

Advance directive   the various methods by which a patient has the right to self-determination prior to a medical necessity; includes living wills, healthcare proxies, and durable power of attorney. (5)

Affirmative Action program   to remedy discriminating practices in hiring minority group members. Also covered under Title VII. (8)

Affirmative defense   allows the defendant (usually physician or hospital) to present evidence that the patient's condition was the result of factors other than the defendant's negligence. (6)

Against medical advice (AMA)   when a noncompliant patient leaves a hospital without physician's permission. (5)

Age Discrimination in Employment (ADEA)   protects persons forty years or older against employment discrimination because of age. (8)

Agent   person authorized to act on behalf of a patient. (5)

Alleges   to assert or declare without proof. (11)

Alternative dispute resolution (ADR)   methods for resolving a civil dispute that do not involve going to court. (6)

Americans with Disabilities Act (ADA)   prohibits employers who have more than fifteen employees from discriminating against disabled individuals. (8)

Amniocentesis   a test for the presence of genetic defects in which a needle is used to withdraw a small amount of amniotic fluid that surrounds the fetus in the uterus. (12)

Amoral   lacking or indifferent to moral standards. (1)

Anencephalic   missing a brain and spinal cord. (12)

Applied ethics   the practical application of moral standards to the conduct of individuals involved in organizations. (1)

Arbitration   submitting a dispute for resolution to a person other than a judge. (6)

Arbitrator   a person chosen to decide a disagreement between two parties. (6)

Artificial insemination   the injection of seminal fluid that contains male sperm into the female's vagina from her husband, partner, or donor by some means other than sexual intercourse. (12)

Artificial insemination donor (AID)   a procedure in which a donor's sperm is used. (12)

Artificial insemination husband (AIH)   a procedure in which sperm from the woman's husband or partner is used. (12)

Assault   imminent apprehension of bodily harm. (2)

Associate practice   a legal agreement in which physicians agree to share a facility and staff but do not, as a rule, share responsibility for the legal actions of each other. (4)

Assumption of risk   a legal defense that prevents a plaintiff from recovering damages if the plaintiff voluntarily accepts a risk associated with the activity. (6)

Autonomy   independence. (8)

Autopsy   a postmortem examination of organs and tissues to determine the cause of death. (7)

Battery bodily harm and unlawful touching (touching without consent of patient). (2)

Beyond a reasonable doubt evidence that is almost an absolute certainty that a person did commit a crime. (2)

Bias unfair dislike or preference for something. (8)

Bioethicists persons who specialize in the field of bioethics. (1)

Bioethics also called biomedical ethics, the moral dilemmas and issues of advanced medicine and medical research. (1)

Bloodborne pathogens disease-producing micro-organisms transmitted by means of blood and body fluids containing blood. (8)

Bonding a special type of insurance that covers employees who handle financial statements, records, and cash. (3)

Borrowed servant doctrine a special application of *respondeat superior* in which an employer lends an employee to someone else. (6)

Brain death an irreversible coma from which a patient does not recover; results in the cessation of brain activity. (13)

Breach neglect of an understanding between two parties; failing to perform a legal duty. (2)

Breach of contract the failure, without legal excuse, to perform any promise or to carry out any of the terms of an agreement; failure to perform a contractual duty. (2)

Bureau of Narcotics and Dangerous Drugs (BNDD) an agency of the federal government responsible for enforcing laws covering statutes of addictive drugs. (7)

Cap limit. (6)

Capitation rate a fixed monthly fee paid by an HMO to health care providers for providing medical services to patients who are members of that HMO. (4)

Cardiac death death in which the heart has stopped functioning. (13)

Cardiopulmonary pertaining to heart and lung function. (13)

Case law also called common law, case law is based on decisions made by judges. (2)

Censure to find fault with, criticize, or condemn. (11)

Certification a voluntary credentialing process usually offered by a professional organization. (4)

Checks and balances designed by the framers of the Constitution so that no one branch of government would have more power than another and so that each branch of government is scrutinized by other branches of government. (2)

Child Abuse Prevention and Treatment Act prohibited withholding of medical treatment solely because the infant is disabled. (12)

Chromosomes threadlike structures within the nucleus (center) of a cell that transmit genetic information. (11)

Civil law relationships between individuals or between individuals and the government, which are not criminal. (2)

Civil Rights Act permits the court to award both compensatory damages and punitive damages to mistreated employees. (8)

Claims-made insurance liability insurance that covers the insured party for only the claims made during the time period the policy is in effect (or policy year). (6)

Class action lawsuit lawsuit filed by one or more people on behalf of a larger group of people who are all affected by the same situation. (2)

Clearinghouse a private or public healthcare entity that facilitates the processing of non-standard electronic transactions into HIPAA transactions (e.g., a billing service). (10)

Clinical Laboratory Improvement Amendment (CLIA) established minimum quality standards for laboratories. (8)

Clone group of identical matching cells that come from a single common cell. (11)

Closing argument closing speech or summary made by the attorneys for both the plaintiff and the defendant. (2)

Comatose vegetative condition. (13)

Common law also called case law, common law is based on decisions made by judges. (2)

Comparable worth also known as pay equity, the theory that extends equal pay requirements to all persons doing equal work. (1)

Comparative negligence a defense, similar to contributory negligence, that the plaintiff's own negligence helped cause the injury; not a complete bar to recovery of damages but only damages based on the amount of the plaintiff's fault. (6)

Compassion ability to have a gentle, caring attitude toward patients and fellow employees. (1)

Compensatory damages an amount of money awarded by the court to make up for loss of income or emotional pain and suffering. (6)

Competent capable of making a decision without mental confusion due to drugs, alcohol, or other reasons. (2)

Compounding the combination and mixing of drugs and chemicals. (7)

Confidentiality refers to keeping private all information about a person (patient) and not disclosing it to a third party without the patient's written consent. (3)

Conscience clause legislation or regulation stating that hospitals and healthcare professionals are not required to assist with such procedures as abortion and sterilization. (4)

Consent the voluntary agreement that a patient gives to allow a medically trained person the permission to touch, examine, and perform a treatment. (5)

Consideration in contract law, consideration is something of value given as part of the agreement. (2)

Consolidated Omnibus Budget Reconciliation Act (COBRA) offers government financing for health insurance coverage continuation after an employee has been laid off a job. (8)

Constitutional law the inviolable rights, privileges, or immunities secured and protected for each citizen by the Constitution of the United States or by the constitution of each state. (2)

Contraception birth control. (12)

Contract law that division of law that includes enforceable promises and agreements between two or more persons to do or not to do a particular thing. (2)

Contributory negligence conduct on the part of the plaintiff that is a contributing cause of injuries; a complete bar to recovery of damages. (6)

Control group research subjects who receive no treatment. (11)

Controlled Substances Act of 1970 a federal statute that regulates the manufacture and distribution of the drugs that are capable of causing dependency. (7)

Copayment an agreed-upon fee paid by the insured for certain medical services; usually $10 to $20. (4)

Coroner a public health officer who holds an investigation (inquest) if a person's death is from an unknown or violent cause. (7)

Corporation a type of medical practice, as established by law, which is managed by a board of directors. (4)

Cost/benefit analysis also called utilitarianism, an ethical approach in which the benefit of the decision should outweigh the costs. (1)

Covered entities healthcare organizations covered under HIPAA regulations such as public health authorities, healthcare clearinghouses, and self-insured employers, life insurers, information systems vendors, and universities. (10)

Covered transactions certain electronic transactions of healthcare information that are mandated under HIPAA. (10)

Credibility gap an apparent disparity between what is said or written and the actual facts. (9)

Credible believable or worthy of belief. (9)

Creditor person or institution to whom a debt is owed. (8)

Criminal case one in which court action is brought by the government against a person or groups of people accused of committing a crime, resulting in a fine or imprisonment if found guilty. (2)

Criminal laws set up to protect the public from the harmful acts of others. (2)

Curative care attempt is made to cure the patient; the opposite of palliative care. (13)

Damages any injuries caused by the defendant; usually a monetary award is given as compensation. (6)

Data statistics, figures, or information. (7)

Debtors persons who owe money. (8)

Defamation of character making false and/or malicious statements about another person; includes libel and slander. (2)

Defendant person or group of people sued civilly or prosecuted criminally in a court of law. (2)

Defensive medicine ordering more tests and procedures than are necessary in order to protect oneself from a lawsuit. (6)

Deidentifying removing descriptive information about the patient. (10)

Deposition oral testimony that is made before a public officer of the court to be used in a lawsuit. (2)

Dereliction neglect, as in neglect of duty. (6)

Diagnostic related groups (DRGs) designations used to identify reimbursement per condition in a hospital; used for Medicare patients. (4)

Direct cause the continuous sequence of events, unbroken by any intervening cause, that produces an injury and without which the injury would not have occurred. (6)

Disclosed made known. (9)

Discovery the legal process by which facts are discovered before a trial. (2)

Discovery rule legal theory that provides that the statute of limitations begins to run at the time the injury is discovered or when the patient should have known of the injury. (3)

Discrimination unfair or unequal treatment. (8)

Dispensing distribution, delivery, disposing, or giving away a drug, medicine, prescription, or chemical. (7)

Doctrine of professional discretion means that a physician may determine, based on his or her best judgment, if a patient with mental or emotional problems should view the medical record. (9)

Do not resuscitate (DNR) a designation placed on a patient's medical record indicating that in the case of cessation of circulation and breathing, artificial resuscitation (CPR) is not to be done. (5)

Double-blind test a research design in which neither the experimenter nor the patient knows who is getting the research treatment. (11)

Drug Enforcement Administration (DEA) a division of the Department of Justice that enforces the Controlled Substances Act of 1970. (7)

Drug Free Workplace Act employers must certify that they maintain a drug free workplace. (8)

Due process the entitlement of all employees to have certain procedures followed when they believe their rights are in jeopardy. (1)

Durable power of attorney a legal agreement that allows an agent or representative of the patient to act on behalf of the patient. (5)

Duty obligation or responsibility. (6)

Duty-based ethics focuses on performing one's duty to various people and institutions. (1)

Electroencephalogram (EEG) test to measure brain activity. (13)

Electronic Medical Record (EMR) fully computerized method of record-keeping. (9)

Embezzlement the illegal appropriation of property, usually money, by a person entrusted with its possession. (2)

Embryo unborn child between the second and twelfth week after conception. (12)

Emergency Medical Treatment and Active Labor Act (EMTALA) a section of COBRA dealing with patient dumping. (8)

Empathy the ability to understand the feelings of another person without actually experiencing the pain or distress that a person is going through. (1)

Employee Assistance Program (EAP) a management-financed, confidential counseling referral service designed to help employees and/or their family members assess a problem such as alcoholism. (7)

Employee Retirement Income Security Act (ERISA) regulates employee benefits and pension plans. (8)

Employer Identification Number (EIN) a number assigned to an employer for purposes of identification. (10)

Employer Identifier Standard a standard number based on an employer's tax ID number or EIN that is used for all electronic transmissions. (10)

Employment-at-will the employment takes place at either the will of the employer or the employee. (8)

Encryptions scrambling and encoding information before sending it electronically. (9)

Endorsement an approval or sanction. (3)

Equal Credit Opportunity Act prohibits businesses (including hospitals) from denying or granting credit based on race and gender—unfair treatment referred to as discrimination. (8)

Equal Employment Opportunity Act (EEOA) authorizes the EEOC to sue employers in federal court on behalf of people whose rights have been violated under Title VII. (8)

Equal Employment Opportunity Commission (EEOC) the group that monitors Title VII of the Civil Rights Act. (8)

Equal Pay Act makes it illegal for an employer to discriminate on the basis of gender in payment to men and women who are performing the same job. (8)

Ethics the branch of philosophy relating to morals and moral principles. (1)

Ethnocentric a belief that one's cultural background is better than any other. (8)

Eugenic (involuntary) sterilization sterilization of certain categories of persons, such as the insane, in order to prevent them from passing on defective genes to their children. (12)

Eugenics   the science that studies methods for controlling certain characteristics in offspring. (12)

Euthanasia   the administration of a lethal agent by another person to a patient for the purpose of relieving intolerable and incurable suffering. (11)

Exclusive provider organization (EPO)   a type of managed care that combines the concepts of the HMO and PPO. (4)

Expert witness   a medical practitioner or other expert who, through education, training, or experience, has special knowledge about a subject and gives testimony about that subject in court, usually for a fee. (2)

Expired   died. (13)

Expressed contract   an agreement that is entered into orally or in writing. (2)

Expulsion   the act of forcing out. (11)

Fair Credit Reporting Act   establishes guidelines for use of an individual's credit information. (8)

Fair Debt Collection Practices Act   prohibits unfair collection practices by creditors. (8)

Fair Labor Standards Act (FLSA)   establishes the minimum wage, requires payment for overtime work, and sets the maximum hours employees covered by the act may work. (8)

Family and Medical Leave Act (FMLA)   allows both the mother and the father to take a leave of absence for up to twelve weeks, in any twelve month period, when a baby is born. (8)

Feasance   doing an act or performing a duty. (6)

Federal Insurance Contribution Act (FICA)   requires employers to contribute to Social Security for employees. (8)

Federal Rules of Evidence   rules that govern the admissibility of evidence into federal court. (6)

Federal Wage Garnishment Law   restricts the amount of the paycheck that can be used to pay off a debt. (8)

Fee splitting   an agreement to pay a fee to another physician or agency for the referral of patients; this is illegal in some states and is considered to be an unethical medical practice. (4)

Felony   a serious crime that carries a punishment of death or imprisonment for more than one year. Examples are murder, rape, robbery, and practicing medicine without a license. (2)

Fetus   unborn child from the third month after conception until birth. (12)

Fidelity   loyalty and faithfulness to others. (1)

Firewalls   software to prevent unauthorized users. (8)

Fixed-payment plan   a payment plan for medical bills that offers subscribers (members) complete medical care in return for a fixed monthly fee. (4)

Food and Drug Administration (FDA)   an agency within the Department of Health and Human Services that ultimately enforces laws regarding oversees drug sales and distribution. (7)

Forensic medicine   Branch of medicine concerned with the law, especially criminal law. (7)

Franchise   a business run by an individual to whom a franchisor grants the exclusive right to market a product or service in a certain market area. (4)

Franchisee   person or company who holds a franchise. (4)

Fraud   the deliberate concealment of the facts from another person for unlawful or unfair gain. (6)

Fraudulent   deceitful. (2)

Garnishment   court order that requires an employer to pay a portion of an employee's paycheck directly to one of the employee's creditors until the debt is resolved. (8)

Gatekeeper   the person, such as a primary care physician, or entity, such as an insurance company, that approves patient referrals to other physicians or services. (4)

Gene markers   list of genes that are responsible for disease. (11)

Gene therapy   the replacement of a defective or malfunctioning gene by splicing or connecting onto the DNA of body cells to control production of a particular substance. (11)

Gestational period   time before birth during which the fetus is developing, usually nine months. (12)

Good Samaritan laws   state laws that help protect healthcare professionals and ordinary citizens from liability while giving emergency care to accident victims. (3)

Group practice   three or more physicians who share the same facility and practice medicine together. (4)

Guardian ad litem   court-appointed guardian to represent a minor or unborn child in litigation. (3)

Habituation the development of an emotional dependence on a drug due to repeated use. (7)

Harvested removed organs or embryos. (11,12)

Health Care Quality Improvement Act provides for peer review of physicians by other physicians and healthcare professionals. (4)

Health Insurance Portability and Accountability Act of 1996 (HIPAA) regulates the privacy of patients' health information. (10)

Health Maintenance Organization (HMO) a type of managed care plan that offers a range of health services to plan members for a predetermined fee per member by a limited group of providers. (4)

Healthcare Integrity and Protection Data Bank (HIPDB) a national data bank that collects and reports disclosures of actions taken against healthcare practitioners, providers, and vendors for noncompliance and fraudulent activities. (10)

Healthcare plan an individual or group plan that provides or pays for medical care. (10)

HIPAA-defined permissions permission to use information based on the reason for knowing, or use of, the information. (10)

Hospice a multi-disciplinary, family-centered care designed to provide care and supportive services to terminally ill patients and their families. (13)

Human genome the complete set of genes within the 23 pairs of human chromosomes. (11)

Human Genome Project a research program funded by the federal government to "map" and sequence the total number of genes within the 23 pairs, or 46 chromosomes. (11)

Human immunodeficiency virus (HIV) the virus that causes the immune system to break down and can eventually result in the disease AIDS. (5)

Hypothermia state in which body temperature is below normal range. (13)

Implied consent an agreement that is made through inference by signs, inaction, or silence. (5)

Implied contract an agreement that is made through inference by signs, inaction, or silence. (2)

Incident report a means of documenting problem events within a hospital or other medical facility. (3)

Indictment a written charge presented to the court by the grand jury against a defendant. (2)

Indigent a person who is impoverished and without funds. (1,4)

Induced abortion an abortion caused by artificial means such as medications or surgical procedures. (12)

Informed (or expressed) consent consent granted by a person after the patient has received knowledge and understanding of potential risks and benefits. (5)

In loco parentis a person assigned by a court to stand in place of the parents and who possesses their legal rights and responsibilities toward the child. (5)

Inquest an investigation held by a public official, such as a coroner, to determine the cause of death. (7)

Institutional Review Board (IRB) a hospital or university board of members who oversee any human research in that facility. (11)

Integrity the unwavering adherence to one's principles; dedication to maintaining high standards. (1)

Intentional torts occur when a person has been intentionally or deliberately injured by another. (2)

In-vitro fertilization the process of combining ovum and sperm outside of a woman's body. (12)

Joint Commission on Accreditation of Healthcare Organizations (JCAHO) an agency that oversees hospital accreditation standards. (39)

Jurisdiction the power to hear a case. (2)

Just cause legal reason. (8)

Justice-based ethics based on the moral restraint of "the veil of ignorance." (1)

Law of agency the legal relationship formed between two people when one person agrees to perform work for another person. (6)

Laws rules or actions prescribed by a governmental authority that have a binding legal force. (1,4)

Liable legal responsibility for one's own actions. (6)

Libel any publication in print, writing, pictures, or signs that injures the reputation of another person. (2)

Licensure a mandatory credentialing process that allows an individual to perform certain skills. (4)

Life-support systems systems such as ventilators/respirators and feeding tubes, that allow medical practitioners to sustain a patient's life. (13)

Litigation   a dispute that has resulted in one party suing another. (2)

Litigious   excessively inclined to sue. (1)

Living will   a legal document in which a person states that life-sustaining treatments and nutritional support should not be used to prolong life; a type of advance directive. (5)

Malfeasance   performing an illegal act. (6)

Malpractice   professional misconduct or demonstration of an unreasonable lack of skill with the result of injury, loss, or damage to the patient. (6)

Managed care organization (MCO)   a type of medical plan that pays for and manages the medical care a patient receives. (4)

Material Safety Data Sheet (MSDS)   an information sheet which provides specific information on handling and disposing of chemicals safely. (7)

Mediation   using the opinion of a third party to resolve a civil dispute in a nonbinding decision. (6)

Medicaid   federal program, implemented by the individual states, to provide financial assistance for the indigent. (4)

Medical ethics   moral conduct based on principles regulating the behavior of healthcare professionals. (1)

Medical etiquette   standards of professional behavior that physicians use for conduct with other physicians. (1)

Medical informatics   the application of communication and information to medical practice, research, and education. (10)

Medical practice acts   laws established in all fifty states that define the practice of medicine as well as requirements and methods for licensure in a particular state. (1)

Medical record   all the written and computer-generated documentation relating to a patient. (9)

Medicare   federal program that provides healthcare coverage for persons over 65 years of age as well as for disabled persons or those who suffer kidney disease or other debilitating ailments. (4)

Mercy killing   another term for voluntary euthanasia. (13)

Microfiche   miniaturized photographs of records. (9)

Minimum necessary standard   means that the provider must make a reasonable effort to limit the disclosure of patient information to only the minimum amount that is necessary to accomplish the purpose of the request. (10)

Minor   a person who has not reached the age of maturity, which in most states is 18. (5)

Misdemeanors   less serious offenses than felonies; punishable by fines or imprisonment of up to one year. These include traffic violations and disturbing the peace. (2)

Misfeasance   the improper performance of an otherwise proper or lawful act. (6)

Morality   the quality of being virtuous or practicing the right conduct. (1)

Morbidity rate   the rate of sick people or cases of disease in relationship to a specific population. (7)

Mortality rate   death rate. (7)

National Labor Relations Act   prohibits employer actions, such as attempting to force employees to stay out of unions, and labels these actions as "unfair labor practices." (8)

National Organ Transplant Law of 1984   federal law that forbids the sale of organs in interstate commerce. (11)

National Practitioners Data Bank (NPDB)   a listing of names that assists with peer review of physicians. (4)

Negligence   an unintentional action that occurs when a person either performs or fails to perform an action that a "reasonable person" would or would not have committed in a similar situation. (6)

Nominal damages   a slight or token payment awarded by the court. (6)

Nonfeasance   the failure to perform an action when it is necessary. (6)

Nontherapeutic research   research conducted that will not directly benefit the research subject. (11)

Notice of Privacy Practices (NPP)   a written statement that details the provider's privacy practices. (10)

Occupational Safety and Health Act (OSHA)   requires an employer to provide a safe and healthy work environment; the employer must protect the worker against hazards. (8)

Occurrence insurance   also called claims-incurred insurance, liability insurance that covers the insured party for all injuries and incidents that occurred while the policy was in effect (policy year), regardless of when they are reported to the insurer or when the claim is made. (6)

Office of Civil Rights (OCR) the federal office that investigates violations of HIPAA. (10)

Open-record laws state freedom of information laws that grant public access to records maintained by state agencies. (9)

Palliative care care for terminally ill patients consisting of comfort measures and symptom control. (13)

Parens patriae authority occurs when the state takes responsibility from the parents for the care and custody of minors under the age of 18. (5)

Parenteral medication route other than the alimentary canal (oral and rectal) including subcutaneous, intravenous, and intramuscular routes. (8)

Partnership a legal agreement in which two or more physicians share the business operation of a medical practice and become responsible for the actions of the other partners. (4)

Passive euthanasia allowing a patient to die by forgoing treatment. (13)

Patient dumping a slang term for transferring patients from one hospital to another if the patient is unable to pay for services. (8)

Per diem daily rate (4)

Permission HIPAA defined areas in which permission must be granted in order to use or disclose patient health information (PHI). (10)

Persistent vegetative state (PVS) an irreversible brain condition in which the patient is in a state of deep unconsciousness. (13)

Placebo group research in which an inactive or alternative type of treatment is given. (11)

Plaintiff a person or group of people suing another person or group of people; the person who instigates the lawsuit.(2)

Pleadings formal written statements. (2)

Posthumous after death. (11)

Postmortem after death. (7)

Precedent a ruling of an earlier case that is then applied to subsequent cases. (1)

Preempt overrule. (8)

Preferred Provider Organization (PPO) a managed care concept in which the patient must use a medical provider who is under contract with the insurer for an agreed-upon fee in order to receive copayment from the insurer. (4)

Pregnancy Discrimination Act employers must treat pregnant women as they would any other employee, providing they can still do the job. (8)

Preimplantation genetic diagnosis (PGD) genetic testing on embryos for genes that cause untreatable or severe diseases. (12)

Preponderence of evidence evidence showing that more likely than not the incident occurred. (2)

Primary care physician (PCP) HMO-designated physician to manage and control an enrolled patient's medical care. (4)

Principle of autonomy right to make decisions about one's own life. (1)

Principle of beneficence action of helping others and performing actions that result in benefit to another person. (1)

Principle of double-effect when an action can have two effects: one that is morally good or desirable and one that is not. (13)

Principle of justice warns us that equals must be treated equally. (1)

Principle of nonmalfeasance means "First, do no harm." (1)

Privacy Rule a requirement that all covered entities under HIPAA must be in compliance with the privacy, security, and electronic-data provisions by April 14, 2003. (10)

Privileged communication confidential information that has been told to a physician (or attorney) by the patient. (5,9)

Probable cause a reasonable belief that something improper has occurred. (7)

Prognosis prediction for the course of a disease. (5)

Prosecutor a person who brings a criminal lawsuit on behalf of the government. (2)

Prospective payment system the payment amount or reimbursement with a set rate for certain procedures is known in advance. (4)

Protected Health Information (PHI) any individually identifiable information that relates to the physical or mental condition or the provision of healthcare to an individual. (10)

Proximate the injury was closely (proximately) related to the defendant's negligence. (6)

Proxy a person who acts on behalf of another person. (5)

Prudent person rule also called the responsible person standard, means the healthcare professional must provide the information that a prudent, reasonable person would want before making a decision about treatment or refusal of treatment. (3)

Public duties responsibilities the physician owes to the public. (7)

Public Health Services Act protects patients who are receiving treatment for drug and alcohol abuse. (9)

Punitive damages also called exemplary damages, monetary award by a court to a person who has been harmed in an especially malicious and willful way; meant to punish the offender. (6)

Quality assurance gathering and evaluating information about the services provided as well as the results achieved and comparing this information with an accepted standard. (1)

Quality of life the physiological status, emotional well-being, functional status, and life in general of the individual. (13)

Reciprocity the cooperation of one state in granting a license to practice medicine to a physician already licensed in another state. Reciprocity can be applied to other licensed professionals such as nurses and pharmacists. (3)

Registration indicates that the person whose name is listed on an official record or register has met certain requirements in that particular profession. (4)

Regulations rules or laws made by agencies. (2)

Rehabilitation Act prohibits employers from discriminating against the handicapped. (8)

Res ipsa loquitur Latin phrase meaning "the thing speaks for itself." (6)

Res judicata Latin phrase meaning "the thing has been decided." (6)

Respite care providing the family with relief from the responsibilities of patient care. (13)

Respondeat superior Latin phrase meaning "let the master answer"; means the employer is responsible for the actions of the employee. (3)

Restraining or protective order court order that prohibits an abuser from coming into contact with the victim. (7)

Retailing the legal act of selling or trading a drug, medicine, prescription, or chemical. (7)

Revocation the act of taking away or recalling, such as taking away a license to practice medicine. (11)

Revoke take away, as in revoke a license. (3)

Rider additional component to an insurance policy. (6)

Rights-based ethics a natural rights ethical theory that places the primary emphasis on a person's individual rights. (1)

Rigor mortis stiffness that occurs in a dead body. (13)

Risk management a practice to minimize the incidence of problem behavior that might result in injury to the patient and liability for the organization. (3)

Safe Haven Laws are safe alternatives to leaving babies in unsafe places when a parent voluntarily gives up custody. (12).

Sanctions penalties or fines. (10)

Sanctity of life sacredness of human life; all human beings must be protected. (1)

Scope of practice the activities a healthcare professional is allowed to perform as indicated in their licensure, certification, and/or training. (3)

Settlement the act of determining the outcome of a case outside a courtroom; settling a case is not an indication of legal wrongdoing. (6)

Sexual harassment unwelcome sexual advances or requests for sexual favors. (1)

Slander speaking false and malicious words concerning another person that brings injury to his or her reputation. (2)

Social Security Act federal law that covers all private and most public sector employees. (8)

Social utility method of allocation a method of determining the allocation of organs by giving them to people who will benefit the most. (11)

Sole proprietorship a type of medical practice in which one physician may employ other physicians. (4)

Solo practice a medical practice in which the physician works alone. (4)

Spontaneous abortion termination of pregnancy that occurs naturally before the fetus is viable. (12)

Standard of care the ordinary skill and care that medical practitioners use and that is commonly used by other medical practitioners in the same locality when caring for patients; what another medical professional would consider appropriate care in similar circumstances. (3)

Stare decisis   Latin phrase meaning "let the decision stand." (2)

State's preemption   when the state privacy laws are stricter than the privacy standards established by HIPAA. (10)

Statute of limitations   the period of time that a patient has to file a lawsuit. (3)

Statutes   laws enacted by state and federal legislatures. (2)

Stem cells   master cells in the body that can generate specialized cells. (11)

Stereotyping   negative generalities concerning specific characteristics about a group are applied to an entire population. (8)

Sterilization   the process of medically altering reproductive organs so as to terminate the ability to produce offspring. (12)

Subpoena   court order for a person or documents to appear in court. (2)

Subpoena *duces tecum*   Latin phrase meaning, "under penalty take with you"; a court order requiring a person to appear in court and to bring certain records or other material to a trial or a deposition. (2)

Subpoenaed   ordered by the court. (9)

Substitute judgment rule   used when decisions must be made for a person who cannot make his or her wishes known. (13)

Summary judgment   judge's ruling to end a lawsuit without a trial based on a matter of law presented in pleadings. (2)

Surrogate mother   a woman who agrees to bear a child for another couple. The husband's sperm is implanted into the woman's uterus. (12)

Sympathy   pity for someone else. (1)

Telemedicine   the use of communications and information technologies to provide healthcare services to people at a distance. (10)

Terminally ill   one whose death is determined to be inevitable. (13)

Therapeutic research   a form of medical research that might directly benefit the research subject. (11)

Therapeutic sterilization   sterilization undertaken to save the mother's life or protect her health. (12)

Third-party payers   a party other than the patient who assumes responsibility for paying the patient's bills (for example, an insurance company). (4)

Timeliness of documentation   all entries into a medical record should be made as soon as they occur or as soon as possible afterward. (9)

Title VII of the Civil Rights Act   prohibits discrimination in employment based on five criteria: race, color, religion, gender, or national origin. (8)

Tolerance   a respect for those whose opinions, practices, race, religion, and nationality differ from our own. (1)

Tolling   also known as running of the Statute of Limitations, means the time has expired. (3)

Tort   a civil injury, or wrongful act, committed against another person or property that results in harm and is compensated in money damages. (2)

Tort law   that division of law that covers acts that result in harm to another; covers wrongful acts. (2)

Treatment, payment, and healthcare operations (TPO)   functions that a healthcare provider can perform. (10)

Truth in Lending Act (Regulation Z)   requires a full written disclosure about interest rates or finance charges concerning the payment of any fee that will be collected in more than four installments. (8)

Unborn Victims of Violence Act   law that provides legal penalties for any harm done to an unborn child at federal facilities such as military bases or in crimes that cross state lines. (12)

Unemployment Compensation   provides for temporary weekly payments for the unemployed worker. (8)

Uniform Anatomical Gift Act   a state statute allowing persons 18 years of age and of sound mind to make a gift of any or all body parts for purposes of organ transplantation or medical research. (5)

Unintentional torts   such as negligence, occur when the patient is injured as a result of the healthcare professional's not exercising the ordinary standard of care. (2)

United Network for Organ Sharing (UNOS)   the legal entity in the United States responsible for allocating organs for transplantation. (11)

Utilitarianism   an ethical theory based on the principle of the greatest good for the greatest number. (1)

Vesting   a point in time, such as after ten years of employment, when an employee has the right to receive benefits from a retirement plan. (8)

Viable   in the case of a fetus, ability to survive outside the uterus. (12)

Viatical settlements   allows people with terminal illnesses, such as AIDS, to obtain money from their life insurance policies by selling them. (13)

Virtue-based ethics   a character trait based on a concern for the person. (1)

Vital statistics   major events or facts from a person's life, such as live births, deaths, induced termination of pregnancy, and marriages. (7)

Waive   give up a right. (2)

Wireless Local Area Networks (WLANs)   a wireless system that is used by physicians and nurses to access patient information. (10)

Withdrawing life-sustaining treatment   discontinuing a treatment or procedure, such as artificial ventilation, after it has started. (13)

Withholding life-sustaining treatment   failing to start a treatment or procedure such as artificial ventilation. (13)

Worker's Compensation Act   protects workers and their families from financial problems resulting from employment related injury, disease, and death. (8)

Wrongful discharge   when an employee believes that the employer does not have a just-cause, or legal reason, for firing the employee. (8)

Index

Numbers in *italics* indicate figures; those with a *t* indicate tables.

A

Abandonment of patients, 105
Abernathy v. Sisters of St. Mary's, 143
AbioCor, 339
Abortion, 302–9
  Baby Doe regulations, 307–8
  Baby K case, 308
  Conscience Clause in, 308–9
  employee's right to refuse participation in, 306
  ethical issues concerning, 274–75, 307, 307*t*
  funding for, 306–7
  historical progression of cases, 304
  incompetent persons and, 305
  induced, 303
  mandatory parental consent to, 268*t*
  Medicaid and, 305, 306
  opposition to, 306
  partial birth, 305
  Plan B contraceptive pill and, 305–6
  Roe v. Wade, 303, 304
  spontaneous, 303
Abuse
  child, 170–71
  elder, 171–72
  gathering evidence in cases of, 173–74
  Safe Haven Laws and, 314
  signs of, 172–73, 172*t*
  spousal, 172
  substance, 173
Accreditation, 60–61
Accrediting Bureau of Health Education Schools
  (ABHES), 90
Acquired immune deficiency syndrome
  (AIDS), 179
  Americans with Disabilities Act and, 198
  blood exposure to, 108
  duty to report, 169
  duty to treat, 107–9
  ethical considerations and, 107
  HIV-infected employees and, 108–9
  improper disclosure and, 233
  on-the-job protection for healthcare workers, 109
  privacy and, 242–43
  viatical settlements for, 337
Active euthanasia, 328
Addiction, 175
Administrative law, 43–44
Adolescent medicine, 87*t*
Advance directives, 337–38. *See also* Self-determi-
  nation acts (advance directives)
Affirmative action programs, 196
Affirmative defense, 143
Against medical advice (AMA), 106

Age Discrimination in Employment Act (ADEA),
  197–98
Agent, 114
Agnew-Watson v. County of Alameda, 206
AID. *See* Artificial insemination donor (AID)
AIDS. *See* Acquired immune deficiency syndrome (AIDS)
AIDS-related complex (ARC), 169
AIH. *See* Artificial insemination husband (AIH)
Alabama
  state court system case, 45
  Tuskegee syphilis research study in, 264
Alcohol abuse patients, medical records and, 229
Alleges, 266
Allen v. Mansour, 273
Allergy and immunology, 87*t*
Allied health professionals, 89–93
  code of ethics, 267–269
  conscience clause and, 93
  healthcare professions, 90–91
  licensure and certification, 89
  practicing without license, 60
Allocation
  of organs, 272–74
  social utility method of, 272
Alterations, to medical records, 222–24
Altered medical records, 147–48
Alternative dispute resolution (ADR), 150–51
Alzheimer's disease
  duty to tell truth and, 110
  euthanasia and, 328
  gene markers for, 279
  genetic testing and, 312
  patient identification and, 110
AMA. *See* Against medical advice (AMA); American
  Medical Association (AMA)
American Academy of Neurology, 327
American Academy of Orthopedic Surgeons, 108, 125
American Association of Medical Assistants (AAMA), 89
  code of ethics, 269, 347–48
American Bar Association, 327
American Board of Allergy and Immunology, 86
American Board of Anesthesiology, 86
American Board of Emergency Medicine, 86
American Board of Internal Medicine, 86
American Board of Medical Specialists, 86
American Board of Pediatrics, 87
American Board of Surgery, 86
American Board of Urology, 86
American Civil Liberties Union (ACLU), 331
American College of Physicians, 88
American College of Surgeons, 88
American Dietetic Association, 269
American Health Information Management Association
  (AHIMA), 230, 269

American Hospital Association (AHA), 112, 113
American Medical Association (AMA), 12,
    265, 275
  abortion and, 303
  direct killing, opposition to, 332
  HIV-infected healthcare workers and, 108
  judicial council opinions of, 267, 268t
  Principles of Medical Ethics and, 103t, 267
  Uniform Determination of Death Act and, 327
American Medical Technologists (AMT) association, 89
American Nurses Association (ANA), 269, 275
  code of ethics, 347
American Society for Medical Technology, 269
American Society of Radiologic Technologists, 269
Americans with Disabilities Act (ADA) of 1990, 107,
    198–99, 253
Amniocentesis, 310
Amorality, 9
AMT Institute for Education (AMTIE), 89
Amyotrophic lateral sclerosis (ALS), case of, 100
Analysis, cost/benefit, 10
Anencephaly, 308
Anesthesiology, 87t
Angiogram, case of, 322
Appellate court system, 50
Applied ethics, 3
Arbitration, 150
Arbitrator, 150
Arizona, life-support case in, 327
Arkansas, Plan "B" contraceptive pill and, 305–6
Armstrong v. Flowers Hosp., 197
Arthritis Measurement Scale (AIMS), 334
Artificial conception, 294–98
  artificial insemination, 294–95
  ethical considerations in, 295
  fertility drugs, 298
  in-vitro fertilization, 295–96
  legal status of offspring, 295
  selective reduction or harvesting embryos, 298
  surrogate motherhood, 296–97
Artificial insemination (AI), 294–95
Artificial insemination donor (AID), 294
  consent for, 294
  legal status of offspring and, 295
Artificial insemination husband (AIH), 294
Assault, 37
Assisted conception. See Artificial conception
Assisted suicide, argument of, 329–32
Associate practice, 84
Assumption of risk, 143–44
Autonomy, 189
  principle of, 21
Autopsy, 168

B

Baby Doe regulations, 307–8
Baby K case, 308
Baby M case, 296–97
Bankruptcy, 209
Barnes Hospital v. Missouri Commission on Human
    Rights, 151
Battered child syndrome, 170
Battery, 37
Bedside charting, 232
Behavior ethics, 266. See also Ethics
  principles (values) and, 12–15
Bench trial, 36
Bendiburg v. Dempsey, 146

Beneficence
  defined, 13
  principle of, 21
Benefits regulations. See Compensation and benefits
    (federal regulations)
Beyond a reasonable doubt, 42
Bias, 189
Big Town Nursing Home v. Newman, 38
Bioethical issues, 269–74
  organ and tissue donation, 271
  transplant rationing, 272–74
Bioethicists, 22
Bioethics (biomedical ethics), 3, 21–22, 265, 270t
  reasons to study, 3–7
Biomedical research, ethics of, 275–78
  conflicts of interest, 277–78
  consent in, 275–76
  debate over treatment and, 276–77
  double-blind tests, 278
  randomized test trials, 278
  researcher and, 275
Birth and life issues. See also specific issues
  abortion and, 302–9
  assisted (artificial) contraception, 294–98
  choices in, 338–39
  conscience clause and, 308–9
  contraception and, 299
  fetal development and, 293–94
  genetic engineering and, 279–82
  genetics and, 309–12
  Human Genome Project and, 278–79
  sterilization and, 299–302
  wrongful-life suits, 312–14
Birth certificates, 165–66
Birth control, ethical issues surrounding, 302
Blank v. Palo Alto-Stanford Ctr., 86
Bloodborne pathogens, 200
Blue Cross and Blue Shield, 140
BNDD. See Bureau of Narcotics and Dangerous Drugs
    (BNDD)
Bondu v. Gurvich, 230
Bonding, 67
Borrowed servant doctrine, 144–45
Bouvia v. Superior Court, 328
Brain death, 326
Brain-oriented death, 325–27
Brandeis, Louis, 242
Breach
  of contract, 40, 41
  defined, 40
Brinson v. Axelrod, 172
Buckley v. Hospital Corp. of America, Inc., 198
Burden of proof, 47
Bureau of Narcotics and Dangerous Drugs (BNDD), 175
Bush, George W., 281
Bush, Jeb, 332

C

CAAHEP. See Commission on Accreditation of Allied
    Health Education Programs (CAAHEP)
California
  artificial insemination case in, 308
  completeness of medical records, case, 225
  liability case in, 151
  reporting laws in, 169
  stem cell research and, 270
  withdrawing life-sustaining treatment, case, 328
  workers' compensation case in, 206

Canterbury v. Spence, 122
Cap, 138
Capitation rate, 78
Cardiac death, 325
Cardiology, 87*t*
Cardiopulmonary, 323, 325
Cardiopulmonary resuscitation (CPR), 19, 37, 64,
    106, 114, 118, 135, 152, 337, 338
Cardiovascular surgery, 88*t*
Cardoza, Benjamin, 330
Carson, Benjamin, 339
Case law. *See* Common law
Catholicism
    birth control and, 299
    brain death and, 327
    direct killing, opposition to, 332
    euthanasia and, 328
    Plan "B" contraceptive pill and, 305
Censure, 266
Centers for Disease Control and Prevention (CDC),
    165, 264
    HIV-infected healthcare workers and, 109
Certification, for allied health professionals, 89
Certified medical assistant (CMA), 90*t*, 223
Certified medical transcriptionist (CMT), 90*t*
Chain of custody, for abuse, 174
Charitable organizations, immunity for, 143
Charting
    bedside, *232*
    guidelines for, 222*t*
    notations, *223*
Checks and balances, 31
Chemical waste, 179
Child abuse, 170–71
    reporting, 171
Child Abuse Prevention and Treatment Act of 1974, 170
Child Abuse Prevention and Treatment Act of 1987, 307
Child Protection Group v. Cline, 229
Chromosomes, 279
Circuit courts. *See* Court of appeals
Civil liability cases, 145–46
Civil (private) law, 36–42
    class action lawsuit, 41–42
    contract law, 39–41
    defined, 36
    tort law, 36–39
Civil (public) law, components of, 42
Civil Rights Act of 1964, 191
    Title VII of, 17, 195–96
Civil Rights Act of 1991, 196–97
Civil trial, procedure for, 48
Claims, against estates, 210
Claims-made insurance, 149
Class action lawsuit, 41–42
Clearinghouse, 246
Cline v. Lund, 67
Clinical Laboratory Improvement Act (CLIA) of 1988,
    202
    requirements, 201*t*
Clinton, Bill, 279
Cloning, 279–80
Closing arguments, 47–48
Codes of ethics, 345–48
    American Medical Association, 103*t*
Collection agency, using, 208
Colorectal surgery, 88*t*
Comatose state, 323, 331
Commission on Accreditation of Allied Health
    Education Programs (CAAHEP), 61, 90

Committees, ethics, 22
Common law, 35
Communicable diseases, reporting cases of, 168–69
Communication, malpractice prevention and, 156
Comparable worth, 17
Comparative negligence, 144
Compassion, 15
Compensation and benefits (federal regulations),
    203–6, 204*t*
    Employee Retirement Income Security Act, 206
    Equal Pay Act, 204
    Fair Labor Standards Act, 204
    Family and Medical Leave Act, 206
    Federal Insurance Contribution Act, 205
    Social Security Act, 203
    unemployment compensation, 205
    Workers' Compensation Act, 205–6
Compensatory damages, 138
Competency, 40
Compounding, 176
Comprehensive Omnibus Budget Reconciliation Act
    (COBRA), 104, 205
Conception, wrongful, 313
Confidentiality, 268*t*. *See also* Health Insurance
    Portability and Accountability Act (HIPAA)
    in AAMA code of ethics, 348
    AIDS and, 169, 242–43
    case of, 240
    defined, 16
    duty to respect, 110
    legal obligations, 231
    maintaining, 227*t*
    medical records and, 226–29
    patient, 239–62
    patient rights and, 62–63, 112–13
    right to privacy, 242
Conflicts of interest, 277–78
Conjoined twins, 339
Connecticut
    contraception, ban in, 299
    emergency room and, 313
Conscience Clause, 93
Consent, 119–24
    for artificial insemination donor, 294
    biomedical research and, 275–76
    exceptions to, 124
    under HIPAA, 246
    implied, 123–24
    informed, 120–23, 278
    refusal to grant, 124
    for sterilization, 300
Consideration, 40
Consolidated Omnibus Budget Reconciliation Act
    (COBRA), 203, 207
Constitutional law, 33
Consumer Protection Act, 207
Consumer protection and collection practices, 206–10,
    207*t*
    claims against estates, 210
    Emergency Medical Treatment and Active Labor Act,
    207
    Equal Credit Opportunity Act, 207
    Fair Credit Reporting Act, 207
    Fair Debt Collection Practices Act, 208–9
    Federal Wage Garnishment Law, 209
    guidelines for collection, 209*t*
    statute of limitations, 210
    Truth in Lending Act, 207–8
Continuing education (CE), 89

Contraception, 299
  Conscience Clause in, 308–9
Contract law, 36, 40–41
Contracts
  breach of, 40, 41
  expressed, 40
  implied, 41
  termination of, 41
  types of, 40–41
Contributory negligence, 144
Control group, 264, 275
Controlled substances, 174–77
  Controlled Substances Act of 1970, 175
  prescriptions of, 175–77
  schedule for, 176*t*
Controlled Substances Act of 1970, 175, 176
Cooley's anemia, 310*t*
Copayment, 79
Coroner, 167, 167*t*
Corporation, 85
  professional, 85
Corrections, to medical records, 222–24
Cosmetic/plastic surgery, 88*t*
Cost/benefit analysis, 10
Council on Ethical and Judicial Affairs (AMA),
    267, 268*t*
Court, use of medical records in, 233–34
  improper disclosure, 233
  subpoena *duces tecum*, 233–34
Court of appeals, 45
Court system, 44–45
  appellate, 50
  federal, 45
  state, 45
  structure of federal, 33
  testifying in, 49
  types of courts, 45
Covered entities, 246, 247*t*
Covered transactions, 247
Creative care, 337
Credibility, of medical records, 225
  defined, 225
Credibility gap, 225
Creditor, 209
Criminal case, 42
Criminal (public) law, 42–43
Cruzan, Nancy, 330–31
Cruzan v. Director, Missouri Dept of Health, 331
Cultural issues, 189–90
Cystic fibrosis, 298, 310*t*

D

Damages, 138–39
  compensatory, 138
  nominal, 139
  punitive, 139
Darling v. Charleston Community Memorial Hospital,
    65, 66
Data, 165
Davis v. Davis, 296
DEA. *See* Drug Enforcement Administration (DEA)
Death and dying, 321–44
  active *versus* passive euthanasia, 328–29
  advance directives, 337–38
  assisted suicide, argument of, 329–32
  brain-oriented death, 325–27
  cardiac death, 325
  choices in, 338–39

conjoined twins, 339
criteria for death, 324–25
death certificates, 166–68
direct *versus* indirect killing, 332
hospice care, 335–36
legal definition of death, 323–33
mechanical heart recipient, 339
medications, use of, 334–35
ordinary *versus* extraordinary means, 332–33
palliative care, 336–37
process of, 323
quality-of-life issues, 334
Quinlan, Karen Ann, case, 323–24
right to die legislation, 333
right to refuse treatment, 333
stages of dying, 333, 333*t*
suicide, 338–39
Uniform Determination of Death Act, 327
viatical settlements, 337
withdrawing *versus* withholding treatment, 327–28
Debtors, 209
Defamation of character, 37, 38
Defendant, 35, 46
Defensive medicine, 7
  defined, 149
  practicing, 149–50
Deidentifying, 248
DeMay v. Roberts, 112
Denial defense, 143
Dental assistant, 91*t*, 151
Dental hygienist, 91*t*
Deontological theory, 10
Department of Children and Families (DCF), 314
Department of Clinical Bioethics, 277
Department of Health and Human Services, 44, 79,
    141, 177, 254, 275
Deposition, 47
Dereliction of duty, 136–37
Dermatology, 87*t*
Diagnostic related groups (DRG), 80
Die with Dignity Act (Washington), 328
Dilation and evacuation (D&E), 305
Direct cause, 137–38
Direct killing, indirect *versus*, 332
Disclosure, 229
  improper, 233
  permitted incidental, 250, 250*t*
  requirements, medical records and, 232
Discovery rule, 63
Discrimination
  employment, 194–99, 195*t*
  Title VII of the Civil Rights Act and, 195
  in workplace, 188
Disease leg, case of, 30
Dispensing, 176
District court, 45
Doctrine of professional discretion, 226
Documentation
  malpractice prevention and, 156–57
  timeliness of, 224
Doe v. Borough of Barrington, 107
Dolly (cloned sheep), 279–80
Donor siblings, conceiving, 311
Do not resuscitate (DNR), 114, 338
Double-blind test, problems with, 278
Double-effect, principle of, 332
Douglas, William O., 299
Downs v. Sawtelle, 301
Down syndrome, 310, 310*t*, 313

Drug abuse patients, medical records and, 229
Drug Enforcement Administration (DEA), 175
Drug-Free Workplace Act of 1988, 203
Drugs
  controlled, 175
  fertility, 298
  illegal sale of, 146–47
Duchenne's muscular dystrophy, 310*t*, 311
Duenwald, Jay, 281
Due process, 16–17
Durable power of attorney, 114, 114*t*, *116–17*, 118
Duty
  defined, 136, 136*t*
  dereliction of, 136–37
  negligence and, 136
Duty-based ethics, 11, 13

E

EIN. *See* Employer Identification Number (EIN)
Elder abuse, 171–72
Electrocardiograph technologist, 91*t*
Electroencephalogram (EEG), 323, 326
Electronic medical records (EMR), 231
Emanuel, Ezekiel, 277
Embezzlement, 38, 67
Embryo, 281, 293, *293*
  harvesting, 298
Emergencies (medical)
  consent and, 122
  duties during, 104
Emergency medical technicians (EMT/paramedic), 64,
  91*t*, *92*, 106, 153, 255
Emergency Medical Treatment and Active Labor Act
  (EMTALA), 104–5, 203, 207, 308
Emergency medicine, 87*t*
Emergency room (ER), 313
Emotional issues, 20–21
Empathy, 15, 16
Employee Assistance Program (EAP), 177–78
  warning signs for, 178*t*
Employee health and safety (federal regulations)
  Clinical Laboratory Improvement Act, 202
  Consolidated Omnibus Budget Reconciliation
    Act, 203
  Drug-Free Workplace Act, 203
  Health Maintenance Organization Act, 202
  Occupational Safety and Health Act, 200–201
Employee Retirement Income Security Act (ERISA) of
  1974, 194, 206
Employees
  abortion, right to refuse participation in, 274, 306
  employer's duty to, 67
  protection for, 177–79
  respondeat superior and, 66
  safety (*See* Employee health and safety (federal regu-
    lations))
  scope of practice for, 66–67
  under Title VII of Civil Rights Act, 196
  "troubled," 177
Employer Identification Number (EIN), 248
Employer Identifier Standard, 248
Employers
  duty to employees, 67
  liability and, 148
  under Title VII of Civil Rights Act, 196
Employment-at-will doctrine, 195
Employment discrimination, 194–99
  equal employment opportunity and, 195*t*

EMR. *See* Electronic medical records (EMR)
EMTALA. *See* Emergency Medical Treatment and
  Active Labor Act (EMTALA)
Encryptions firewalls, 231
Endorsement, 59
Environment, protection of, 177–79
Environmental Protection Agency (EPA), 282
EPA. *See* Environmental Protection Agency (EPA)
Epilepsy, case of, 186
Equal Credit Opportunity Act of 1975, 207
Equal Employment Opportunity Act (EEOA) of 1972,
  196, 197
Equal Employment Opportunity Commission (EEOC),
  193, 196, 197
Equal employment opportunity (federal regulations)
  Age Discrimination in Employment Act, 197–98
  Americans with Disabilities Act, 198–99
  Civil Rights Act of 1991, 196–97
  employment at-will concept, 195
  employment discrimination laws and, 195*t*
  Equal Employment Opportunity Act, 197
  National Labor Relations Act, 199
  Pregnancy Discrimination Act, 197
  Rehabilitation Act, 198
  Title VII of Civil Rights Act, 195–96
Equal Pay Act of 1963, 204
Erickson v. Dilgard, 124
ERISA. *See* Employee Retirement Income Security Act
  (ERISA) of 1974
Estate of Berthiaume v. Pratt, 39
Estates, claims against, 210
Ethics, 8–17, 263–89
  abortion and, 274–75, 307, 307*t*
  AIDS and, 107
  applied, 3
  artificial conception and, 295
  of biomedical research, 275–78
  birth control and, 302
  codes of, 267, 269, 345–48
  committees, 22
  common sense approach to, 17
  defined, 8
  duty-based, 11, 13
  early history, 265
  emotions and, 20–21
  of fee splitting, 86
  genetic engineering and, 279–82
  genetic testing and, 311–12
  healthcare reform and, 282–84
  Human Genome Project, 278–79
  information technology and, 256–57
  interpersonal, 15–17
  justice-based, 11, 13
  life and, 291–319
  Lo's clinical model, 19–20
  managed care and, 81–82
  medical, 9
  medical etiquette and, 23–24
  models and, 18–20
  personal choice and, 274–75
  principles of medical ethics (AMA), 103*t*
  principles or values driving behavior, 12–15
  quality assurance programs and, 23
  reasons to study, 3–7
  religious beliefs and, 20, 21
  rights-based, 10–11, 13
  seven-step decision model, 19
  standards and behavior, 266
  sterilization and, 302

Ethics, (*continued*)
  surrogate motherhood and, 297
  theories of, 9–12
  three-step model, 18–19
  utilitarianism, 10, 13
  virtue-based, 12, 13
Ethnocentrism, 189
Etiquette, medical, 23–24
Eugenic (involuntary) sterilization, 301
Eugenics, 302
Euthanasia, 275
  active *versus* passive, 328–29
  arguments against, 329
  arguments in favor of, 329
Evidence
  chain of custody for, 174
  Federal Rules of Evidence, 147
  gathering in abuse cases, 173–74
  preponderance of, 36, 137
Examination for licensure, 58
Exclusive provider organization (EPO), 79
Expert witness, 49
Expired, defined, 323
Expressed consent. *See* Informed consent
Expressed contract, 40
Expulsion, 266
Extraordinary means, ordinary *versus*, 332–33

F

Fair Credit Reporting Act of 1971, 207
Fair Debt Collection Practices Act of 1978, 208–9
  bankruptcy and, 209
  collection agency, 208
Fair Labor Standards Act (FLSA) of 1938, 204
Fairness, 15
Fair v. St. Joseph's Hospital, 206
False claims, 142t
False imprisonment, 37, 38
Falsification, of medical records, 223–24
Family and Medical Leave Act (FMLA) of 1994, 206, 253
Family practice, 87t
FDA. *See* Food and Drug Administration (FDA)
Feasance, 135
Federal assistance (healthcare) programs, 79–81
  diagnostic related groups, 80
  Medicaid, 80–81
  Medicare, 79
Federal Communications Commission (FCC), 208
Federal court system, 45
Federal Insurance Contribution Act (FICA) of 1935, 205
Federal Licensing Examination (FLEX), 58
Federal Patient Self-Determination Act of 1991, 337
Federal regulations
  compensation and benefits, 203–6
  consumer protection and collection practices, 206–10, 207t
  employee health and safety, 200–203
  affecting medical professional, 194
Federal Rules of Evidence, 147
Federal Wage Garnishment Law of 1970, 209
Fee-for-service (FFS) basis, 79
Fee splitting, 86, 268t
Fellow of American College of Physicians (FACP), 88
Fellow of American College of Surgeons (FACS), 88
Felony, 42
  case process, 43
Fertility drugs, 298

Fetal development, 293–94
Fetus, 293
Fidelity, 13
Fifth Amendment, 16
Fixed-payment plan, 77
Fletcher, Joseph, 111
FLEX. *See* Federal Licensing Examination (FLEX)
Florida
  liability case in, 152
  missing medical records case, 230
Food, Drug, and Cosmetic Act of 1938, 174, 177
Food and Drug Administration (FDA), 174, 179, 202, 281, 282
Forensic medicine, 174
Fourteenth Amendment, 16
Franchise, 86
Franchisee, 86
Fraud, 37, 38
  defined, 38
  documentation and, 226
  malpractice and, 139–41
  Medicare and, 38, 139, 250
Fraudulent practices, 38
Functional Living Index: Cancer (FLIC), 334

G

Garcia v. Elf Atochem, 196
Garnishment, 209
Gatekeeper, 78
Gender harassment, 17
Gene markers, 279
Gene therapy, 268t, 280
Genetic engineering, 279–82
  cloning, 279–80
  gene therapy, 280
  human stem cell research, 281–82
  whistle blowing, 282
Genetics
  conceiving donor siblings, 311
  counseling/testing and, 309–12
  embryo harvesting, 298
  ethical questions regarding, 311–12
  hereditary disorders, 310t
  prenatal testing, 310–11
  testing of newborns, 311
Gentleness, 13–14
Geriatric medicine, 87t
Gestational period, 293
Ghost surgery, 268t
Goff v. Doctors General Hospital, 65
Goforth v. Porter Med. Assoc., Inc., 302
Good Samaritan laws, 64, 143
Grand jury, 46
Grijalva v. Shalala, 79
Griswold v. Connecticut, 299
Grodin, Michael, 339
Group practice, 84–85
Grubbs v. Medical Facilities of America, Inc., 198
Guardian ad litem, 63, 305, 333
Guilmet v. Campbell, 147
Gunshot wounds, reporting, 174

H

H. influenzae type B vaccine (HiB), 168
Habituation, 175
Hackett, Thomas, 111
Hand surgery, 88t

Hardship, 198
  undue, 198
Harris v. McRae, 304
Harvard Criteria for a Definition of Irreversible Coma, 326
Harvard Medical School, 326
Harvest, defined, 272
Harvesting, embryo, 298
Harvet v. Unity Medical Ctr., 192
Hayes v. Shelby Memorial Hosp., 197
Hazard Communication Standard (HCS), 201
Healthcare consumer, role of, 124–25
Healthcare environment, 76–97
  allied health professionals, 89–93
  federal assistance programs, 79–81
  Health Care Quality Improvement Act, 82
  managed care, 77–79, 81–82
Healthcare Integrity and Protection Data Bank (HIPDB), 251
Healthcare plan, 247
Healthcare professions, 90*t*–91*t*
Health Care Quality Improvement Act (HCQIA) of 1986, 82
Healthcare reform, 282–84
Health Insurance Portability and Accountability Act (HIPAA) of 1996, 63, 188, 241, 244–56
  affected parties, 246–48
  confidentiality and, 112
  covered transactions, 247
  denial of request for privacy, 248
  identifiers for healthcare providers, 248
  misconceptions about, 254–55
  Notice of Privacy Practices, 245
  obligations to patient under, 249
  patient rights under, 246*t,* 251, 251*t*
  penalties for noncompliance, 250–51
  permissions, 252*t*–253*t*
  permitted incidental disclosures, 250, 250*t*
  precautions relating to, 256*t*
  Privacy Rule, 244, 245, 250
  problems relating to implementation of, 253–54
  Protected Health Information, 245, 248
  recommendations, 255–56
  release of information and consent, 246
  release of medical records under, 228
  rules relating to research, 253
  state's preemption, 248
Health Maintenance Organization (HMO) Act of 1973, 202
Health maintenance organizations (HMOs), 77, 78–79, 85, 102, 153
  case of, 132
Heller v. Ambach, 153
Hematology, 87*t*
Hemophilia, 310*t*
Hepatitis A vaccine, 168
Hepatitis B vaccine, 200
Hereditary disorders, 310*t*
Hickman v. Sexton Dental Clinic, 151
HIPAA-defined permissions, 251, 251*t*–253*t*
HIPDB. *See* Healthcare Integrity and Protection Data Bank (HIPDB)
Hippocrates, 265
Hippocratic Oath, 241, 265, 345
Hiring practices, 191–92
  recommendations for, 192*t*
Hitler, Adolph, 280
HIV. *See* Human immunodeficiency virus (HIV)
HIV-infected employees, restrictions of, 108–9

H.L. v. Matheson, 304
Honesty, 15
Honor, in AAMA code of ethics, 348
Hospice care, 335–36
Human dignity, in AAMA code of ethics, 348
Human genome, 278
Human Genome Project, 278–79
Human immunodeficiency virus (HIV), 107, 169, 179
Humility, 14
Huntington's chorea, 310*t*
Huntington's disease, 298, 311
Hurlock v. Park Lane Med. Ctr., 224
Hyde, Henry, 305
Hyde Amendment, 304, 306
Hypothermia, 324

I

Illinois, retention of records case, 230
Immunity, for charitable organizations, 143
Implied consent, 123–24
Implied contract, 41
Improper disclosure, 233
Incident report, 68
Incompetent patients, 106
Incompetent persons, abortion and, 305
Independent practice association (IPA), 85
Indiana, Baby Doe regulations and, 307
Indictment, 46
Indigent, 10, 80
  duty to treat, 104–5
Indirect killing, direct *versus,* 332
Induced abortion, 303
Infection control, 87*t*
Infectious materials, 201*t*
Infectious waste, 179
Informatics, 256–57
Information technology (informatics), 256–57
Informed consent, 120–23, 278
In loco parentis, 119
Inquest, 167
In re Axelrod, 172
In re Baby M, 297
In re Doe, 305
In re Quinlan, 324
In re Schroeder, 170
Institutional Review Board (IRB), 275
Insurance
  claims-made, 149
  fixed-payment plan, 77
  liability, 149
  malpractice, 149–50
  occurrence, 149
  private, 77
  third-party payers, 77
Insurance Co. of N. America v. Prieto, 151
Integrity, 15
Intentional torts, 37–39
  assault, 37
  battery, 37
  defamation of character, 37, 38
  false imprisonment, 37, 38
  fraud, 37, 38
  invasion of privacy, 37, 38–39
Internal medicine, 87*t*
Internal Revenue Service (IRS), 167
Interpersonal ethics, 15–17
Interview questions, 193, 193*t*
Invasion of privacy, 37, 38–39

In-vitro fertilization (IVF), 295–96
Involuntary sterilization, 301
Iowa, wrongful-death statutes in, 139
Irreversible coma, 326

J

Jackovich v. A.L. Yocum, Jr., 124
James v. Johnson, 295
JCAHO. *See* Joint Commission on Accreditation of Healthcare Organizations (JCAHO)
Jeczalik v. Valley Hospital, 93
Jenkins v. Bogalusa Community Medical Center, 144
Jespersen, Mackayala, 324
Joint Commission on Accreditation of Healthcare Organizations (JCAHO), 60, 89, 220, 224
Journal of the American Medical Association, 334
Jurisdiction, 45
Just cause, 195
Justice, 14
　principle of, 21
Justice-based ethics, 11, 13

K

Keene v. Brigham & Women's Hosp., Inc., 232
Kern v. Gulf Coast Nursing Home, Inc., 152
Kevorkian, Jack, 328, 330
Kobler, William, 254
Korman v. Mallin, 121
Kübler-Ross, Elisabeth, 333

L

Laboratory or medical technologist (MT), 91*t*
Laboratory technician, 151
Laboratory technologists, *202*
Lambert v. Bessey, 35
Landau v. Medical Board of California, 151
Landeros v. Flood, 170
Law
　administrative, 43–44
　civil (private), 36–42
　class action lawsuit, 41–42
　classification of, 36–44
　common (case), 35
　constitutional, 33
　contract, 36
　criminal (public), 42–43
　defined, 7
　Good Samaritan laws, 64
　medical, 7–8
　public, 34
　reasons to study, 3–7
　regulatory, 34
　right-to-know, 200
　sources of, 33–35
　state open-record, 229
　statutory, 34
　tort, 36–39
Law of agency, 147
Legal system, 29–53
　branches of, 32
　classification of laws in, 36–44
　court system and, 44–45
　federal court structure in, 33
　separation of powers in, 32
　sources of law, 33–35
　trial process, 46–50 (*See also* Trial process)

Liability insurance
　claims-made, 149
　occurrence, 149
Liability (personal), 145–50
　altered medical records, 147–48
　alternative dispute resolution, 150–51
　civil liability cases and, 145–46
　of health professionals, 151–54
　illegal sale of drugs, 146–47
　law of agency, 147
　liability insurance and, 149
　malpractice insurance and, 149–50
　physical conditions of premises, 146
　promise to cure, 147
　responsible party for, 148
Libel, 38. *See also* Defamation of character
Licensed practical nurse (LPN), 89, 91*t*
Licensure process
　accreditation and, 60–61
　allied health professionals and, 89
　endorsement in, 59
　examination for, 58
　for physicians, 58–61
　practicing without a license and, 60
　reciprocity and, 59
　registration in, 59
　revocation and suspension, 60, 266
Life, ethics and, 291–319
Life-support systems, 323
Litigation
　defined, 46
　example, 30
　procedure, 46–47
Litigious society, 4
Living will, 114, 114*t*, *115*
Lo, Bernard, 19–20
Lo's clinical model for decision making, 19–20
Loss, of medical records, 231–32
Lovelace Medical Ctr. v. Mendez, 313
Love v. Heritage House Convalescent Center, 205
Loyalty, 15

M

Maher v. Roe, 304
Malfeasance, 135
Malpractice insurance, defensive medicine and, 149–50
Malpractice issues, 48, 131–62
　communication and, 156
　defined, 39, 134
　documentation and, 156–57
　fraud, 139–41
　negligence, 134–39
　Office of Inspector General and, 141–43
　prevention, 154–57
　tort reform, 154
Malpractice suits
　borrowed servant, 144–45
　comparative negligence, 144
　contributory negligence, 144
　defense to, 143–45
　res judicata, 145
　statute of limitations and, 145
Managed care, 77–79
　ethical considerations in, 81–82
Managed care organizations (MCOs), 78, 81, 82
Mandel v. Doe, 153

Massachusetts
  health insurance legislation in, 283
  liability case in, 152
  religious beliefs case in, 191
  stem cell legislation in, 281
Material Safety Data Sheet (MSDS), 179, 201
Matter of Baby K, 308
McCullough, Dennis, 337
McLaughlin v. Cooke, 302
Mechanical heart recipient, 339
Mediation, 150
Medicaid, 77, 141–42
  abortion and, 304, 305, 306
  advance directives and, 337
  confidentiality and, 242
  as federal assistance program, 80–81
  fraud and, 38, 139, 250
  managed care ethics and, 81–82
  medical records and, 225
  minimum health insurance and, 284
  organ transplants and, 273, 274
  Rehabilitation Act and, 198
  sterilization and, 300
  Title VII of the Civil Rights Act and, 195
  viatical settlements and, 337
Medical assistant, 151
Medical ethics, 9
Medical etiquette, 23–24
Medical informatics, 256
Medical law, 7–8
Medical Patients Rights Act, 62, 112
Medical practice
  associate practice, 84
  group, 84–85
  partnership, 83
  professional corporations, 85
  solo, 82–83
  types of, 82–85, 85*t*
Medical practice acts, 8, 57–58
Medical records, 217–38
  alcohol and drug abuse patients and,
    229
  altered, 147–48
  birth certificates, 165–66
  case of, 164
  case of lost, 218
  completeness of entries in, 224–25
  confidentiality and, 226–29
  contents of, 220–25
  corrections and alterations to, 222–24
  credibility of, 225
  death certificates, 166–68
  defined, 219
  electronic, 231
  example of, 221*t*
  falsification of, 223
  filing system for, *219*
  guidelines for charting, 222*t*
  improper disclosure of, 233
  loss of, 231–32
  ownership of, 226
  Privacy Act and, 228–29
  purpose of, 219–20
  release of information, 227–28
  reporting and disclosure requirements, 232
  retention and storage of, 229–32, *231*
  state open-record laws, 229
  subpoena *duces tecum,* 233–34
  timeliness of documentation, 224
  time periods for retaining, 230*t*
  use of, in court, 233–34
Medical records technician (ART), 91*t*
Medical specialty boards, 86–88
  American College of Physicians, 88
  American College of Surgeons, 88
  physician abbreviations and, 88*t*
Medical waste, 178–79
Medicare, 10, 77, 141–42
  accreditation and, 60
  advance directives and, 337
  card, example of, 80
  confidentiality and, 242
  diagnostic related groups and, 80
  as federal assistance program, 79
  fee splitting and, ethics of, 86
  fraud and, 38, 139, 250
  managed care ethics and, 81–82
  medical records and, 220, 225
  minimum health insurance and, 284
  noncompliance, 250
  organ transplants and, 273
  Rehabilitation Act and, 198
  Social Security Act and, 203
  Title VII of the Civil Rights Act and, 195
Medicare Act, 10
Medicare-Medicaid Antifraud and Abuse
  Amendments, 38
Medications, use of, 334–35
Mendel, Gregor, 309
Mengele, Josef, 267
Mercy killing. *See* Euthanasia
Michigan
  Baby M case, 296–97
  organ transplant case in, 273
  physician-assisted suicide laws in, 328
  promise to cure case and, 147
Minimum necessary standard, 249
Minnesota
  child abuse case in, 170
  reporting laws in, 169
  telemedicine in, 257
  wrongful discharge suit in, 192
Minors
  abortion and, 304
  rights of, 119
  sterilization (voluntary) of, 300
Misdemeanors, 42
  case process, 44
Misfeasance, 135
Mississippi, liability case in, 152
Missouri
  completeness of medical records, case, 224
  liability case in, 151
  passive euthanasia law in, 330
  wrongful-death statutes in, 139
Modified Rights of the Terminally Ill Act, 19, 37,
  106, 114
Mohr v. Williams, 122, 123
Molinari, Susan, 242, 243
Moon Lake Convalescent Center v.
  Margolis, 152
Morality, 9
Morbidity rate, 165
Morena v. South Hills Health Systems, 153
"Morning after" pill, 306
Morrison v. MacNamara, 39
Mortality rate, 165
Murray v. Vandevander, 300

N

National Board of Medical Examiners (NBME), 58
National Childhood Vaccine Injury Act of 1986, 168
National Conference of State Legislatures, 154
National Council Licensure Examination (NCLEX), 91t
National Institute of Health Clinical Center, 277
National Labor Relations Act of 1935, 199
National Labor Relations Board (NLRB), 199
National Organ Transplant Law of 1984, 273
National Practitioner Data Bank (NPDB), 82
NBME. See National Board of Medical Examiners (NBME)
Nebraska, abortion laws in, 305
Needlesticks, 109
Neglect of duty, 136–37
Negligence, 39, 134–39
    comparative, 144
    contributory, 144
    damages, 138–39
    defined, 134
    dereliction or neglect of duty, 136–37
    direct or proximate cause, 137–38
    duty and, 136
    four Ds of, 136–39, 136t
    sterilization suits, 301–2
    tort of, 135–39
Negligent torts. See Unintentional torts
Nephrology, 87t
Neurology, 87t
Neurosurgery (CNS), 88t
New Jersey
    Baby M case, 296–97
    brain-oriented death and, 325
New York
    Baby M case, 296–97
    child abuse case in, 170, 188
    falsification of medical records, case of, 223–24
    liability case in, 153
    organ donation in, 272
    sex crimes legislation in, 242
The New York Times, 278
Nixzmary's Law, 188
Nominal damages, 139
Noncompliance issues
    patients and, 106
    penalties under HIPAA, 250–51
Nonfeasance, 135
Nonmalfeasance, principle of, 21
Nontherapeutic research, 275
Noonan, John T., 293
Norton v. Argonaut Insurance Company, 61, 220
Notations, chart, 223
Notice of Privacy Practices (NPP), 245
    refusal to sign, 245t
Nuclear medicine, 87t
Nuremberg Code, 267, 346
Nurse practitioner (NP), 91t
Nurses, 152
    code of ethics, 269, 347
Nursing assistants, 152

O

O'Brien v. Cunard, 123
Obstetrics and gynecology, 87t
Occupational Safety and Health Act (OSHA) of 1970, 11, 200–201
    whistle blowing and, 282

Occupational therapist (OT), 91t
Occurrence insurance, 149
OCR. See Office of Civil Rights (OCR)
Odomes v. Nucare, Inc., 204
Office of Civil Rights (OCR), 255
Office of Inspector General (OIG), 141–43
    immunity for charitable organizations and, 143
    violation of statutes and, 142
Oken, Donald, 110
Oklahoma
    consent for artificial insemination donor in, 294
    sterilization case in, 300
Older Americans Act, 171
Oncology, 87t
O'Neill v. Montefiore Hospital, 41
On-the-job AIDS protection, employees and, 109
Open-record laws, 229
Ophthalmology, 87t
Oral surgery, 88t
Ordinary means, extraordinary versus, 332–33
Oregon
    euthanasia case in, 328
    organ transplant case in, 274
Organ donation, 268t, 271
Organ donor card, 273
Organ transplants, 274
Orthopedics, 87t
Orthopedic surgery, 88t
Osborne v. McMasters, 142
OSHA. See Occupational Safety and Health Act (OSHA) of 1970
OSHA Occupational Exposure to Bloodborne Pathogens Standards rules, 200
OTC. See Over-the-counter medications (OTC)
Otorhinolaryngology (ENT), 87t
Over-the-counter medications (OTC), 124, 132
Ownership, of medical records, 226

P

Pacemaker, case of, 76
Palliative care, 336–37
Paramedics, 153. See also Emergency medical technicians (EMT/paramedic)
Pardazi v. Cullman Med. Ct., 196
Parens patriae authority, 119
Parenteral, defined, 200
Parrish v. Clark, 152
Partial birth abortion, 305
Partnership, 83
Passive euthanasia, 328
    Cruzan, Nancy case, 330–31
Pathology, 87t
Patient dumping, 207
Patient Protection Act. See Patient Protection and Affordable Care Act (Patient Protection Act)
Patient Protection and Affordable Care Act (Patient Protection Act), 284
Patients. See also Acquired immune deficiency syndrome (AIDS); Physician-patient relationship
    abandonment of, 105
    alcohol and drug abuse, 229
    confidentiality and, 14, 110, 112–13, 239–62
    duty to properly identify, 110
    incompetent, 106
    noncompliant, 106
    obligations to under HIPAA, 249
    "A Patient's Bill of Rights," 113, 113t
    responsibilities of, 119–24

rights of, 112–18
rights under HIPAA, 246*t*
rights under privacy standards, 251, 251*t*
self-determination acts, 113–18
terminally ill, 327
Patient Self-Determination Act (PSDA), 118
Pediatrics, 87*t*
Pennsylvania
   abortion case in, 304
   liability case in, 153
   stem cell legislation in, 281
   wrongful-death statutes in, 139
People v. Gandotra, 140
People v. Scofield, 140
People v. Smithtown Gen. Hosp., 224
Per diem, 81
Permission, 245
   HIPAA-defined, 251, 251*t*–253*t*
Permitted incidental disclosures, 250, 250*t*
Perseverance, 14
Persistent vegetative state (PVS), 326, 331
PGD. *See* Preimplantation genetic diagnosis (PGD)
Pharmacists, 91*t*, 153
Pharmacy technician, 91*t*, 92
Pharmacy technician code of ethics, 15
Phenylketonuria (PKU), 310*t*, 311
Phlebotomist, 91*t*
Physical medicine/rehabilitative medicine, 87*t*
Physical therapists (PT), 91*t*, 153
Physical therapy patient, example, 56
Physician assistants (PA), 91*t*, 153
Physician-assisted suicide (PAS), 93, 268*t*, 328
Physician-patient relationship, 99–129
   consent and, 119–24
   minor rights and, 119
   professional practice responsibilities and, 103–12
   role of healthcare consumer in, 124–25
   standard of care and, 61–62
Physicians
   American Medical Association principles, 103*t*
   designation and abbreviations of, 88*t*
   duties of, 104–12, 104*t*
   licensure of, 58–61
   malpractice insurance and, 149–50
   practicing medicine without license, 60
   primary care, 78–79
   public duties of, 163–84
   respondeat superior and, 65–67
   responsibilities of, 102
   revocation of licensure, 60
   rights of, 101–2
   standard of care and, 61–62
Pius XII (Pope), 332
Placebo group, 275
Plaintiff, 35, 46
Plan "B" contraceptive pill, 305–6
Planned Parenthood of Central Missouri v. Danforth, 304
Planned Parenthood of Southeastern Pennsylvania v. Casey, 304
Pleadings, 47
Pneumococcal (pneumonia) vaccine (PCV7), 168
Polonsky v. Union Hospital, 152
Poor Sisters of St. Francis v. Catron, 153
Posthumous, 272
Postmortem, 168
Precedent, 8
Preempt, 194
Preferred provider organization (PPO), 79

Pregnancy
   prenatal testing, 310–11
   wrongful-life, 313
Pregnancy Discrimination Act of 1978, 196, 197
Preimplantation genetic diagnosis (PGD), 298
Premises, physical conditions of, 146
Prenatal testing, 310–11
Preponderance of evidence, 36, 137
Prescriptions, controlled drugs and, 175–77
Preventive medicine, 87*t*
Primary care physician (PCP), 78–79, 227
Prince v. Commonwealth of Massachusetts, 191
Principle of double-effect, 332
Principles of Medical Ethics (AMA), 267
Privacy. *See also* Confidentiality
   AIDS and, 242–43
   denial of request for, 248
   forms protecting, 245*t*
   invasion of, 37, 38–39
   right to, 242
   workplace and, 188–89
Privacy Act of 1974, 228–29
Privacy Rule, 244, 245, 250
Privacy standards, patients' rights under, 251, 251*t*
   HIPAA-defined permissions, 251, 251*t*–253*t*
Privileged communication, 113, 226
Probable cause, 170
Probate court, 45
Professional corporations, 85
Professionalism, 187
Prognosis, 110
Project Bioshield, 270
Promise to cure, 147
Prosecutor, 46
Prospective payment system, 81
Protected Health Information (PHI), 245, 247, 256
   deidentification of, 248, 249*t*
Protective order, 172
Proximate cause, 137–38
Proxy, 113
Prudent person rule, 62
Psychiatry, 87*t*
Public duties, 165
Public health records. *See* Vital statistics and public health records
Public Health Service, 278
Public Health Services Act, 229
Public law, 34
Punitive damages, 139

Q

Quality assurance (QA) programs, 23, 60
Quality-of-life issues, 334
Quinby v. Morrow, 152
Quinlan, Karen Ann, 323–24, 330, 331

R

Radioactive waste, 179
Radiologic technologist, 91*t*
Radiology, 87*t*
Randomized test trials, 278
"Reasonable person standard," 62
"Reasonable physician standard," 121
Reciprocity, 59
Reform, healthcare, 282–84
Registered Medical Assistant (RMA), 89
Registered nurse (RN), 91*t*, 152, 223. *See also* Nurses

Registration
  for allied health professionals, 89
  for licensure, 59
Regulations, 34
Regulation Z. *See* Truth in Lending Act (Regulation Z) of 1969
Regulatory law, 34
Rehabilitation Act of 1973, 198
Release of information, 227–28
  under HIPAA, 246
Religious issues, 20, 21, 171, 189–92, 302
Reporting, medical records and, 232
Research
  control group in, 275
  nontherapeutic, 275
  placebo group in, 275
  rules relating to, 253
  therapeutic, 275
Res ipsa loquitur (RIL), 137–38, 143
Res judicata, 145
Respect, 15
Respiratory therapists (RT), 91*t*, 153–54
Respite care, 336
Respondeat superior, doctrine of, 64–67
  altered medical records and, 148
  borrowed servant doctrine and, 144–45
  civil liability cases and, 145
  employer-employee responsibilities and, 66, 67
  malpractice insurance and, 149
  role of supervisor concerning liability, 147, 148
  scope of practice and, 66–67
Responsibility, 14
Restraining (protective) order, 172
Retailing, 176
Retinoblastoma, 310*t*
Revocation, of licensure, 60, 266
Rheumatology, 88*t*
Rider, 149
Rights
  of minors, 119
  patient, 112–18
  physician, 101–2
Rights-based ethics, 10–11, 13
Right to die legislation, 333
Right-to-know laws, 200
Right to refuse treatment, 333
Rigor mortis, 324
RIL. *See Res ipsa loquitur* (RIL)
Risk, assumption of, 143–44
Risk management, 67–68
Rodgers v. St. Mary's Hospital, 230
Roe v. Wade, 39, 93, 299, 303, 304, 306
Rowland v. Christian, 146
Rust v. Sullivan, 304

S

Safe Haven Laws, 313–14
Safety, malpractice prevention, 155–56
Saint Christopher's Hospice, London, 335
Sanctions, 250
Sanctity of life, 14
Satler v. Larsen, 171
Saunders, Cicely, 335
Schiavo, Terri, 331–32
Scope of practice, 66–67
Selective reduction, 298
Self-determination acts (advance directives), 113–18, 114*t*

durable power of attorney, 114, 114*t*, 118
  living will, 114, 114*t*
  Uniform Anatomical Gift Act, 114*t*, 118
Settlement, 147
Seven-step decision model, 19
Sexual harassment, 16, 17
Sexually transmitted diseases (STD), 168
Sick days, 204
Sickle cell anemia, 298, 310*t*
Simkins v. Moses H. Cone Hospital, 196
Skinner v. Oklahoma, 300
Slander, 38
Smith v. Cote, 313
Social Security Act of 1935, 203
Social utility method of allocation, 272
Social worker, 91*t*
Sole proprietorship, 83
Solid Waste Disposal Act, 282
Solo practice, 82–83
South Carolina, liability case in, 151
Specialties, medical, 87*t*–88*t*
Spontaneous abortion, 303
Spousal abuse, 172
St. John's Reg. Health Center v. American Cas. Co., 148
Standard of care, 61–62
Standards of proof, 48–49
Standing medical orders (SMOs), 140
Stare decisis, 35
Starks v. Director of Div. of Employment Section, 205
State Board of Medical Examiners, 57
State Board of Registration, 57
State court system, 45
State Dep't. of Human Services v. Northern, 333
State open-record laws, 229
State's preemption, 248
Statute of limitations, 63, 145
  consumer protection and collection practices, 210
  retaining records and, 229
Statutes, 34
  violation of, 142
  wrongful-death, 139
Statutory law, 34
Stem cell research, 270, 281–82
Stem cells, 281
Stereotyping, 189
Sterilization, 299–302
  consent for, 300
  defined, 299
  ethical issues, 302
  eugenic (involuntary), 301
  negligence suits related to, 301–2
  therapeutic, 300
  voluntary, 300
Storage, of medical records, 229–32, *231*
Subpoena, 47
Subpoena *duces tecum*, 47, 233–34
Subpoenaed, defined, 219
Substance abuse, 173
Substitute judgment rule, 338
Suicide, 338–39
Summary judgment, 47
Surgery, 88*t*
Surgical specialties, 88*t*
Surgical technician, 91*t*
Surrogate motherhood, 296–97
  ethical considerations with, 297
Suspension, of licensure, 60

Swanson v. St. John's Lutheran Hospital, 93
Sympathy, 15

T

Tarasoff v. Regents of the University of California, 111
Tay-Sachs disease, 310, 310t
Teeters v. Currey, 63
Telemedicine, 256–57
Teleological theory, 9
Tennessee
  ownership of embryos, case, 296
  right to die legislation and, 333
Terminally ill patients, 327
Texas, *Roe v. Wade,* 303
Therapeutic research, 275
Therapeutic sterilization, 300
Third-party payers, 77
Thompson, James A., 281
Thompson v. Brent, 61, 65
Thoracic surgery, 88t
Thor v. Boska, 225
Three-step ethics model, 18–19
Timeliness of documentation, 224
Tissue donation, 271
Title VII of the Civil Rights Act of 1964, 195–96
Tolerance, 14
Tolling, 63
Tools, Robert, 339
Tort law, 36–39
  defined, 36
  intentional, 37–39
  unintentional, 39
Tort reform, 154
Transplant rationing, ethics of, 272–74
Treatment, payment, and healthcare operations
  (TPO), 247
Treatment (medical)
  biomedical research debates and, 276–77
  right to refuse, 333
  withdrawing life-sustaining, 327–28
  withholding life-sustaining, 327–28
Trial process, 46–50
  appellate court system, 50
  closing arguments, 47–48
  expert witness, 49
  grand jury and, 46
  procedure, 46–47, 48
  standards of proof, 48–49
  subpoena, 47
  summary judgment, 47
  testifying in court, 49
Truth, 110–12
Truth in Lending Act (Regulation Z) of 1969, 41,
  207–8
Tubal ligation. *See* Sterilization
Tugg v. Towney, 199
Tuskegee syphilis research study, case of, 264, 278

U

UDDA. *See* Uniform Determination of Death Act
  (UDDA)
Ultrasound technologist (ARRT), 91t
Unborn Victims of Violence Act, 306
Undue hardship, 198
Unemployment compensation, 205
Uniform Anatomical Gift Act, 118, 338
Uniform Business Records Act, 147

Uniform Determination of Death Act (UDDA), 327
Unintentional torts, 39, 40
United Network for Organ Sharing (UNOS), 271
*United States v. Busse, Dey, Lupulescu, and
  Failla,* 140
United States v. NME Psychiatric Hospitals, 102
UNOS. *See* United Network for Organ Sharing
  (UNOS)
U.S. Medical Licensing Examination (USMLE), 58
USMLE. *See* U.S. Medical Licensing Examination
  (USMLE)
Utah, abortion case in, 304
Utilitarianism, 10, 13

V

Varicella (chicken pox) vaccine, 168
Vesting, 206
Viable (survival), 302
Viatical settlements, 337
Virtue-based ethics, 12, 13
Vital statistics and public health records, 165–74
  birth certificates, 165–66
  completing forms, 166t
  death certificates, 166–68
  defined, 165
Voluntary sterilization, 300
  of unwed minors, 300

W

Waive, 46
Walsh, Patrick, 276
Washington, euthanasia case in, 328
*Watson v. Idaho Falls Consolidated Hospitals,
  Inc.,* 192
Weaver v. Ward, 35
Whistle blowing, 207, 282
Whitehead, Mary Beth, 296
Williams v. Summit Psychiatric Ctrs., 38
Willowbrook State Hospital, case of, 292–93
Wireless local area networks (WLANs), 256
Wisconsin, improper disclosure in, 233
Withdrawing life-sustaining treatment, 327–28
Withholding life-sustaining treatment, 327–28
Witness, expert, 49
WLAN. *See* Wireless local area networks
  (WLANs)
Womble, Larry, 301
Woolfolk v. Duncan, 198
Work, defined, 14–15
Workers' Compensation Act, 205–6
Workmen's Compensation Boards, 43–44
Workplace
  compensation and benefits regulations, 203–6
  consumer protection and collection practices,
    206–10
  cultural considerations, 189–90
  discrimination in, 188
  employee health and safety in, 200–203
  equal employment opportunity and employment
    discrimination, 194–99
  federal regulations affecting professional in, 194
  hiring practices, 191–92
  interview questions in, 193
  privacy and, 188–89
  professionalism in, 187
  religious considerations in, 190–91
Wrongful-death statutes, 139

Wrongful discharge, 192, 195
Wrongful-life suits, 312–14
    Safe Haven Laws, 313–14
    wrongful conception/pregnancy, 313
    wrongful life, 312–13

X

X-ray technologist (radiologic technologist), 91*t*

Y

Yale-New Haven Children's Hospital, 276

Z

Zatarain v. WDSU-Television, Inc., 197
Zoterell v. Repp, 123
Zucker v. Axelrod, 153